Gilly Ford

Helen Stewart

HAIRDRESSING

with Barbering &
African Type Hair units

2nd edition

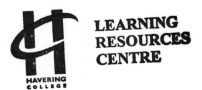

LEARNING
RESOURCES
CENTRE

HAVERING
COLLEGE

www.heinemann.co.uk

✓ Free online support
✓ Useful weblinks
✓ 24 hour online ordering

0845 630 4444

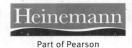

Heinemann

Part of Pearson

Heinemann is an imprint of Pearson Education Limited, a company incorporated in England and Wales, having its registered office at Edinburgh Gate, Harlow, Essex, CM20 2JE. Registered company number: 872828

www.heinemann.co.uk

Heinemann is a registered trademark of Pearson Education Limited

Text © Gilly Ford and Helen Stewart, 2009

First published 2009 12 11 10 09
10 9 8 7 6 5 4 3 2

British Library Cataloguing in Publication Data
A catalogue record for this book is available from the British Library

ISBN 978 0 435468 60 6

Edited by Caroline Broughton
Designed by Wooden Ark
Produced by Kamae Design, Oxford
Original illustrations © Pearson Education Ltd, 2009
Illustrated by Kamae Design / Rosa Dodd c/o NB Illustration
Cover design by Wooden Ark
Picture research by Susi Paz
Cover photo/illustration © Anne Veck Salon, photographer Marco Loumiet
Printed in Spain by Graficas Estella

Websites
The websites used in this book were correct and up to date at the time of publication. It is essential for tutors to preview each website before using it in class so as to ensure that the URL is still accurate, relevant and appropriate. We suggest that tutors bookmark useful websites and consider enabling students to access them through the school/college intranet.

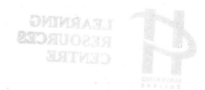

Contents

Foreword by Andrew Barton

For a lad from a small working-class town in Yorkshire, I've not done too badly! I've recently been named the most expensive and sought after hairdresser in the UK... pretty impressive to think that I started in a village salon! There is no such thing as a typical day. One day my life involves working with celebrities or a glamorous photo shoot, the next I could be travelling the world flying the British hairdressing flag with Saks at glitzy hair shows and educational seminars. I'm also recognised as TV's favourite hair expert and love spending time making clients happy at the Saks flagship salon in London. So how did all this come about...

I started a very traditional hairdressing apprenticeship in my home town of Barnsley, Yorkshire, which was tough and very disciplined, but years later I'm forever grateful for it. Along with attending college to study for my hairdressing qualifications it was the best possible start.

Learning all the key skills to the best standard has undoubtedly helped me further down the line in my career at Saks. Whether it's been working on everyday clients, supermodels, super stars or creating hair for super designers at the catwalk shows, it's always important to have a good foundation of knowledge.

I think I have the best job in the world and I'm amazed by just how much excitement I get from my work every day. Working with a great team is possibly the best advice I can offer anyone. Never accept an OK standard and always push your own creativity through experimentation and trial and error.

Hairdressing is competitive, it's fast, ever changing and of course it's about providing a service...but the service of making someone feel great about themselves through their hair is wonderful. I swear the smile a client shows you on her face when you've done her hair is magical and addictive!

Because hairdressing is always changing, there's always something to learn and discover, whether new products or techniques. You'll never be bored and as British hairdressing and training are widely acknowledged as the best in the world, you're guaranteed to have the best start for the career of your dreams!

Level 3 for me was the icing on the cake. It's time for you to connect the many facets of being a hairdresser together and to be really proud of the knowledge you have gained so far.

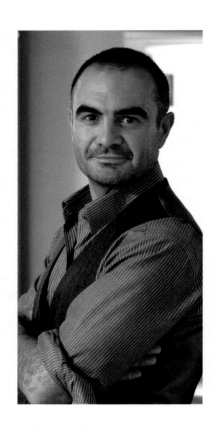

Andrew Barton x

Saks International Creative Director
www.saks.co.uk

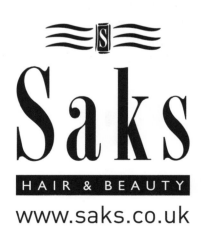

www.saks.co.uk

About the authors

Helen Stewart has been a practising hairdresser for 30 years and a lecturer for 20 years. She works at Trafford College and is responsible for both the Level 2 and the Level 3 hairdressing programmes. She trains, assesses and Internationally verifies across all levels. In addition, she also delivers the assessors award. Helen is a member of the Association of Hairdressers and Therapists.

Helen wishes to thank the following people: To Ade, Paul and Mike for their love and continued support. To Katie Woodman and Sharon Sawyer for their colouring knowledge and expertise. To Natalie Mitchell, Sophie Drake-Thomas and Judith Hughes for their help and guidance throughout the African type hair units.

Gilly Ford has been working in the Hairdressing industry for 26 years and has been teaching for 17 years. She works at Bolton Community College and coordinates the provision of Literacy, ICT and Numeracy across the Hair and Beauty section. Gilly works with learners from Salon Services Certificate level up to Level 3. She has been an internal verifier for 10 years and is a Senior State Registered Hairdresser.

Gilly wishes to thank the following people: To Pete, Natalie, Nick, Sammy and Jessica — it's all about you! x To Kaye Volante, Jennifer Warrington and Samantha Pickup from Gregory Couzens salon, many thanks for adding your expert cutting and colouring skills to the book. To Jiggy Madhavji with thanks for his knowledge and skills in designing patterns in hair. To Siobhain Gleeson-D'Attorre for her help and guidance throughout the hair extensions unit, her expert hairdressing services and her salon realia (Claddagh Hair) used within the book. To Jill Shovelton and Mandy Molyneaux, your valued input and professional critique in developing the Level 3 book has been very much appreciated.

Acknowledgements

The authors and publisher would like to thank the following copyright holders for permission to reproduce photographs and realia:

Guy Kremer p 3; Kateryna Govorushchenko/iStockphoto p 17 (bottom), 192, 194 (bottom), 212, 215, 222, 245, 270 (left), 334 (bottom), 382 (bottom); Dr P. Marazzi/Science Photo Library p 22, 46 (top and image 3), 47 (image 3), 49 (top and image 3), 50 (top), 145; Anne Veck/Photographer: David Howard p 27, 303, 319; Jim Franco/Stone/GettyImages p 43 (bottom), 343; Andrew Syred/Science Photo Library p 44 (left); Eye of Science/Science Photo Library p 44 (right), 49 (image 2); Photo Insolite Realite/Science Photo Library p 46 (image 2); John Hadfield/Science Photo Library p 46 (bottom); St Bartholomew's Hospital/Science Photo Library p 47 (top), 48 (bottom); Science Photo Library p 47 (image 2), 49 (bottom); Getty Images/Giulio Marcocchi p 47 (bottom); Mrs M C Sherlock FIT MAE/The Institute of Trichologists/www.trichologists.org.uk p 48 (top); Wellcome Trust p 48 (image 2 and 4); Bsip Chassenet/Science Photo Library p 48 (image 3); Alex Bartel/Science Photo Library p 49 (image 4); Mr.K_Hobbs_FIT/The Institute of Trichologists/www.trichologists. org.uk p 50 (image 2 and 4); Cut2White p 50 (image 3), 55 (top), 149, 252 (image 3), 274 (top), 280, 394; Krista Kennell/ Corbis p 55 (bottom); Butch Martin/Alamy p 56 (top); Agencja FREE/Alamy p 56 (middle); Famke Backx/iStockphoto p 56 (bottom); Darren Ambrose p 67, 81, 139, 191, 211, 229, 232 (left), 265; Wella System Professionals p 69, 261; Jeff Greenberg/Alamy p 71; Scissors p 73; Images by TONI&GUY p 114, 140, 152 (bottom); Image provided by label.m professional haircare p 83 (left); JFK p 95; Chris Pearsall/Alamy p 96; Kérastase Soleil p 99; Parlux p 103; Wella p 106, 133, 163, 185, 205, 206, 224, 353 (right), 392 (right); Goldwell p 113, 116 (bottom), 160, 180, 255 (top left); Photographs supplied by Saks (High Definition Collection) www.saks.co.uk, photography by Pete Webb p 117 (top), 124, 125, 388, 389; WAHL p 118, 119 (bottom left), 277 (left), 366 (left), 383 (image 2); ForFex p 119 (top); Tim McGuire/Corbis p 148; Cut2White p 157 (colouring fork); Royston Blythe 2008/9 p 169, 285; Ana Abejon/iStockphoto p 177; iStockphoto p 178; Keith Hall p 195; RonaldGrantArchive p 202; Babyliss p 203 (top and image 7), 335; www.hairtools.co.uk p 203 (image 6); SalonsDirect p 204; Bela Tibor Kozma/iStockphoto p 214; Mario Anzuoni/Reuters/Corbis p 219 (left); Hair: Michael Barnes for Goldwell, Make up: Marco Antonio, Photo: Kyoko Homma, Styling: Chiyono Minagawa p 219 (right); Anita Cox p 230; John Carne p 232 (right), 235 (top); Trip p 235 (bottom); Getty Images p 236, 255 (top right), 311 (top left), 390 (top right); Mayk Azzato p 237; Famke Backx/iStockphoto p 243; Racoon p 270, 276; WireImage/GettyImages p 309 (top left), 311 (middle); camilla wisbauer/iStockphoto p 275 (left); Joe Hawkins Photography/Alamy p 286; Arcaid/Alamy p 288; Avlon p 307, 326, 337 (left); Wire Image p 309 (bottom); Purely Natural. RickyB @ Media Image p 309 (top right); Camera Press/True Love p 310, 314; Andreas Kuehn/Stone/GettyImages p 311 (bottom); PYMCA/Alamy p 320; Savagelily.com p 323 (electric heater); Black Like Me p 337 (right); Alamy/Danny Clifford p 345; DBURKE/Alamy p 355; Popperfoto/ GettyImages p 362; Clinique p 371; Matthias Clamer/Stone+/ GettyImages p 372 (bottom); GettyImages/Stone p 390 (left); Jiggy p 405 (left); Matt Carr/GettyImages p 412 (bottom). Wella p 8; L'Oréal Professionnel UK p 59; Antonio Tramontana @ Fratelli's p 86; HQ Professional Hairdressing www.hqprofessional.co.uk p 89; Clynol p 100 (top); Claddagh Hair (Salon: Claddagh Hair www.claddaghhair. co.uk, Designers: Forum Media Limited www.forummedia.org, Business Management Consultants: RDA Business Services Limited www.rda247.com) p 289.

All other photos: Pearson Education Ltd/Mind Studio; Pearson Education Ltd/Chris Honeywell; Pearson Education Ltd/Gareth Boden, Pearson Education Ltd 2004/Gareth Boden, Pearson Education Ltd 2007/Jules Selmes, Pearson Education Ltd 2007/ Lord & Leverett.

For their help and expertise at the Level 3 photoshoot, the authors and publisher would like to thank Trafford College, Carlton Alexander, Lorraine Chaisty-Wilson, Sophie Clarke, Sophie Drake-Thomas, Siobhain Gleeson-D'Attorre, David Fielding, Amanda Gaffey, Grace Granfield, Jignesh Madhavji (www.jiggyzdesignz.com), Yaasin Malik, Natalie Mitchell, Natalie Myers, Reanne Nelson, Pesh, Sharon Sawyer, Jacqueline Schofield, Michelle Schofield, Andrea Sommerville, Kaye Volante, Jennifer Warrington, Fay Williams. For their help with make-up at the shoot: Emma Fairfield, Amanda Gaffey, Emma-Jane Copeland, Aysha Rauf, Jade Thorley, Lauren Wright

For their assistance with sourcing images from the Institute's archives for the section on hair and scalp disorders, and for the expert advice given in the confirmation of captions, the authors and publisher would like to thank the Institute of Trichologists. www.trichologists.org.uk

Introduction

This book has been written to help you achieve your Level 3 (NVQ/SVQ) Diploma in Hairdressing. It also includes a range of Barbering and African type hair units, to help you develop your skills further in these areas. The book is designed to provide you with all the information you need in an accessible format including all the necessary technical guidance with illustrations to support the text.

Throughout the book, reference is made to maintaining, improving and personalising your professional skills, as this is an essential part of your vocation. Each technical unit is supported by step-by-step photographs, to help you both understand the content and give you ideas to help develop your current skills.

Hairdressing is an ever-changing industry that requires creativity, confidence and inspirational ideas. The Level 3 standards reflect that current direction; nothing short of perfection is good enough and this should be reflected in your passion to be the best! We wish you every success in achieving your Level 3.

Key features

In the salon — case studies based on real-life events that you may face in the salon. They are designed to allow you to consider how you would respond to situations that may actually arise. Questions are provided to enable you to explore the key issues and decide on your own course of action.

Be professional — tips and suggestions for promoting good practice in the salon and in your working methods.

Check it out — activities to help you to apply theory to practical situations. These can also be used to provide evidence for your portfolio, key skills or customer service.

Remember — highlights specific areas that you need to pay particular attention to and to remind you of the important legal and professional issues within the hairdressing business.

Check your knowledge — a set of questions provided at the end of each unit to help you check your understanding of that unit.

Assessment guidance — guidance provided at the end of each unit to help you understand what you are required to do in order to successfully complete it.

Salon life — a full-page magazine-inspired feature covering a key issue or topic, with expert guidance relating to problems that may be encountered in the salon.

Diploma/NVQ/SVQ

NVQ stands for **National Vocational Qualification** and SVQ for **Scottish Vocational Qualification** (for those training in Scotland). This means that it is a nationally recognised qualification in a vocational area. If you are doing this qualification with City & Guilds it will be called Level 3 Diploma. These qualifications are based on the National Occupational Standards (NOS) for Hairdressing. The NOS are written by HABIA including representatives from industry, trainers and teaching staff.

How to gain your Level 3 in Hairdressing

In order to gain the Level 3, you will need to collect the evidence required for each unit. Many forms of evidence are acceptable including observed work, oral questions, witness statements and assignments.

To achieve a Level 3 in Hairdressing, candidates must be able to:
- show competence in a broad range of hairdressing skills and activities, for example, cutting and re-styling, and be able to perform in a wide variety of contexts, including non-routine tasks
- demonstrate considerable responsibility for their work and the ability to work independently
- guide and train others, as is required of the job.

Who is the qualification for?

This qualification is designed for hairdressers who work independently in the salon and support others in their role. You may have already achieved Levels 1 and 2 in Hairdressing. However, if you have sufficient practical experience working as a hairdresser, but have not yet achieved a formal qualification, you may also be at the right stage to study at Level 3.

How the qualification is structured

To complete the full award you must achieve a total of nine units. These nine units are made up of four mandatory units and five optional units, chosen from the two option groups. The path you wish to follow in your hairdressing work will determine which optional units you choose.

A **unit** is the term given to each separate area of competence, whether that is a technical or non-technical area, for example, cutting, thermal styling, consultation or health and safety.

We have included the following Barbering and African type hair units to help you broaden your skills and knowledge further: Design and create patterns in hair; Provide shaving services; Creatively cut hair using a variety of barbering techniques; Design and create a range of facial hair shapes; Design and create intricate styles using plaiting techniques; Style African type hair using thermal styling techniques.

Assessment of the qualification

You may provide a range of sources of evidence to prove competence as listed below; however, most of your evidence will be derived from direct observation of your work by your assessor/s. All of the evidence must be recorded in your candidate logbook and a portfolio of evidence should be built over time to prove your competence.

Types of evidence

- **Observation**: Direct observations by your assessor watching you produce the work.
- **Witness testimony**: A detailed record of the work you have produced which must be signed by both yourself and a witness.

- **Oral questions**: Questions asked directly by your assessor to check your understanding.
- **Written questions**: Questions that you must answer in order to check your understanding of the subject area.
- **Assignments**: A piece of written work that must be produced to assess your knowledge of the subject area.
- **Mandatory written test paper**: A written test that must be taken under controlled conditions.
- **GOLA** (Global Online Assessment) testing (applicable only if you are doing your qualification with City & Guilds): Questions that are answered online. These may be taken under controlled conditions.
- **Product evidence**: Any evidence that is a product of the assessment, for example, a consultation sheet or record card.
- **Simulation**: Simulation of an activity may be used only under specific circumstances and for particular units.
- **Accreditation of prior learning**: This enables you to claim knowledge and skills you have already acquired from previous work or study. Evidence must be produced to prove your competence and knowledge in a particular area. This could be statements from employers and clients, or photos of work you have completed.

Assessment and quality

While you are working towards your Level 3 Hairdressing, you may be assessed by all or just a few of the above methods. Your assessor/s will judge your competence against the standards as written and you have a right to appeal against any assessment decision made. The quality of assessment is controlled by measures which are set in order to standardise assessment decisions, and these are regularly checked and monitored by internal verifiers and external verifiers employed by the awarding body.

1

The workplace
environment

Unit G22

Monitor procedures to safely control work operations

What you will learn:

- How to ensure that healthy and safe practices are being followed within work areas

- The appropriate action to be taken to control workplace hazards.

Guy Kremer

3

Introduction

Health and safety is an essential aspect of any workplace environment and especially so within the hairdressing salon. Without a thorough understanding of the importance of health and safety in your work and working practices, you could become a danger to yourself and those around you.

As a senior member of staff, you will be expected to monitor health and safety procedures in the workplace. Your responsibilities are not just to other salon staff, but also to anyone else that enters the business premises, for example, clients, representatives, maintenance staff, etc.

This unit is about making sure that statutory and workplace instructions are being carried out.

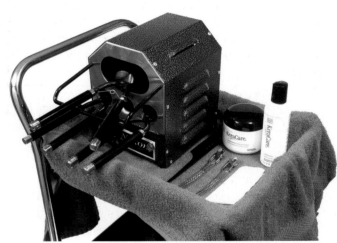

Health and safety should be a key factor when preparing for a service

You the stylist

As a stylist, you should have a good awareness of health and safety to ensure that your working practices are sound and comply with current legislation. To do this you need to be aware of the everyday hazards that are present in your place of work and also the ones that may occur more infrequently. However, being aware of such hazards is not enough; you must be able to decide how much of a threat they pose and act accordingly. You will be expected to check that health and safety instructions are being followed and any risks are controlled safely and effectively. It is also your responsibility to liaise with the relevant person and inform them of any breaches of health and safety.

You must ensure your health and safety knowledge is up to date, relating to both statutory and workplace instructions to ensure you are always promoting good practice and adhering to any relevant legislation.

> **Check it out**
>
> Try visiting the HSE website (www.hse.gov.uk). The website publishes practical guidance on where hazards occur and how to control them.

How to ensure that healthy and safe practices are being followed within work areas

Before you begin to address issues such as hazards and risks, it is helpful to first define a few key terms. This will help you to clarify how they relate to your salon environment.

Hazard: a hazard is anything that has the potential to cause harm, for example, a hairdryer flex, water on the floor, or a heavy box that needs moving.

Risk: a risk is the chance, either high or low, that the harm caused by the hazard will occur.

Control measure: something that reduces and/or controls the risks to health and safety.

Workplace: the workplace refers to all areas of the business premises including the staff rooms, toilets, and so on. This means every area of the salon and not just the part where hairdressing is carried out.

Statutory instructions: covers all health and safety legislation applicable to running and working in a salon.

Workplace instructions: covers the salon's policies and procedures.

Policy: a statement that directs the present and future decisions of an organisation.

Procedure: a series of clearly defined steps (and decisions) that explains or describes how to go about completing a specific task.

Have a look around your workplace and see if you can identify any hazards. If you can, what are the potential risks to health and safety?

It is vital that you are aware of current health and safety legislation and how it relates to you and your responsibilities within the salon. Your working life is controlled by two sets of external laws known as acts and regulations. An act is laid down by Parliament and, after going through the parliamentary process, becomes law. It usually contains general objectives that employers, employees and others must achieve. A regulation is a statutory instrument — in other words, a detailed means of meeting the general objectives of an act.

Risk assessment

Risk assessments should be carried out at regular intervals. A risk assessment is a careful examination of the areas of your work that could cause harm to people in the salon. All workers (and others that enter the place of business) have a right to be protected from harm. No one can pre-empt every eventuality; however, so long as people are protected as far as is 'reasonably practicable', business owners have fulfilled their responsibility.

Five steps to risk assessment:
1. Identify the hazards.
2. Decide who might be harmed.
3. Evaluate the risks and decide on precautions.
4. Record the results and ensure they are implemented.
5. Review risk assessments and update them if and when necessary.

Although it may not be your responsibility to carry out risk assessments, you should ensure that you monitor the workplace at regular intervals (this should be agreed between yourself and your employer) following workplace instructions. All staff should be adequately trained in health and safety, but you need to ensure they are compliant and any training needs are identified and acted upon. This will ensure the salon environment is run in a safe and effective manner.

Remember

Regular staff meetings are an excellent way of discussing health and safety issues and getting valuable feedback from other workers. This can help confirm competence and identify training needs, thus helping you to fulfil your obligations.

You should keep a log of any accidents or incidents that occur in the salon, as these may be used when reviewing health and safety practices. These records must be legible, up to date and available to anyone who is authorised to see them.

It is essential that you liaise with the person who is responsible for health and safety for a number of reasons, which include:
- making recommendations for changes to the workplace policies in your salon
- reporting hazards
- confirming your understanding of preventative measures
- reporting any acts or omissions that could prove to be detrimental to health and safety in the workplace.

Check it out

Devise a log sheet to record any workplace hazards that you have identified or those that have been reported to you. This will help you to remember when you need to give the information to the relevant person who is responsible for health and safety.

 Key Skills Links: Level 2 Communication

Health and safety legislation

The Health and Safety at Work Act 1974

Most health and safety law is derived from the Health and Safety at Work Act 1974. This Act requires employers to:
- provide and maintain a safe working environment
- provide adequate welfare facilities
- provide safe systems of work
- provide information, training and supervision
- ensure the safe handling, storage and transportation of goods and materials
- provide and maintain safe equipment.

These requirements are also included in other regulations, some of which will be discussed later in this unit.

The enforcement of health and safety regulations is carried out by inspectors who are employed by the Health and Safety Executive (HSE), a government-appointed body. Inspectors may enter and inspect a workplace at any reasonable time, following an accident or complaint, and can do so without forewarning. For example, they may:
- offer informal advice
- offer informal advice supported by a formal letter
- issue an improvement notice
- issue a prohibition notice
- recommend prosecution.

An improvement notice will recommend actions to be completed by the employer within a certain period of time, whereas a prohibition notice will require immediate action and may well involve the removal of a process or item of equipment until these actions have been completed. Failure to comply with either of these notices will result in a criminal prosecution in either a Magistrates or Crown Court, depending on the gravity of the offence. Courts have the power to fine or even imprison for such offences.

As an employee, you also have duties under this Act. You must:
- not endanger yourself or others by your acts or omissions
- cooperate with your employer in order for their duties to be fulfilled
- not misuse anything provided in the interests of health and safety
- report all accidents, incidents and unsafe conditions or practices.

As you progress through this unit, you will see that many of your workplace activities relate to this Act.

Check it out

What welfare facilities are provided in your salon?

Electricity at Work Regulations 1989

These regulations are concerned with ensuring safety when using electrical equipment. All employers must ensure:
- all electrical equipment is properly maintained and in good working order
- regular tests are made by a qualified electrician on each piece of equipment, as appropriate
- records are kept regarding the testing of all electrical equipment and may be provided for inspection purposes if required.

As an employee, it is your responsibility to remove and label any faulty equipment and then report it to the relevant person. You must also cooperate with your employer to comply with these regulations.

Check it out

Look at the statements that outline your responsibilities within the Electricity at Work Regulations. What should you be doing to fulfil your obligations relating to this piece of legislation?

Personal Protective Equipment at Work Regulations 1992

These regulations require an employer to provide their employees with protective equipment if they may be exposed to any risk to health or injury during their working hours. The risks will have been assessed during the risk assessment your employer has to carry out under related regulations. All employers have the responsibility to:
- assess the need for the use of personal protective equipment
- supply protective clothing or equipment free of charge
- train staff in the use of personal protective equipment
- ensure the equipment is properly maintained
- ensure it is fit for purpose.

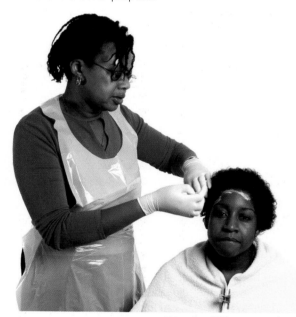

Wearing PPE ensures that both you and your client are protected

Personal protective equipment for you may include gloves, an apron and a facemask for asthmatics when mixing powder bleach, but not of the 'dust free' variety. Personal protective equipment for your clients includes a gown, towels and plastic capes. These should be used to ensure the client's skin and clothes are protected.

Be professional ★★★

- It is your responsibility to look after personal protective equipment and report its loss or demise to your employer so it can be replaced.
- It should be noted, however, that personal protective equipment is considered to be a last resort when implementing measures designed to reduce or control an identified risk. It is essential that other control measures be used before, or in addition to, the provision of such items.

Control of Substances Hazardous to Health Regulations (COSHH) 2002

In the salon you will use many substances that may put your health at risk. The COSHH regulations require all employers to assess the health risks that arise from the use of hazardous substances within the workplace and to provide the controls that will be most effective in protecting staff and members of the public. The regulations apply to substances that have been classified as corrosive, explosive, harmful, highly flammable, irritant, oxidising or toxic. The COSHH classification symbols are shown below.

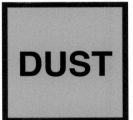

Dust

Flammable

Corrosive

Toxic

Irritant

Oxidising agent

COSHH classification symbols

All employers are required to:

- assess the risk to health from the use of hazardous substances at work and what precautions are needed
- design and introduce appropriate measures to prevent or control your exposure to hazardous substances
- ensure that control measures and safety procedures are followed and protective equipment is used when appropriate
- monitor exposure to hazardous substances and carry out appropriate forms of surveillance to ensure everyone maintains good health
- inform and instruct all staff about the risks and precautions that need to be taken and to carry out training, so everyone is able to work in a safe way when dealing with hazardous chemicals.

Storage of hazardous chemicals

Products that are identified as hazardous must be stored in a cool dark place, with good ventilation and away from direct sunlight. Always read the manufacturer's instructions with regard to storing hazardous substances.

Handling and using hazardous substances

When using hazardous products, for example, colour, perm lotion, neutraliser or relaxing products, disposable gloves and an apron (personal protective equipment) must be worn. Some cleaning materials are classed as hazardous products and therefore gloves and an apron may be necessary. Look out for the COSHH classification symbols on the bottle or packaging and always read the labels to ensure your own safety.

Aerosols should be used away from any source of heat, especially from a lit cigarette or naked flame. Many styling and finishing products are classed as flammable substances and should not be used near any heat source.

Disposal of hazardous substances

Hazardous substances may cause harm to our environment and other people if they are not disposed of in the correct way. Always read the manufacturer's instructions regarding the safe disposal of these substances. If you have any doubts, you can telephone the manufacturer and they will advise you on safe methods of disposal. Your salon may have its own policy for disposing of salon waste – ask the designated person within your salon.

Cosmetic Products (Safety) Regulations 2008

These regulations are specifically concerned with the ingredients contained within hairdressing preparations and their safe usage. The regulations state that hair products supplied to the salon must comply with the UK Cosmetic Products (Safety) Regulations. Under the Health and Safety at Work Act 1974, product manufacturers are required by law to supply health and safety information on any products used in a hairdressing salon that contain potentially hazardous substances. They must also provide information on the precautions to be taken to reduce any risks. This information can be found in the booklet *A Guide to Health and Safety in the Salon*.

In addition to the booklet, your product manufacturer should also supply your salon with a list of their products that specifies which section of the booklet is relevant to each individual product.

These regulations ensure that products sold in the UK are safe when used correctly. The products covered include:

- hair tints and bleaches or lightening products
- products for waving, straightening and fixing
- setting products
- cleansing products (shampoos, powders, lotions)
- conditioning products (lotions, creams and oils)
- hairdressing preparations (lotions, lacquers and brilliantines)
- shaving products (creams, foams and lotions).

These regulations have a direct link with COSHH legislation and should be used by all employers when carrying out a COSHH risk assessment.

10A HAIR COLORANT-DIRECT DYE NON-OXIDATIVE (NON-AEROSOL)

Composition
Solutions of direct colorants in a shampoo or conditioner base which may be liquid, cream or gel.

Ingredients
Colorants	up to 10%
Solvents (e.g. glycols or glycol ethers)	up to 10%
Ethanol	up to 50%

Hazards Identification
Refer to manufacturer's pack for list of declarable colorants which, if present, may require a skin allergy test before use. Liquids products may be flammable.

First-Aid Measures
Eyes: Rinse eyes immediately with plenty of water. If irritation persists seek medical advice.
Skin: Wash skin immediately. If irritation persists seek medical advice.
Ingestion: Drink 2–3 glasses of water or milk. Seek medical advice immediately.

Accidental Release Measures
Use plenty of water to dilute and mop up spillages.

Fire Fighting Measures
Use a carbon-dioxide or dry powder extinguisher.

Handling & Storage
Avoid contact with eyes and face. Do not use on damaged or sensitive skin. Store in a cool place away from direct sunlight and other sources of heat. Use away from sources of ignition. Liquid products may contain alcohol which makes the product flammable; keep small quantities in the salon for immediate use only.

Exposure Controls/Personal Protection
Apply in a well ventilated area. Always wear suitable protective gloves.

Other Information
Do not allow lotion to come into contact with eyes, face or surrounding area.
Do not use on damaged scalp. Follow manufacturer's specific instructions if advised to carry out a skin allergy test before use.

Disposal of Residues
Do not burn. Wash down the drain with plenty of water.

Check it out

Do you have a copy of the booklet, *A Guide to Health and Safety in the Salon*? If not, you can order a copy from The Hairdressing and Beauty Suppliers Association, tel. 01707 649 499 or online at www.hbsa.uk.com.

Manual Handling Operations Regulations 1992

These regulations are concerned with the manual handling of loads, for example, equipment or stock. This includes the way we lift things and move them from place to place. Employers have specific duties under these regulations which involve assessing the risks when manually handling loads. To do this, the employer must look at:

- the task to be undertaken
- the capabilities and limitations of the staff (e.g. pregnant women or staff who have recently returned to work after an illness may not be back to full strength)
- the type of load to be handled
- the working environment (if the atmosphere is damp, your hands may be wet and the load may slip).

Once your employer has assessed the risks, it is necessary to put systems in place to control the likelihood of them occurring. Training and information should be provided to all staff who are involved in manual handling activities.

You also have responsibilities as follows:

- To take reasonable care for your own and others' health and safety who may be affected by your actions.
- To cooperate with your employer so that they can carry out their health and safety duties.
- To use any equipment provided by your employer to enable you to move or handle loads — this could include a sturdy stepladder for placing stock on a high shelf or a trolley device for moving heavy boxes.
- To follow the safe systems of work that your employer has laid down.

Check it out

What are the potential risks of carrying a heavy box with smaller boxes balanced on the top? Practise good manual handling techniques in the salon.

Fire Precautions Act 1971

The Fire Precautions Act 1971 is concerned with fire prevention and the provision of escape routes in the event of an evacuation. The employer is responsible for fire safety in the workplace and ensuring the workplace complies with the fire regulations. Your employer should have a fire certificate if:

- there will be more than twenty people working on the premises at any one time
- there are more than ten people working anywhere other than the ground floor.

Fire Precautions (Workplace) Regulations (Amendment) 1999

Your employer is responsible for undertaking an assessment of the fire risks on the premises, to produce an emergency plan, and to inform, instruct and train you about the fire precautions in your workplace. Your employer should also nominate a designated person to help them.

You also have responsibilities to ensure your own health and safety and that of your colleagues and others who may be affected by your actions.

- You should cooperate with your employer so that they are able to carry out their statutory duties.
- You must inform your employer/health and safety representative of any situation within the workplace that you feel may constitute a risk to health and safety.
- You must use all equipment correctly, following the training and instruction guidance you have received.

Check it out

Ask your employer to confirm the salon's policy relating to the use of extinguishers, as some insurance policies do not allow this.

Be professional ★★★

- Make sure you understand and comply with the health and safety policies in your workplace.
- Know what you should do if you discover a fire, including calling for the fire brigade.
- Be familiar with the evacuation routes within your salon and any fire exit signs.
- Know the locations of all fire fighting equipment.
- Keep fire doors closed to stop the spread of fire, heat and smoke.
- Make sure all cigarettes are extinguished properly and only smoke in designated areas.
- Report any ideas you may have for reducing the risk of fire in your workplace.

Remember

You should not be fighting fires unless you have been trained to do so. If you have already received training, can you remember which type of fire extinguisher you should use for the different types of fires?

Health and Safety (First Aid) Regulations 1981

These regulations require your employer to provide adequate and appropriate equipment, facilities and personnel to enable first aid to be given to you if you are injured or become ill at work. The minimum first aid provision within a hairdressing salon is a suitably stocked first aid box and an appointed person to take charge of first aid arrangements.

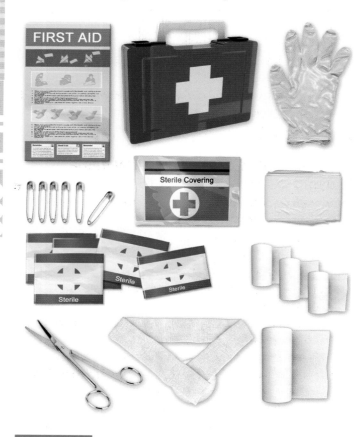

> **Check it out**
>
> If you want to obtain a first aid qualification, do you know where you could find an appropriate course?

Your employer should have chosen an appointed person within the salon to take charge when someone is injured or becomes ill at work (this includes calling an ambulance if necessary). The appointed person should look after the first aid equipment and ensure the first aid box is restocked at regular intervals. He or she should not give first aid unless they have been trained and hold a current first aid at work certificate. As there should be an appointed person in the workplace at all times, your employer may have chosen two people to carry out this role to ensure there is always one appointed person in the salon.

Reporting of Injuries, Diseases and Dangerous Occurrences Regulations (RIDDOR) 1995

These regulations are the responsibility of your employer, but also include self-employed people. Your employer, or self-employed person, must report:

- a death or major injury
- an over-three-day injury
- a dangerous occurrence
- a work-related illness, which may include dermatitis, skin cancer and occupational asthma.

All workplace accidents or incidents, however trivial they may seem at the time, should be reported to your employer. In addition, under the RIDDOR regulations, employers have a legal duty to report any workplace accidents, diseases or dangerous occurrences to the Health and Safety Executive (HSE). This information enables the HSE and local authorities to identify where and how risks arise, and to investigate any serious accidents.

Environmental Protection Act 1990

This Act is relevant to hairdressers, as you have to dispose of waste products, including chemicals. The part of this Act that affects you is concerned with your duty of care when disposing of waste. All salon waste should be disposed of in a manner that will not pollute the environment or cause harm to others.

Your employer's responsibilities within this Act are to:

- dispose of all waste in a safe manner
- provide training for all employees in the safe disposal of waste
- contact product manufacturers for information regarding the safe disposal of products, including out-of-date stock.

Your employer should have a commercial waste contract, which should include sharps.

> **Check it out**
>
> What is the correct procedure for disposing of sharps?

10

Local Government (Miscellaneous Provisions) Act 1982

The Local Government (Miscellaneous Provisions) Act 1982 has its own set of by-laws relating to hairdressers and barbers. These may also be referred to as 'local by-laws' and are specific to the area where the business is situated. Both you and your employer have responsibilities under this Act.

The Act is primarily concerned with cleanliness and hygiene. It covers the salon, tools and equipment, and people working there. If you do not comply with these regulations, you could be liable to a fine.

Check it out

> Contact your local authority to get a copy of the Local Government (Miscellaneous Provisions) Act 1982, relating to hairdressers and barbers, if your salon does not already have one.

The Management of Health and Safety at Work Regulations 1999

These regulations are considered to be the most important legislation relating to health and safety since the Health and Safety at Work Act 1974. This is because they legally require all employers to effectively manage health and safety within their business.

Your employer is obliged to:

- carry out risk assessments to determine what health and safety measures are needed to protect you, the employee, and others who may enter the business premises
- plan, implement, and control whatever measures are deemed necessary
- review these measures on a regular basis
- provide health and safety training to all employees.

Check it out

> How often does your salon give health and safety training?

The Provision and Use of Work Equipment Regulations 1998

Under these regulations your employer is required to prevent or control the risks to your health and safety from any equipment you use at work. This applies to both new and second-hand equipment. The regulations state that equipment used at work must be:

- suitable for use and used for the purpose for which it is intended
- maintained in a safe condition for use
- inspected on a regular basis, by a competent person, and records kept
- used only by people who have been trained and instructed in its correct usage.

Written instructions must be provided if and when necessary.

Workplace (Health, Safety and Welfare) Regulations 1992

Your employer should ensure your workplace complies with the requirements of these regulations by:

- maintaining the workplace and all equipment and systems used there
- ensuring adequate ventilation
- keeping the workplace at a reasonable temperature (minimum 16°C)
- making sure you have sufficient light to work comfortably
- keeping your workplace clean and tidy
- ensuring you have enough room to work comfortably
- keeping floor and 'traffic routes' in a reasonable condition (no holes, slopes or uneven surfaces)
- ensuring the workstations and seating are suitable
- providing you with suitable washing and toilet facilities (with soap and a means of drying your hands)
- making sure you have accommodation for clothing (worn at work) and changing facilities
- providing you with facilities for resting and eating (if meals are to be eaten on the premises)
- providing you with clean drinking water and cups
- removing waste materials on a regular basis
- keeping you safe from falling objects
- making sure all doors and gates are suitably constructed and fitted with any necessary safety devices
- making sure windows are protected against breakage and incorporate signs (or similar) where there is a danger of someone walking into them
- making sure escalators and moving walkways have safety devices fitted so they can be stopped in an emergency.

It should be noted that there is amendment legislation to a number of the above Acts and Regulations.

The appropriate action to be taken to control workplace hazards

In this section, we will identify the hazards in your workplace, evaluate the risks and look at ways to control them.

A hazard is something that can cause harm. You must remain alert to the presence of hazards in the workplace to help prevent accidents or damage to property. Under the Health and Safety at Work Act 1974, you have a duty of care not to intentionally harm yourself, your colleagues, or other people by your acts or omissions. You must be vigilant at all times and act accordingly when you identify a hazard.

Hazards occur in all areas of everyday life, from crossing the street to boiling the kettle. All you need to do is look around the workplace and see how many things have the potential to harm you or other people around you. Stairs or steps in the salon could be deemed a hazard, but what is the likelihood of anyone actually falling? If the stairs are well maintained and have a handrail, the likelihood of an accident is reduced. However, if the stairs are wet after mopping or the handrail becomes loose, the risk would be much higher.

The backwash area may also be classed as a hazardous area, as there is the possibility of spillages, which would leave the floor wet and slippery. However, if immediate action is taken, the risk will be reduced.

Hazards in the workplace

'Staff only' areas in the workplace are often forgotten when it comes to health and safety as the clients do not see this part of the business premises.

Check it out

Look around your staff room. Using the same format as in the table below:
1 Identify any additional hazards.
2 State the risk involved.
3 What should you do about it?
4 How could you prevent the hazard from becoming a risk?

Some of the substances used in the salon are hazardous, especially those used for chemical treatments, for example, colours, bleach or relaxers. These products are potentially very dangerous. However, if used with protective equipment, good training and following the manufacturer's instructions, they should not pose a threat. Used in untrained hands, the outcome could be very different — the client could suffer chemical burns to the scalp or skin.

As part of your job role you will be carrying out numerous activities, including chemical work, styling hair (using electrical equipment, sharps and styling/finishing products) and stock control. Within each of these areas there is an element of risk. However, if policies and control measures are followed, it should greatly reduce the risks involved.

Check it out

Look at the table below. How could you prevent the hazards from becoming risks?

Identify the hazard	What is the risk?	What should I do?
Water on the floor	Slipping	• Inform everyone in the salon • Cone off the area and wipe up the spillage • Do not remove the cones until the floor is dry
Perm lotion on the floor	Slipping	As above, but the spillage must be diluted first and PPE worn
Shampoo on the floor	Slipping	• Inform everyone in the salon • Cone off the area and wipe up the spillage • Mop the floor using a detergent to remove any slippery residue • Do not remove cones until the floor is dry
Mirror smashed on floor	Cuts from broken glass	Carefully pick up the glass and either: 1. Wrap in several layers of newspaper and place into a cardboard box. Seal the box and label it with 'broken glass' or 2. Place the glass into the sharps box. On completion, sweep the floor to make sure there are no shards of glass left on the floor

Your employer will have various procedures and policies in place, all of which are there to protect you, your colleagues, and others who enter your place of work. The policies should cover:

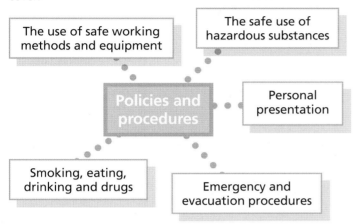

The use of safe working methods and equipment

The safe use of hazardous substances

Policies and procedures

Personal presentation

Smoking, eating, drinking and drugs

Emergency and evacuation procedures

Remember

You should always report or deal with any hazards identified as soon as possible to ensure the salon is a safe environment for everyone.

Firstly, you need to establish who is responsible for health and safety in your salon, as certain hazards will need to be reported to this person. If you do not know who to report to, how can these problems be rectified? Secondly, you will need to find out who is the appointed person for first aid and who acts as designated person in the event of an evacuation. This is usually the owner, but it could be the salon manager, the senior stylist, or even you!

Check it out

Within your salon, identify who is responsible for the following:
- health and safety
- first aid
- evacuating the premises in the event of an emergency.

The use of safe working methods and equipment

Sterilisation

It is vital that you look after your equipment by keeping it clean and well maintained. One way of doing this is to ensure that equipment is sterilised. Sterilisation is the complete destruction of living organisms to prevent cross-infection. All tools should be cleaned before sterilising to remove traces of hair, dirt and dust. Brushes, combs and rollers should be cleaned with hot soapy water. Scissors and razors should be wiped with alcohol or spirit.

Autoclave

The autoclave is the most effective method of sterilisation. The principle is the same as a pressure cooker. Sterilisation takes place as the water inside the autoclave is heated to 121°C (due to a build up of pressure).

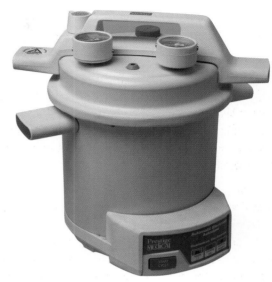

An autoclave

Chemical sterilisers

Many salons sterilise tools in a chemical jar. The chemicals must be prepared according to the manufacturer's instructions, using PPE if stated. Tools must be completely immersed in the chemical for the specified length of time for sterilisation to take place. Check with the manufacturer that fluid is suitable for metal tools, otherwise they may rust. Remember that the fluid will need to be changed periodically to ensure it is of the correct strength.

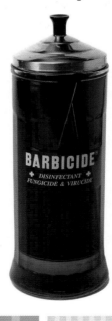

A chemical jar

Ultra-violet radiation cabinet

This is used in many salons as a means of sterilisation. The ultra-violet light rays come from the top of the cabinet and will sterilise the surfaces that they hit. You must remember to turn the tools over to ensure all surfaces are sterilised. Each side of your tools should be sterilised for at least twenty minutes.

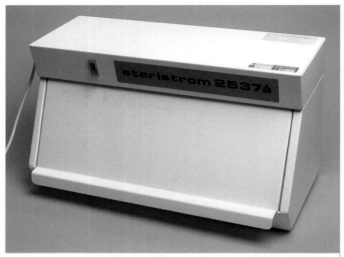

A UV cabinet

Moist heat sterilisation

Towels and gowns should be washed on a hot wash cycle. The temperature of the water should reach 95°C.

Cleaning detergents

Whilst cleaning detergents will ensure work surfaces and floors are clean, they are unlikely to sterilise them.

> **Check it out**
>
> Why should all tools be clean and sterilised before use?
> What kind of infection could be carried on unsterilised tools?

Risk of infection

As part of your duty of care towards your clients, you must be aware of the risk of infection when using sharps. Think about the implications of accidentally cutting your client with dirty scissors. What if your client has the HIV virus or hepatitis B or C, which is passed through body fluids such as blood? Can you afford to take the risk?

To evaluate the risks, think of the worst thing that could possibly happen. This will help you to decide whether the hazard presents a high, medium or low risk. Once you have established this, you need to decide how to reduce the risk, remove it completely, or report it to the designated person for them to take action.

Identify the hazard	What is the risk?	What should I do?
Use of sharps	• Cutting the client • Cross-infection	• Check cutting tools prior to use and only use cutting tools that you have been trained to use • Use extreme care • Dispose of sharps in the 'sharps bin' • Ensure all tools are sterile before use

Safe working methods

You need to look at all aspects of your job role and decide whether your working methods are safe or a liability. For example, you may be responsible for ordering and receiving stock. The stock may arrive in a large heavy box, which you then need to move to the stockroom. This could prove to be hazardous; if you try to lift the box, you may drop it on your foot, causing bruising or possibly broken bones. It may cause disc or ligament injuries, which would necessitate you taking time off work. The situation may be avoided by using a mechanical device, for example, a trolley, to move the box. If you do not have access to such a device, then unpack the box and move the stock in workable loads. This may take longer, but the risk of injury should lessen considerably. You could ask a colleague for help and between you it may be possible to move the box.

> **Remember**
>
> If moving objects manually, remember to bend your knees, keep your back straight and stand up using the muscles in your legs, rather than those in your back.

1 Think about the lift. Where is the load to be placed? Do you need help? Are handling aids available?

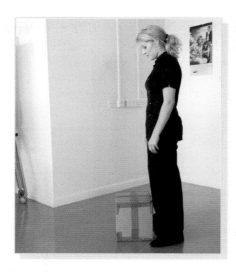

2 Bend your knees and keep your back straight. Tuck in your chin. Lean slightly forward over the load to get a good grip.

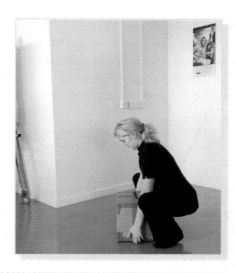

3 Once you are confident with your grip on the load, lift smoothly from the legs remembering to keep your back straight.

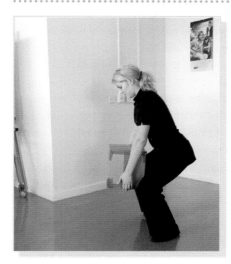

4 Carry the load close to your body as you walk.

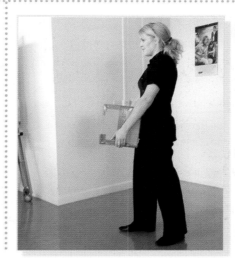

Identify the hazard	What is the risk?	What should I do?
Moving heavy or awkwardly shaped boxes of stock	• Over-stretching muscles, possibly straining your back • Dropping the box onto your feet or toes	• Unpack the box until you are able to lift it comfortably and then stand using your leg muscles, keeping your back straight • Ask for help from a colleague • Use a trolley or other mechanical devise
Storing/reaching stock on a high shelf	• Over-stretching muscles, possibly straining your back, shoulders or arms • Dropping stock, causing breakages and/or spillages	• Use a sturdy stepladder • Store frequently used stock at eye level or below

When undertaking any task within the salon, your posture is important. Many hairdressers suffer with back problems due to incorrect posture, stooping or leaning over the client. This is most common in taller people and can be avoided by using hydraulic chairs, which can be adjusted in height to accommodate the stylist. As your work requires you to stand for long periods of time, you need to ensure you are standing correctly with your weight evenly distributed. This will prevent unnecessary stress and strain on your body and should help to prevent fatigue.

Monitor procedures to safely control work operations **Unit G22**

Preventing dermatitis

It is believed that approximately 50% of hairdressers will suffer from work-related **dermatitis** at some point in their career. Therefore it is essential you are aware of the causes of work-related dermatitis and how to prevent it.

> **Dermatitis**
>
> this is the name given to inflammation of the skin, usually affecting the hands. Dermatitis can result in dryness of the skin, itching, redness, flaking, swelling and blistering.

There are two types of dermatitis that can affect hairdressers:

- Irritant contact dermatitis — this is a local inflammation of the skin that develops after either prolonged exposure to chemicals or water, but may also occur after a one-off exposure.
- Allergic contact dermatitis — this is due to exposure to sensitising agents, usually para-compounds found in permanent colouring products. In many cases, the sensitivity to the specific product or preparation will last indefinitely.

> **Be professional ★★★**
>
> - Try to avoid exposure to chemicals and 'wet work' where possible. If it's unavoidable, make sure you are wearing 'single use' gloves (either vinyl or nitrile types with a 300 mm sleeve where possible).
> - Use plenty of hand cream throughout the day, especially after you have washed your hands. If you allow your skin to become dry, this can lead to dermatitis.
> - Make sure you dry your hands thoroughly after washing.
> - Throw away your 'single use' gloves every time you take them off and make sure you change your gloves between clients.
> - Keep a check on your skin, looking out for signs of dryness and cracking which may be early signs of dermatitis.
> - If you have possible symptoms of dermatitis, see your GP as soon as possible.

Using electrical equipment

You will use a number of electrical appliances in the salon. Electricity can kill so do not take unnecessary risks. Using electrical equipment for its intended purpose should minimise the risk of damage. Before using any piece of electrical equipment you should have received training or instruction on its usage. If you know how to use the equipment safely, the risk of accidents is reduced. Check that an appropriate person has tested the equipment so you know it is safe to use.

Visually check each piece of equipment prior to use. You should check the plugs and sockets are not cracked or broken. You could be electrocuted if you touch something live. Ensure the flex is not worn or that bare wires are showing. This will prevent electrocution.

> **Remember**
>
> Knowing how to use electrical equipment safely reduces the risk of accidents in the salon.

> **Be professional ★★★**
>
> - Do not use too many electrical appliances from one socket; this could lead to overloading and possibly fire.
> - Check the air filter on hand dryers to ensure they are free from dust and debris, as they could overheat.
> - Ensure straightening irons or tongs are cool before storing. The heat from the irons or tongs may wear the flex, leaving the bare wires on show.
> - Electrical appliances should be switched off and unplugged after use.
> - If your salon policies differ in any way to those of the manufacturer, you must report it to your employer or designated person immediately, as there could be significant risks attached.
>
> Any risk that you consider to be high risk should be reported to the designated person for health and safety in your salon.

Electrical equipment, such as a hairdryer, roller ball or kettle, can present risks if they are not well maintained and checked regularly. For example, a hairdryer used near water or with wet hands has the potential to cause harm. However, if it is used properly, away from the water and with dry hands, the risk will be considerably less. A hairdryer with trailing wires is also a hazard, as people may trip and hurt themselves, or the plug may become loosened in the socket, which could leave the pins exposed.

Salon life

Burning incompetence

Lisa's story

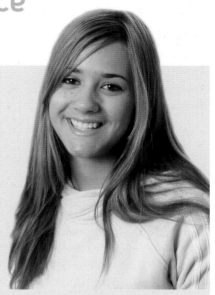

I was new to the salon. My client was having bleached highlights using the cap as she'd had her hair coloured but it was too dark and needed correcting. I pulled through some highlights and then applied the bleach and went to get the climazone, but another stylist was already using it. The client was in a hurry, so I decided to use the old steamer in the back room. I had never used a steamer before, but I sort of knew how to use it as I had seen one being used a few years ago when I was training.

I filled the glass bottle to the brim, put it into the steamer and switched it on. It took a little while to heat up, but as I was busy with my next client I wasn't too worried. Suddenly the client under the steamer let out a cry and when I turned around the steamer was 'spitting' boiling water onto her neck. The client suffered scalding to her neck and has decided to sue the salon for negligence.

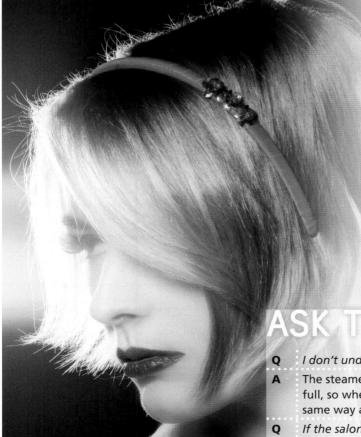

Be professional ★★★

- Remember, ignorance is no excuse – if you don't know how to do something in the salon, ask!!
- If you are responsible for health and safety in the salon, this also includes ensuring all staff have been trained to use electrical equipment. It is your responsibility to monitor the working practices of the staff and suggest additional training if you consider it is necessary.
- If using a steamer, it is best to use distilled water, especially if you live in an area that has hard water. Failure to do this will result in limescale deposits on the heating element, which will affect the steamer's operation and could even cause it to stop working.

ASK THE PROFESSIONALS

Q *I don't understand why the steamer did that?*

A The steamer has a reservoir (that you can't see) which must have been full, so when you put water into it, it overflowed and spat – in the same way as a kettle would if it were overfilled.

Q *If the salon had more climazones, this wouldn't have happened, would it?*

A No it wouldn't. However, you should never use a piece of electrical equipment unless you have had training in its use.

The table below identifies a few hazards associated with using electrical appliances.

Identify the hazard	What is the risk?	What should I do to prevent the hazard from becoming a risk?
Cracked plugs/frayed flexes	Electric shock / electrocution	• DO NOT USE • Report to designated person
Trailing flexes	Trip hazards and possibility of electrocution	• Avoid trailing flexes by using another socket • Take the flex around the outside of the room, thus removing the hazard
Curling tongs left on worktop and switched on after use	• May burn someone • May be knocked off the worktop and broken	• Isolate the power after use and unplug the appliance • Allow to cool, then store safely where applicable
Heated electrical styling tools	Burning the client	• Keep the heated styling tool away from the client's face and protect the skin/scalp by placing a comb underneath (where possible), thus keeping the heat source away from the skin • Use extreme care

The safe use of hazardous substances

In the salon you will use numerous substances that are considered to be hazardous to health. When using chemical substances, ensure you read and follow any instructions the manufacturer gives. If your salon policies differ in any way from the manufacturer's instructions, you must inform your employer or designated person immediately, as there could be significant risks involved.

When dealing with chemicals it is essential that you use the personal protective equipment that has been supplied to you by your employer. This is to prevent marking your clothes and, more importantly, to protect your hands. If your hands become irritated and sore, this will affect your ability to work. Dermatitis is a common complaint amongst hairdressers and in some cases may end a promising career. It is suggested that some colouring products may be carcinogenic (cancer causing) and prolonged use of such chemical products without the appropriate protection may have very serious consequences.

Chemical products should not be used on skin with cuts or abrasions, or be allowed to come into contact with the eyes or face. As some of these products are caustic, for example, relaxers used on African type hair, they may burn the eyes, which may lead to scarring of the delicate tissue in the eye, causing temporary or permanent blindness. In addition, relaxers, if used incorrectly without due care or without sufficient training, can cause skin/scalp burns and hair loss.

Be professional ★★★

- A skin test is required when using quasi and permanent colouring products. This is to safeguard your client from the possibility of an allergic reaction and should be carried out 24–48 hours prior to the colour application. Other pre-service tests should be carried out where applicable to ensure the safety of your client.
- Store chemicals in a cool, dry place away from direct sunlight or heat source.
- When applying PW lotion, do not flood the scalp as this may cause chemical burns. The excess will drip onto the floor and may cause someone to slip.
- Do not mix chemicals together unless stated by the manufacturer. They may give off heat or dangerous fumes.
- Look out for the COSHH symbols on items such as hairspray or even the disinfectant you use to clean the toilet. If the product is stored, handled, used and disposed of correctly, the risk of accident or injury is significantly reduced.

Identify the hazard	What is the risk?	What should I do to prevent the hazard from becoming a risk?
Storing H_2O_2 in a lemonade bottle	Someone may drink it	• Never use food or drink containers to store chemicals • If transferring chemicals to another bottle, ensure it's properly labelled
Storing H_2O_2 near aerosols	In the event of a fire, the oxygen from the H_2O_2 will feed the fire and the aerosols may explode	Move the stock to ensure the H_2O_2 is not stored near the aerosols. If this is not within the scope of your job role, report it to the designated person
Use of styling and finishing products	• Product in client's eyes • Fire if used near naked flame	• Use extreme care • Use a face shield if possible when using finishing sprays • Do not use near naked flame or lit cigarette

Smoking, eating, drinking and drugs

Smoking

Since the introduction of the smoking ban in England, it is not legal to smoke in enclosed public places. Therefore smoking in the salon or other areas of the workplace is not permitted. If this legislation is not adhered to, your employer could face fines of up to £2500. It is your employer's responsibility to display 'no smoking' signs in the salon and also to take reasonable steps to make sure that staff, clients and visitors comply with this.

As part of your job role includes ensuring compliance with legislation, you must make sure that the non-smoking policy is adhered to.

Check it out

If you are a smoker, how much time have you needed to take off work due to smoking-related illnesses, chest infections etc.?

Eating

Eating in the salon is unprofessional and gives a poor impression to clients. The lingering smell of food can be off-putting for clients, especially food that has a strong smell. Food that is dropped on the floor makes the floor slippery and therefore the hazard becomes a risk. The risk becomes greater if you have, for example, a client with impaired sight; the client may not see what is visible to others and slip.

Drinking

Providing drinks in the salon carries its own set of risks. A hot drink may be accidentally spilled onto a client causing scalding or it may be spilled onto the floor, making it slippery and creating a hazard. The effects of alcoholic drinks on the body make them unacceptable within the working environment. Even in low doses, alcohol will:

- aid relaxation
- reduce tension
- lower inhibitions
- impair concentration
- slow reflexes
- reduce coordination.

Even drinking alcohol in small quantities can reduce your effectiveness at work. A few drinks will lower your inhibitions, leaving you open to mistakes. A hangover will also affect your ability to work effectively.

Drugs

Using drugs whilst working in the salon is not recommended. The taking of drugs, depending on the type of drug, may have an effect on your ability to work safely. If you are taking prescribed drugs, it is important that you read the warning information specific to the medication. For example, tranquillisers may leave you slightly drowsy the following day and impair your ability to concentrate. Prescribed or non-prescribed medication for conditions such as hay fever may also affect your ability to work. You should inform your employer of any potential side effects from the medication you are taking and, if necessary, they may adjust your workload accordingly.

The side effects from the use of such drugs are varied and include:

- extreme over-activity (hyperactivity)
- fatigue (resulting from an inability to sleep)
- unexpected changes in mood or behaviour
- a deterioration in performance at work.

It is important to remember that taking recreational drugs is illegal in the UK and, if you have taken recreational drugs the night before, they may still be affecting your actions for up to 48 hours. This has obvious implications for the salon. Firstly, there is the likelihood of an accident or incident occurring due to one of the above contributory factors. Secondly, there is the impact on the business resulting from poor performance and increased absence.

In the salon

A category 'A' mistake

The junior stylist comes to work with a slightly glazed look and smiling much more than usual. She is usually quite morose and sullen. You notice an unusual 'sweet' smell on her breath and clothing. The salon owner asks her to carry out a trim on an elderly client with long hair, a task she is more than capable of carrying out. When you look round, the client's hair is three centimetres long at the back. The junior stylist does not seem concerned in any way and is ready to start on the top.

- What do you think may have happened?

There are other practices in the salon that may be classed as unsafe. The table below identifies a few hazards associated with unsafe practices.

Identify the hazard	What is the risk?	What should I do?
Running in the salon	Slip, trip or fall	Don't run!
Water spray fights	Water on the floor, someone may slip	• Mop up the water immediately and allow the floor to dry • Remember your duty of care

Risks from environmental factors

A carelessly discarded cigarette is one of the most common reasons for 'paper bin' fires. The problem that occurs for hairdressers is that there are likely to be other types of waste in the bin. Cotton wool saturated with PW lotion or plastic gloves may give off toxic fumes on ignition; an empty aerosol of hairspray could explode.

Emergency and evacuation procedures

Emergency situations arise from time to time and may be due to any of the following factors.

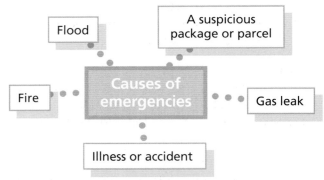

By now you should have identified those people in your salon who are responsible for first aid, health and safety and evacuating the premises.

Illness or accident

In the event of an accident or illness, you should report to the person responsible for first aid. Their responsibility is to take charge of the situation, assess the need for medical intervention and act accordingly. The appointed person should not give first aid unless they have been trained and hold a current first aid certificate. They may call an ambulance if they feel it is necessary.

Fire

In the event of a fire, you should follow the evacuation procedure laid down in policy within your salon. Do not take any unnecessary risks. You should:

- evacuate the premises by the nearest exit, taking your client/s with you
- close doors and windows en-route. A fire needs oxygen to continue burning; by reducing the amount of oxygen, it should contain the fire
- dial 999 for the fire brigade
- meet at the designated assembly point. The appointed person should now be checking to ensure that everyone has left the building.

When leaving the salon, you must not stop to collect your personal items as prolonging your stay in the salon could increase the risk of injury from the fire. Your evacuation policy should include provision for disabled people, as they may not be as mobile as you and should be classed as a higher risk. You should also be familiar with all evacuation routes. There may be instances where one fire exit is inaccessible due to the fire so you must know of other escape routes. Fire exits should be clearly identified and, in larger premises, green fire exit signs should indicate the way to safety.

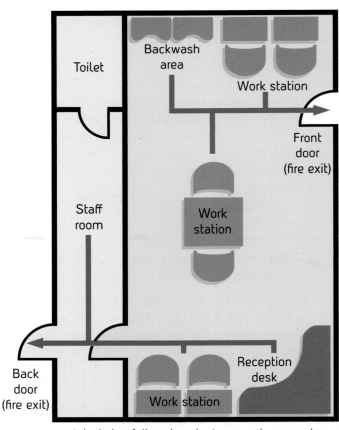

It is vital to follow the salon's evacuation procedure

Fire extinguishers

All new portable fire extinguishers are predominantly red with a zone of colour to indicate the contents of the extinguisher.

- A water extinguisher should be used for fires involving wood, cloth, paper, plastics and coal.
- A foam extinguisher should be used on liquid fires as it forms a blanket of foam over the surface of the burning liquid and smothers the fire.
- A dry powder extinguisher is used for burning liquids such as oil, paint and grease. However, it MUST NOT be used on chip pan fires. The dry powder extinguisher does not cool the fire very well; care must be taken as the fire may re-ignite. A fire blanket will help to cool a fire and prevent re-ignition.
- A carbon dioxide (CO_2) extinguisher may be used on burning liquids (except chip pan or fat pan fires) and electrical fires. Again, these extinguishers have limited cooling properties and a fire blanket may be used to prevent re-ignition.
- A wet chemical extinguisher should be used to tackle fires involving deep fat fryers and chip pan fires. You may not come across this type of fire in the salon; however it is important to be aware of the different types of extinguishers available.

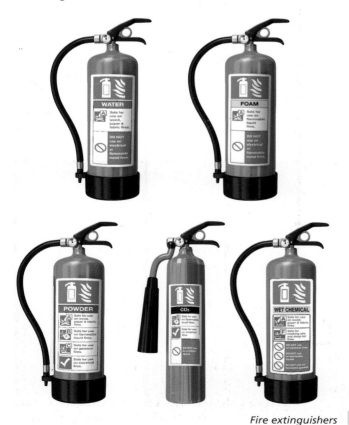

Fire extinguishers

Identify the hazard	What is the risk?	What should I do?
Pouring water onto an electrical fire	Electrocution	• If in doubt, stay out and call the fire brigade • Ask your employer to send you for training

Suspicious parcels or packages

Suspicious parcels or packages should be considered high risk as they may endanger lives. Your salon should have a policy specifically for dealing with suspicious packages in a way that will reduce the risk to health and safety. It should include the following.

- Do not touch the package!
- Evacuate the salon.
- Call 999 for the police.
- Do not re-enter the salon until you have been authorised to do so by the police.

Flood

In the event of the salon being flooded due to a leak or burst pipes, it is necessary to follow your salon's procedures. In particular:

- the electricity must be turned off at the mains to prevent electrocution
- the water should be turned off at the mains supply to prevent further leakage
- call the plumber to fix the leak
- in extreme cases, it may be necessary to call the fire brigade to pump out the water.

Gas leak

In the event of a gas leak or if you suspect you can smell gas, procedures must be followed to prevent a gas explosion. You should evacuate clients and other staff not included in the salon's procedure for gas leaks.

Those remaining must ensure that:

- they do not turn electric switches on or off as they may 'spark' and ignite the gas
- they do not smoke or use naked flames
- they turn the gas supply off at the meter, to prevent any more gas escaping
- they open all doors and windows to get rid of the gas
- the appointed person will call the gas emergency number.

Check it out

If your salon does not have policies in place to cover the above emergencies, how would you rate the risk – high, medium or low?

Personal presentation

Hairdressing is a fashion industry and the way you look is important. Clients will judge you not only on your hairdressing skills but also on the way you look. Personal presentation also has important implications for health and safety, as outlined below.

Clothes

Your clothes should be regularly laundered and preferably made from cotton or a poly-cotton material, as these fabrics will allow your skin to breathe. Cotton fabrics also minimise perspiration and are easy to clean. Avoid wearing woollen clothes, as they may make you too hot; hair tends to stick into the weave and digs into the skin, which can be uncomfortable. You should also try to avoid clothing with 'floaty' sleeves, as these could get caught in equipment.

Shoes

Your shoes should have a low heel and a closed-in toe. Shoes with high heels throw your body out of alignment, which in time will lead to backache due to unnecessary stress put on the muscles and ligaments.

A closed-in shoe will help to prevent hair cuttings from becoming stuck in the soles of your feet. This can be extremely painful as the hairs are not always easy to find and your skin may become infected. Hairdressers tend to stand for most of the day and your feet need to be comfortable. Leather shoes are best as they allow your feet to breathe.

Another potential problem is varicose veins, which can develop as a result of standing for long periods of time. Once they have developed, they are uncomfortable. Wearing 'support tights' may be helpful, especially if you are pregnant.

Jewellery

Ideally, rings shouldn't be worn in the salon, as products may become lodged underneath thus causing contact dermatitis. Large rings with stones or rough edges may scratch the client.

Personal health

Your own health, especially poor health, has serious implications for the people around you. If you have contracted an illness that is infectious or contagious, you run the risk of passing it on to your colleagues or clients. Ideally, you should not attend work if you know there is the possibility of you passing it on to another person. Remember, you have a duty of care towards your clients.

In the salon

Blood and tears

Mr Lewis called into the salon for a beard trim with Shannon, the new stylist. Shannon had a small cut on her right hand from being careless with a bread knife. She didn't think she needed a plaster because the cut was quite small. As Shannon prepared to trim Mr Lewis's facial hair, she accidentally opened the wound on the edge of the workstation. The salon manager noticed what was going on and insisted that Shannon find a plaster in the First Aid box.

- What kind of risk did Shannon pose to her client?
- How could this situation have been avoided?

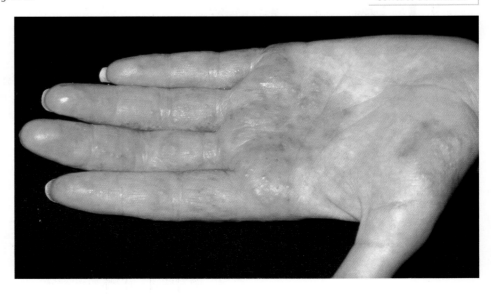

Contact dermatitis

Check your knowledge

The following questions will help you to check your understanding of this unit. The answers can be found on page 417. Take care, as there may be more than one correct answer for some questions.

1 A hazard is defined as:
   a the possibility that harm will occur
   b something that controls the risks to health and safety
   c something that has the potential to cause harm
   d all areas of the salon

2 When using hair colouring products, which legislation is applicable?
   a Electricity at Work Regulations
   b COSHH
   c Manual Handling Operations Regulations
   d Personal Protective Equipment at Work Regulations

3 Which of the following are methods of sterilisation?
   a Infra-red cabinet
   b Ultra-violet cabinet
   c Soap and water
   d Autoclave

4 You discover the fire exit in the salon is blocked with boxes of stock. Do you:
   a move the boxes somewhere else
   b tell the manager
   c ignore them, as somebody will move them eventually
   d call the Fire Brigade

5 You should always be on the look out for hazards in the salon as this will:
   a reduce the risk of accidents
   b ensure you are fulfilling your health and safety obligations
   c ensure you are busy all the time
   d increase the number of accidents that occur

6 Jewellery should be avoided since this will:
   a prevent contact dermatitis
   b prevent scratching the client
   c prevent scalding the client
   d please the manager

7 When lifting heavy or awkward shaped packages, you should:
   a lift it any way you can
   b ask for help from a colleague
   c make sure you keep your back straight and lift using your leg muscles
   d empty some of the items out of the box until you can lift it easily

8 If one of the stylists accidentally cuts a client during a cutting service, you should:
   a ignore it, unless the client complains
   b make sure it's logged in the accident book
   c apologise to the client
   d reprimand the stylist

9 You notice one of the juniors is removing a colour without wearing gloves. Do you:
   a shout at the junior across the salon
   b get her a pair of gloves to use
   c speak to her afterwards, explaining the reasons why gloves should be worn
   d make sure it's logged in the accident book

10 Risk assessments should be carried out:
   a every week
   b if the salon acquires a new piece of equipment
   c every month
   d if a new member of staff starts work

Assessment guidance

For this unit, you are required to prove consistent occupational competence. This should be demonstrated through a variety of relevant work activities.

You should be assessed using a variety of assessment methods and your knowledge should be assessed along with your performance evidence wherever possible.

You must prove that you have monitored the operation of the salon's health and safety procedures, relating to all people that enter the salon.

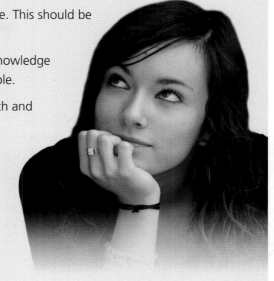

Simulated activity is not allowed for any part of this unit. However, you may be assessed using a combination of assessment methods from the list below:

- Direct observation of the candidate in the workplace.
- Witness testimony by colleagues and line managers of the candidate's successful performance of activities in the workplace.
- Documentary and other product-based evidence.
- A personal report by the candidate endorsed by colleagues.
- Questions.
- Discussion.
- Professional discussion.

Unit G21

Provide hairdressing consultation services

What you will learn:

- How to identify clients' needs and wishes
- How to analyse the hair and scalp
- How to make recommendations to your client
- How to advise clients on hair maintenance and management
- How to agree services with your client.

Anne Veck, photographer: David Howard

Introduction

The consultation is the most crucial part of any service offered in the salon. An effective and comprehensive consultation and advisory service will ensure the clients are satisfied with the service they receive and contribute to the overall professional image the salon is portraying. The consultation/advisory service should not finish when you start the required service, but continue for the duration of the client's visit.

In this unit you will learn the techniques needed to carry out an effective consultation and the importance of giving advice and guidance to your clients. This may include referring them to a specialist for further advice and/or treatment. You will also be encouraged to offer your support to colleagues who may be experiencing difficulties with their own consultations.

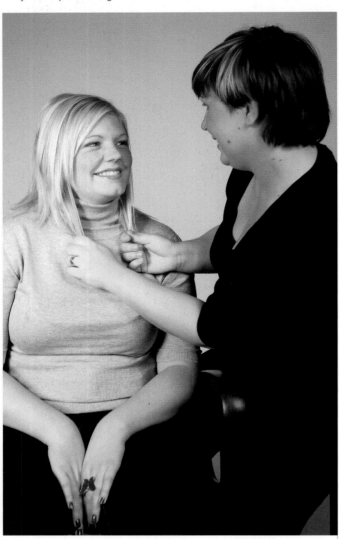

Effective consultation is the key to client satisfaction

You the stylist

As a stylist you must carry out thorough and effective consultations. You need to find out everything about your client's hair before starting work, as this will ensure you make the correct decisions regarding the services that are available to your client. This includes identifying the client's requirements using your communication skills, analysing the hair and scalp (including carrying out pre-service testing when necessary), and then making your recommendations. A good consultation instils confidence in the client and, as a result of this, you will build a good relationship with your client, based on trust. Your clients need to feel you have their best interests at heart, rather than being a means to boost your commission!

Once you have the trust of your clients, they will more readily accept your recommendations, as long as your recommendations are honest. It is not always easy to tell a client that their wishes are unachievable, but as long as you use tact and diplomacy, you will find that honesty is the best policy.

You should also be able to discuss the client's home-care regime and give advice and guidance.

You should be able to participate in discussions with your clients regarding their needs and wishes as well as making general conversation. For many clients their visit to the salon incorporates the hair service and an element of socialising. A silent service can be uncomfortable for some clients as well as the stylist. You must learn to gauge the situation and make openings to encourage your clients to speak.

Hairdressers are renowned for discussing the weather and the client's last or forthcoming holiday, but this does not need to be the case. You should try to find out about your client's interests and bring these into the discussion. A quiet client may become quite animated when discussing an area they are interested in and the things you learn may surprise you! It is also a good opportunity to discuss the client's home hair-care regime. You will, however, come across the silent client, the one who shows no desire to speak once their needs and wishes have been established and the service is underway. You must respect their decision, as it may be the only time that day they have have the opportunity for peace and quiet.

Identifying clients' needs and wishes

Many clients find it difficult to express their requirements, as they do not always know how to explain what they want. As a professional hairdresser, you must be able to establish the exact nature of your clients' needs and wants. This requires you to have excellent interpersonal skills. You will need to use these skills to draw information from the client and also to make sure that both you and the client have a complete understanding before commencing any service.

Communication

Communication is a two-way process that involves both sending and receiving information. As a hairdresser, you are expected to be able to make conversation with your clients. However, good communication is not just about talking; it also involves listening, hearing and interpreting what the other person is saying in a positive manner.

We communicate in a number of ways, as shown below.

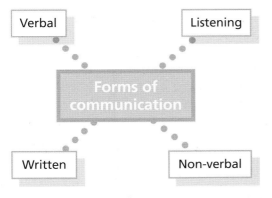

Verbal · Listening · Forms of communication · Written · Non-verbal

Verbal communication

When speaking to clients you must make sure the language you use is suitable for the recipient. You may need to simplify your language to ensure total understanding. Many clients are not familiar with hairdressing jargon and do not always understand what you are saying to them. For example, you might tell your client that you will taper the nape area, graduate the back and leave some weight on the top. Do you think your client really understands exactly what you mean or could this be better explained by using visual aids, for example, style books, colleagues in the salon and so on? Many clients find it easier to relate to a picture than to words, as it conjures up a more realistic mental image and is easier for them to understand.

Some clients find it difficult to express their needs and wishes and require time and encouragement to put their point across. Your clients should never feel hurried as this may prevent them giving you essential information. At intervals you should stop and summarise the information the client has given you. This gives the client the opportunity to either confirm or refute your understanding of the conversation. For example, you could say, 'So do you want your hair to cover your ears?' or 'Do you want a heavy fringe?'

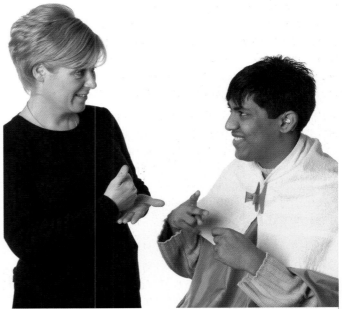

Using sign language can help you communicate with clients with a hearing impairment

Remember

It is essential that you allow the client sufficient time to think and answer, as failure to do this could result in an unwanted outcome and a dissatisfied client.

Once you are both happy with the situation, you should move the conversation along to the next point of discussion. You should be able to initiate and focus on specific areas that need to be developed to ensure you have a total understanding. Remember to summarise when a new topic has been discussed. You may need to use explicit questioning to help draw the information from the client; this questioning should cover both 'factual' and 'feeling' questions.

Provide hairdressing consultation services **Unit G21**

Factual questions

You should use factual questions to find out relevant information about the client's hair such as home-care routine, previous chemical history and so on. Many stylists like to use this type of question to open a conversation, as it is non-threatening to the client. For example, 'How often do you shampoo your hair? Which products do you use at home to style your hair?' This will give you an invaluable insight into their home-care regime, leaving you the opportunity to give them advice and guidance on maintaining their hair and improving it where necessary, thus ensuring their hair is in optimum condition.

Feeling questions

Feeling questions should be used to establish the clients' fears, opinions, doubts or worries. These questions usually include words such as 'feel', 'think' or 'want', and are an excellent tool for finding out how the client really feels. For example, 'You feel a vibrant red colour isn't really you, but what do you think about this smoky, more subdued red?' You must treat your client's worries and doubts as important issues and readily accept their opinions. Ignoring their worries will lead to client dissatisfaction.

Other types of questions

When trying to elicit information from your clients, the way you structure your questions is very important. You should try wherever possible to use open questions. These questions start with words such as 'what', 'why', 'when', 'how', 'where' and 'who', and will require the client to give a more detailed answer. For example, 'How did you feel about your last hair colour?' (This is an open and feeling question.)

Closed questions require either a 'yes' or 'no' answer and are not very good at drawing information from the client, for example, 'Same colour as last time?' This does not readily set the client up to express his or her wishes, but would be seen more as a lost opportunity to convey their views. However, you should use closed questions when closing the consultation or drawing a conversation to its end, for example, 'So you want a very soft curl, just to give the hair body and support the style?' This gives the client the opportunity to answer either yes or no.

When questioning the client, remember to give yourself sufficient time to reflect on what they have just told you. You should then summarise or re-phrase the information to ensure you have fully understood their requirements.

Non-verbal communication

Only a small percentage of the impression you create stems from what you say; the majority comes from your body language. It is very important that you are aware of your non-verbal communication skills.

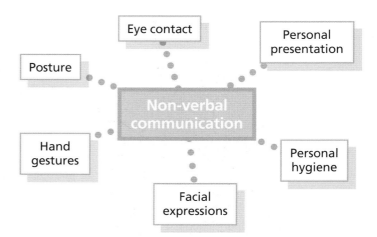

Posture

Try to maintain good posture. If you slouch around the salon, it gives the impression you do not particularly care and clients will assume this is reflected in the work you carry out in the salon.

Eye contact

You should make eye contact with your client frequently enough to show that you are responsive, but avoid staring at the client as this becomes intimidating.

Hand gestures

These are commonly used to convey feelings or to emphasise a point. However, overuse of hand gestures may appear ridiculous to onlookers.

Facial expressions

You should try to maintain positive facial expressions as these are seen as friendly and caring. Smiling at your client will make them feel more comfortable in your company. However, this does not mean walking around with a permanent grin on your face.

Your non-verbal communication should be positive at all times in the salon, for example, smiling, making eye contact and so on. This will help to put others at ease, which includes both clients and other members of staff. When instructing junior members of staff, your body language should be open and unthreatening, as this will again be reflected in the salon's atmosphere and the willingness of others to help you. Other members of staff and clients may be easily offended by negative body language.

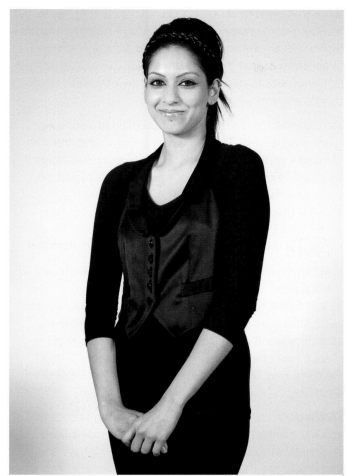

Stylists should maintain their professional image at all times

- Keep in mind the phrase 'actions speak louder than words'. Your body language can tell someone far more about how you are feeling than what you may actually say.
- You may think you can cover up feeling hurt or angry, but those who can read body language will know exactly what you are saying without words!

Written communication

Some salons now use prescription pads to note a client's hair and home-care details. This then leads to a home-care maintenance programme that may be discussed with the client.

Kera-care
CONDITIONING HAIR CARE SYSTEM

Date: _____
Name: _____
Address: _____
City: _____ Country: _____
Postcode: _____ Phone: _____

__Please tick the best response to each of the following__

Scalp Condition:
☐ Dry/Itchy ☐ Normal ☐ Oily

Hair Condition:
☐ Virgin ☐ Relaxed
☐ Colour treated ☐ Permanently waved

Hair Texture:
☐ Fine ☐ Medium ☐ Coarse

Dignosis:
☐ Weak ☐ Dry/Brittle ☐ Damaged
☐ Over processed ☐ Shedding ☐ Healthy
☐ Other

How often do you visit the salon for service?
☐ Every week ☐ Every two weeks
☐ Once a month ☐ Every two months or longer

Do you shampoo at home between visits?
☐ Yes ☐ No

How do you have your hair styled?
☐ Blow dry/Hot curl ☐ Wrap set ☐ Roller set
☐ Rod set ☐ Other

What is you daily active lifestyle?
☐ Aerobics ☐ Swimming
☐ Running/Jogging ☐ Other

How do you select products for home maintenance?
☐ Salon/Stylist ☐ Beauty supplier
☐ Other

Kera-care hairscription

The following Aslone Hair Care Maintenance is suggested for your hair texture, conditioning, and daily styling needs. Follow this recommended hair care regime to restore and maintain healthy looking hair.

SHAMPOOS
☐ Dry & Itchy Scalp Moisturising Shampoo
☐ Hydrating Detangling Shampoo
☐ 1st Lather Shapoo

CONDITIONERS
☐ Leave-In Conditioner
☐ Humecto Cream Conditioner
☐ Dry & Itchy Sclap Moisturising Conditioner

LIGHT OILS
☐ Oil Moisturizer with Jojoba Oil
☐ Conditioning Cream Hairdress
☐ Dry & Itchy Scalp Glossifer
☐ High Sheen Glossifer
☐ Essential Oils for the Hair

STYLING ESSENTIALS
☐ Protein Styling Gel
☐ Finishing Spritz
☐ Setting Lotion
☐ Silken Seal
☐ Silkien Seal Liquid Sheen
☐ Foam Wrap-set Lotion

Next appointment: _____ Time: _____

Comments / Product Usage: _____

A hairscription

Personal presentation/personal hygiene

Personal hygiene is important to hairdressers as they work in such close proximity to clients. Your own hygiene should be excellent, as you do not wish to portray anything other than total professionalism to your clients. Stale breath and body odour will portray a negative impression of you.

Although hairdressing is a fashion industry, many salons now have quite strict dress codes for staff, for example, no sleeveless or cropped tops. It can be quite off-putting to have an armpit in your face or a large expanse of flesh showing. If you make the effort to look smart, clean and tidy, clients will assume you will take the same care and consideration over their hair.

Check it out

Ask a colleague or friend to watch you whilst you are working (or better still, make a video recording) and analyse your body language. Do you appear friendly and approachable? If you do not, now is the time to change!

Completion of client record cards is essential to the smooth running of any salon. The information contained on a client record card should be legible, unambiguous and clear, and leave the reader in no doubt as to its meaning. Record cards that are filled in incorrectly or are incomplete may cause chaos in the salon, as mistakes can occur leaving the client dissatisfied with the service, and the salon in breach of the Data Protection Act (see also page 98).

Listening

Listening plays a large part in any consultation as you need to listen to your client's requirements and act accordingly. Further questioning on your part to ascertain your client's wishes may follow.

As a professional hairdresser, you should adopt an attitude of active participation when listening to your client's wishes. Maintaining positive body language and using words of encouragement may help you do this. You can show this by:

- facing the client
- maintaining eye contact
- leaning towards the client
- acknowledging what has been said
- facing the client at the same level rather than speaking through the mirror.

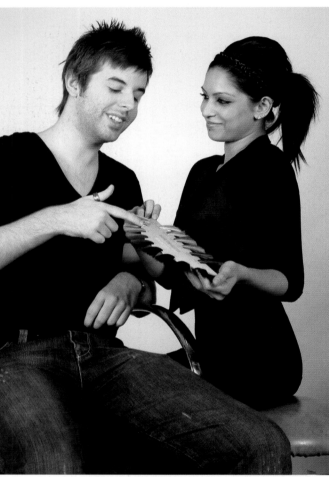

Use positive body language and active listening skills when discussing clients' needs and wishes

People are often heard saying, 'I know you're listening to me, but are you hearing what I'm saying?' meaning you are listening in a half-hearted manner and probably not trying to understand what is being said to you. This type of passive listening leads to mistakes and client dissatisfaction, as the client's requests are often ignored.

You also need to learn the skill of listening to what your client is not saying! This involves learning to read the messages your clients are sending through spoken words, their facial expressions and body posture. You should pay particular attention to:

- what they say
- the way it is said
- what is not being said.

How often have you said something but not really meant it? A friend in an awful outfit asks if you like it and you agree so you do not hurt their feelings, but can you really lie that well? Most clients cannot. You need to take the time and effort to notice these things. You may also notice that the client's tone of voice alters. If the words become 'clipped', the client may not be happily accepting the information you are giving.

Keep a close check on your client's facial expressions. While you will hopefully have mastered the art of maintaining positive facial expressions, your client may not have and you should use this information to your advantage. This will obviously depend on the circumstances, but you may be required to ask further feeling questions to discover what the client is trying not to tell you. Have you ever taken the time to look for indicators such as these?

During your consultations you will be expected to adopt the techniques you have just learned and utilise them to the full. Your questioning and listening techniques, coupled with open and responsive body language, will ensure your client feels comfortable about asking you questions. You may be required to go over things several times to ensure the clients have a full understanding of the service they are to receive.

Check it out

If you have some spare time, study people's body language and their methods of communication. It is sometimes easier to do this when you are sitting on the outside looking in, for example, when the client belongs to another stylist.

Giving the client information on hair maintenance and management

Most clients know little about maintaining and managing their own hair, therefore, as the expert, it's up to you to educate your clients. There is little point in carrying out an elaborate colouring service if the client doesn't have the time or money to maintain it, so it's essential you explain how frequently the client will need to visit the salon and the approximate cost of such visits.

You must also ensure the client is aware of the correct shampoo and conditioning products for their hair type, so the client's hair remains in optimum condition between visits. You may also need to explain to your client that some varieties of '2 in 1' shampoos and conditioners have a silicone base, which can be problematic when carrying out colouring or perming services, as failure to do so could result in an unhappy client!

When you have carried out a re-style, it's essential that you advise the client on the correct styling and finishing products to use, as well as which tools and equipment to use, as this will enable them to recreate the look at home, thus pleasing the client and enhancing the professional image of the salon at the same time!

Remember

Don't forget to inform your client as to how they can protect their hair from the effects of humidity, for example using styling and finishing products will help to prevent the atmospheric moisture from entering the hair and to avoid steamy environments when possible.

You may need to discuss their current home-care routine and explain whether it will have an effect on future services, for example, is the general condition good enough for the required service or should the products or treatment of the hair be changed to allow for future services to take place?

Many clients don't treat their hair very well, so it's essential that you try to instil good practice into the clients. For example, use of home hair colours may lead to problems when the client decides to have a professional colour carried out, or failing to use a heat protection product before using heated styling equipment of any variety will cause the hair to become dehydrated and therefore may prevent the required service from being carried out.

Be professional ★★★

- Use all of your communication skills when identifying clients' wishes.
- Use visual aids whenever possible.
- Thorough and effective consultations prevent mistakes and client dissatisfaction.

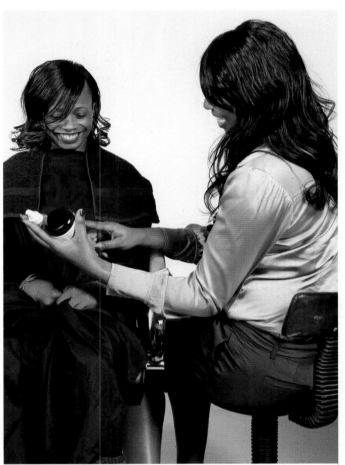

After a re-style, advise your client on the correct styling and finishing products to use to help them recreate their new look at home

Analysing the hair and scalp

Before you are able to accurately analyse the hair and scalp, you should have a thorough understanding of the hair growth and the hair's characteristics, as this will have a considerable bearing on the outcome. To begin with, you should have a good understanding of the basic structure of the hair and skin and how they work.

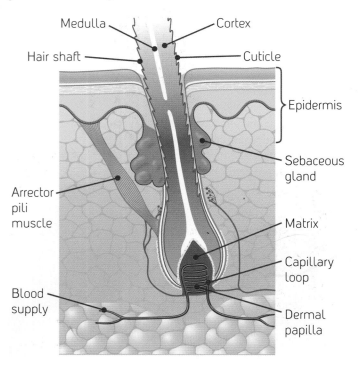

A vertical cross-section of a hair in its follicle

Parts of the hair

Cuticle

The cuticle is the outermost part of the hair and is made up of layers of overlapping scale-like bands. It acts as protection for the rest of the hair, but as keratin — the protein found in skin and hair — is brittle it may be damaged by harsh treatment and overuse of chemicals. The cuticle may not be present towards the ends of the hair, as it may have been damaged or destroyed completely; therefore the ends of the hair will be more porous.

The number of layers of cuticle scales varies depending on the type of hair. Coarse hair has the most layers of cuticle, making it more resistant to chemicals. You may have discovered this already when perming or colouring coarse hair.

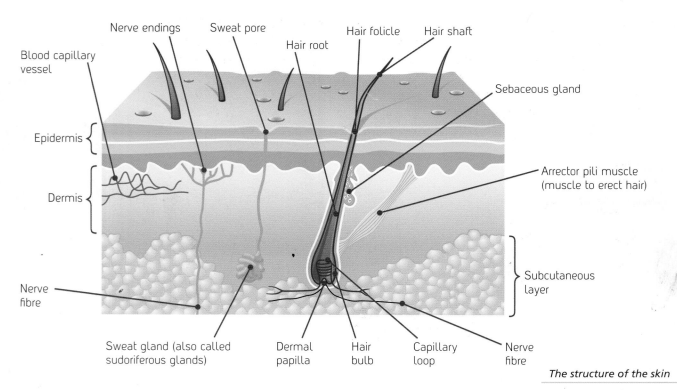

The structure of the skin

Cortex

The cortex makes up the bulk of the hair and gives the hair its strength and elasticity. The cortex is important, as this is where the changes occur during bleaching, perming, relaxing, colouring and styling. The cortex is made up of bundles of parallel fibres, which are in turn made up of smaller fibres.

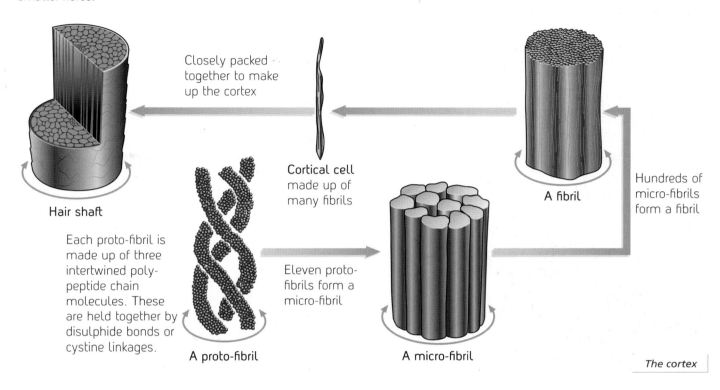

Hair shaft

Closely packed together to make up the cortex

Cortical cell made up of many fibrils

A fibril

Hundreds of micro-fibrils form a fibril

Each proto-fibril is made up of three intertwined poly-peptide chain molecules. These are held together by disulphide bonds or cystine linkages.

A proto-fibril

Eleven proto-fibrils form a micro-fibril

A micro-fibril

The cortex

Melanin and pheomelanin, the hair's natural colour pigment, are found in the cortex. African type hair has two different types of cortex, the ortho-cortex and the para-cortex. The ortho-cortex has a less crowded structure and always lies on the outer curve of a wave. It is less crowded as the hair is stretched at this point. It has a lower sulphur content than the para-cortex. The para-cortex is compressed on the inside of the wave, making this part of the cortex more crowded. When carrying out chemical treatments on curly hair, this must be taken into consideration, as the hair will absorb chemicals at different rates, giving an uneven result.

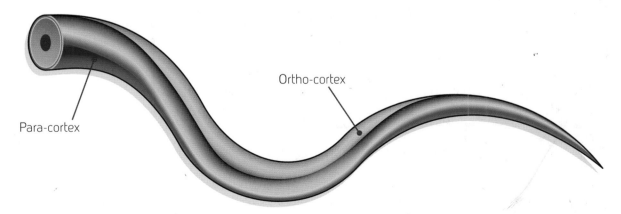

Ortho-cortex

Para-cortex

The para- and ortho-cortex

Medulla

The medulla is the central part of the hair and is made up of small soft cells with air spaces in between. People with very fine hair may not have a medulla.

Sebaceous glands

The sebaceous glands are sac-like structures attached to the hair follicles all over the body. They produce sebum, which is an oily substance used to lubricate and waterproof the hair and skin, and prevent them from drying out. If too little sebum is produced, the skin may become dry and cracked, which could lead to dermatitis. Sebaceous glands are plentiful on the face and scalp.

Arrector pili muscle

The arrector pili muscle is a small involuntary muscle that is attached to each hair follicle. When you are cold or frightened, the muscle contracts making the hair stand on end. It serves no purpose in hairdressing.

Sudoriferous (or sweat) glands

The sudoriferous glands are found in the dermis and look like coiled tubes that extend and lead to the surface of the skin to form a pore. The purpose of these glands is to regulate the body temperature through the excretion of sweat onto the skin surface. When sweat evaporates, it cools the skin and the body temperature becomes lower. Sweat is mainly composed of water, salts and waste products.

Hair follicle

The hair follicles are tiny indentations in the skin. The hair that is below the skin is contained within the follicle. The angle at which the follicle lies will determine the hair's natural fall.

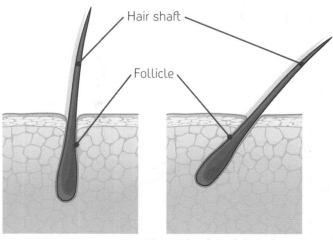

The angle of the follicle determines the natural fall of the hair

Hair shaft

Follicle

Dermal papilla

Often referred to as the growing factory. The base of the hair follicle is pushed upwards, like the bottom of a wine bottle. The papilla is situated in this space. The cells produced in the papilla are pushed upwards into the germinal matrix.

Hair bulb

The hair bulb has two distinctive parts — the upper bulb and the germinal matrix. In the germinal matrix all the cells look the same. In the upper bulb the hair starts to develop into its three layers.

Blood supply

The blood supply enters the papilla, bringing food and nourishment for healthy cell growth. It also takes away waste products.

Nerve supply

The nerve supply is also attached to the papilla. This supply is in addition to other nerves in the area, and it is what enables you to feel your hair being pulled.

Parts of the skin (see page 34)

Epidermis

The epidermis is the outermost layer of the skin. The part of the epidermis that we see is called the stratum corneum and this is made up of flat, horny cells. It is these cells that are constantly being shed and replaced. Skin problems associated with the production and shedding of these cells include dandruff and psoriasis.

Dermis

The dermis is situated below the epidermis and contains blood vessels, sweat and sebaceous glands, nerve endings and hair follicles. The dermis is made up of protein fibres.

Subcutaneous layer

The subcutaneous layer is situated below the dermis and contains fatty tissue, which acts as insulation (to prevent body heat from being lost), and as a defence to protect the internal organs.

The characteristics of different hair types and textures

Hair may be considered fine, medium or coarse in texture, but this may vary at different parts of the scalp and, in the case of curly hair, along the hair shaft. The degree of curl in the hair may also vary. It is essential during your consultation that you consider all the hair you will be working with and not just the part that is easy to see.

Why do some people have straight hair and others curly?

There are currently three schools of thought surrounding this question, but there is little solid evidence to support any particular theory.

1   The first theory suggests that the amount of curl in the hair is determined by the shape of the follicle, for example, a straight follicle will produce straight hair and a bent follicle will produce wavy or curly hair, depending on the degree of curvature.

Straight hair

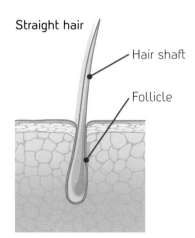

Hair shaft

Follicle

Wavy hair

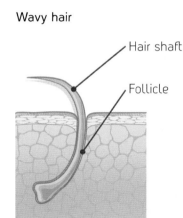

Hair shaft

Follicle

Curly hair

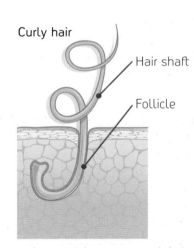

Hair shaft

Follicle

Different-shaped follicles may produce straight, wavy or curly hair

2   The second theory suggests the amount of curl in the hair is due to an uneven rate of mitosis (cell division). Hair grows as a result of cell division in the germinal matrix. As the number of cells increase, they push the old cells upwards into the upper bulb. If the cells on one side of the hair are dividing more quickly than the other, this will make one side of the hair longer than the other, producing a bend in the hair. If the cell division alternates from one side to the other, the result will be curly hair.

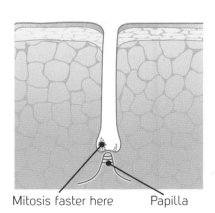

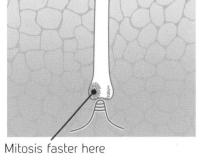

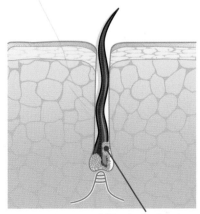

Mitosis faster here   Papilla

Mitosis faster here

Mitosis faster here

Curly hair resulting from an uneven rate of mitosis

To support this theory, think about a person who has undergone chemotherapy. The hair after treatment is often quite straight, whereas beforehand it was curly. The hair returns to being curly at a later date.

During chemotherapy, the whole body's systems are disrupted and mitosis is suppressed. The body would naturally take quite a while to return to normal, even after the treatment has been completed, and this may include mitosis, hence the hair being initially straight but reverting to curly once the body's balance has been restored.

3   The third theory suggests that keratinisation occurs in the cortex asymmetrically. As the hair moves upwards in the follicle, the hair begins the process of keratinisation (where the living cells die and harden). By the time the hair is a third of the way up the follicle, the hair has been fully keratinised. On one side of the cortex, keratinisation occurs early (and becomes the para-cortex) whilst on the other side, keratinisation is delayed (and this becomes the ortho-cortex). Until keratinisation takes place, the hair will continue to grow — so the ortho-cortex will be longer in length than the para-cortex, producing curl.

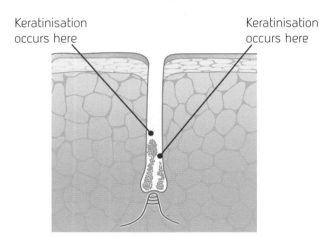

Keratinisation occurs here

Keratinisation occurs here

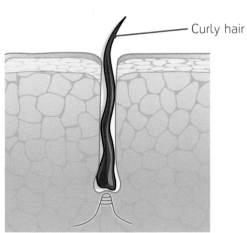

Curly hair

Curly hair resulting from uneven keratinisation

Check it out

Look at the above information and discuss the pros and cons of each theory with your tutor and group members. Then draw your own conclusions.

KS **Key Skills Links**: Level 2 Communication

The hair growth cycle

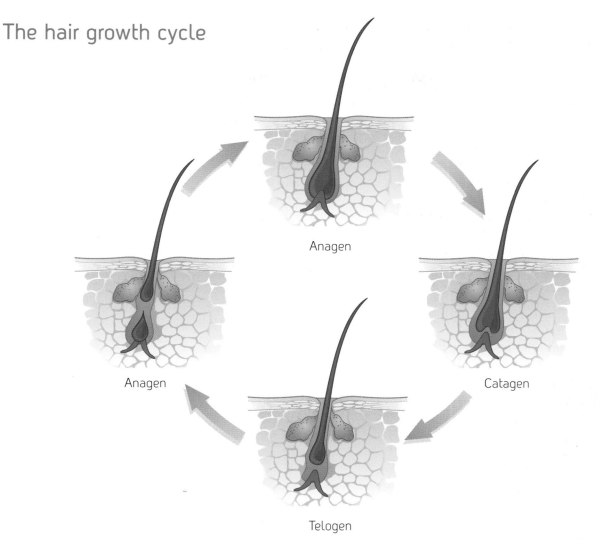

Anagen

Catagen

Telogen

Anagen

The hair growth cycle

At the base of the hair follicle lies the dermal papilla. The dermal papilla is fed by nourishment from the blood stream, which helps to produce new hair. Within each hair follicle there is a period of hair growth, followed by a resting phase. The total cycle goes through three separate phases, which are:

1 anagen – growth or active phase
2 catagen – transitional or changing phase
3 telogen – resting phase.

The hair growth cycle is repeated many times during a person's lifetime. Each hair grows then falls out and a new hair grows in its place.

Anagen

This is the growing or active phase of the growth cycle. There is plenty of activity taking place in the dermal papilla. This average phase lasts from one to six years, but some people have a short anagen cycle and regardless of what they may do, their hair will never grow long as it is predetermined to fall out after a specified time. Some people with very long hair have a much longer anagen cycle than average. The anagen phase is the longest with approximately 85 per cent of hair in this active state at any one time. Some areas of the body have a much shorter phase in the anagen cycle, for example, masculine facial hair.

Catagen

At the end of the anagen phase, hair growth stops and no new cells are produced in the dermal papilla. This phase lasts for approximately two weeks and during this time the follicle shrinks up to one-sixth of its original length.

Telogen

This is a period of rest for both the follicle and the papilla and lasts between ten to twelve weeks. Approximately 10 to 15 per cent of the follicles are in this phase at any one time.

At the end of the telogen phase the hair follicle re-enters the anagen phase, the follicle lengthens downwards and the papilla becomes active again, ready for the growth of a new hair.

As each follicle across the scalp is at a slightly different point in the cycle at any given time, this explains why a client's haircut loses its shape after a few weeks. On a positive note, it keeps hairdressers in business!

During pregnancy, the hormonal changes in the body keep the hair in the anagen phase of the growth cycle for the length of the pregnancy and many women notice their hair becoming thicker during pregnancy. However, after giving birth, the hormone levels change yet again and all the hairs that should have been lost during the pregnancy are shed fairly quickly. This can be very distressing to a client who is not only contending with a new baby, but is also worried she is losing her hair. This condition does rectify itself eventually, but the client will require reassurance from you in the meantime.

Under normal circumstances, the hair growth cycle will continue for the duration of a person's life. However, there are factors that may influence hair growth or cause damage to the hair follicle. These factors include genetic influences (for example, male pattern baldness) or the results of scarring and radiation.

Reference to client records

Reference to clients' previous records should be made whenever possible. This will give you a wealth of information the client may not know or understand, for example, allergic reactions to relaxing products previously used, type of colourants used and so on.

Remember

All information contained on a client's record card should be accurate and up to date to comply with the Data Protection Act, even if the information is handwritten!

Observation

An experienced stylist can tell a lot about a client's hair and scalp just by looking at it, for example, the texture, condition and any previous chemical treatments. Prior to questioning the client, you should have made an initial assessment of your client's hair and scalp and any potential problems that may arise from your observation.

Questioning

You should use questioning as a tool to find out as much as you can from your client, as this will enable you to make an accurate judgement regarding the most suitable service you can then carry out. You should use open questions whenever possible as you will gain more information from your client. However, not all clients are honest when giving information about their hair and the treatments that have been carried out on it, especially those done by a non-professional. If in doubt, carry out any necessary tests, as this will save time in the long run and prevent client dissatisfaction.

Testing

Testing the hair prior to salon services is a practice that should be adopted by all professional hairdressers, especially as litigation is becoming more widespread. It only need take a few minutes to carry out some tests and could save you hours (not to mention money) if the service goes wrong and needs to be corrected, or the client sues the salon for negligence. If you have any worries or concerns regarding the suitability of a client's hair, carry out the necessary tests to eliminate the doubt and ensure the client's hair is suitable for the service they requested. All tests should be carried out following your salon's procedures and the manufacturer's instructions.

The kinds of tests you should be carrying out are shown in the table opposite.

Test	When it should be carried out	Why it should be carried out	How it should be carried out	The expected outcome	The potential consequences if it is not carried out
Porosity (sometimes called a texture test)	Prior to colouring, perming and relaxing	To assess the amount of damage to the cuticle; to check the speed at which products will be absorbed into the hair	It should be carried out on dry hair. Hold a few strands of hair; run your fingers from roots to points and then points to roots. This test cannot be carried out on wet hair as the hair swells when wet and will not give a true indication of the hair's porosity	The hair should feel fairly smooth at the root area, becoming rougher towards the ends	The result may be uneven. The hair will become more porous
Elasticity	Prior to colouring, perming, relaxing, thermal styling and styling hair	To assess the degree of damage to the internal structure	Hold a few strands of hair between the fingers and thumbs and pull gently. Best carried out when the hair is wet	The hair should stretch and return to its original length. If the hair stretches and does not return to its original length, this indicates the presence of internal damage	The hair may overstretch and/or break
Incompatibility	Prior to colouring and perming	To test the hair for the presence of metallic salts or other incompatible substances	Take a cutting of hair from the affected part of the head, secure with cotton or sellotape. Pour 20 ml of liquid 6% H_2O_2 into a non-metallic bowl. Add 5 drops of ammonium hydroxide. Leave for up to 30 minutes	If there are no incompatible substances on the hair, there should be no reaction in the bowl. If the metallic salts are present, the liquid in the bowl will effervesce and become hot. The hair colour may change to green, black or purple	The hair colour may change. Extreme heat will be given off causing the hair to disintegrate and causing scalp burns

Test	When it should be carried out	Why it should be carried out	How it should be carried out	The expected outcome	The potential consequences if it is not carried out
Skin test before colouring	24–48 hours before each colour service	To test for allergic reaction to the product	Cleanse a small area of skin behind the ear. Mix a small amount of the darkest colour with 6% H_2O_2 and apply a small amount to the cleansed area	**A negative reaction:** There has been no reaction at all. The skin looks as it did before the skin test took place. **A positive reaction:** This can vary from redness and mild irritation to severe swelling rendering the client unable to close their eyes, speak or breathe properly	The client may have a severe allergic reaction
Skin test before perming	24–48 hours before a perming service, especially if the client has known sensitivity	As above	Cleanse a small area of skin behind the ear. Apply a small amount of perm lotion to the cleansed skin	As above	As above
Test cuttings (sometimes called a colour test)	Prior to a colouring service	To ensure optimum results. It is also reassuring for the client to see the results	Take a few cuttings from various parts of the head and secure with cotton or sellotape. Mix a small amount of the desired colour/s with the correct strength H_2O_2 and place the cuttings into the colour. Process as normal. Rinse the hair and assess the results. Alternatively, you can apply the chosen colour straight onto a small section of the hair or even weave out a few highlights. This would be carried out on hair that was still attached, rather than cuttings	This test will clearly indicate whether it is safe to proceed with the service.	Client dissatisfaction due to an incorrect result or possible damage/ breakage to the hair

Remember

Always follow your salon's procedures when carrying out pre-service testing. Most of these will reflect the manufacturer's instructions. Remember, they have tried and tested all their products and know how to achieve the best results.

Salon life

Dying for black hair?

Greta's story

Dave and I had been friends for years and he had coloured his hair black for as long as I could remember. He told me he didn't always stick to the same product manufacturer, but bought whatever was cheapest.

I was entering a hairdressing competition the following week and Dave had agreed to be my model. I was really pleased as this meant we would be spending time together and Dave was pleased because he was getting his hair coloured blue/black professionally and was saving money too! A few days before the competition, Dave came into the salon to have his hair coloured. He said he had used the product before and never had any type of reaction, so I thought it would be OK to colour his hair. The result was fantastic. Later that evening, Dave's scalp started to itch and his throat became dry and he found it difficult to swallow. During the night the itch became unbearable and Dave was having trouble breathing, so he got up. As he walked past the mirror he was horrified by what he saw. His face was blue and so swollen that he did not recognise himself. He felt very ill and was really frightened. He called me and I went round to his house immediately. I took one look at him and took him straight to the accident and emergency department at the local hospital. He was admitted to hospital as he had had a severe allergic reaction to the colouring preparation that had been used on his hair. As his face and throat had swelled, he was having trouble breathing and he was placed on a ventilator and given a massive dose of antihistamine. It took quite a few days for the swelling to subside and he was unable to model for the competition.

Be professional ★★★

Even if the client says they've had their hair coloured professionally somewhere else, you still have a duty of care towards every client; therefore a skin test is imperative! Failure to carry out a skin test prior to a colour service could be deemed negligence.

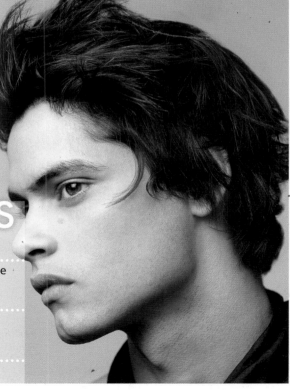

ASK THE PROFESSIONALS

Q *I feel really bad and don't understand why this happened?*

A Although Dave had always coloured his hair and even used the same product before, he had become sensitised to the product and the result was a severe allergic reaction.

Q *Does this mean that I should always carry out a skin test on a client whose hair I haven't coloured before, even if they've had it done somewhere else?*

A Yes, you should.

Unit G21 — Provide hairdressing consultation services

Unit G21 Provide hairdressing consultation services

Healthy hair

Healthy hair is recognised by its shiny appearance. This is because the cuticle scales are closed and the light reflects off the hair giving it lustre. Curly hair, even in good condition, does not always appear shiny, as the light rays hit an uneven surface causing the light rays to scatter. Consequently, shine products may be used to give the illusion of healthy hair.

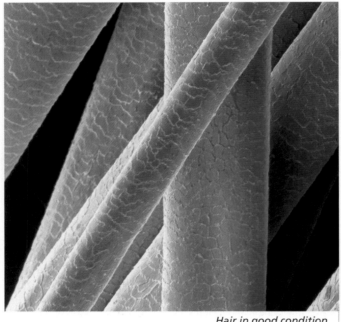

Hair in good condition

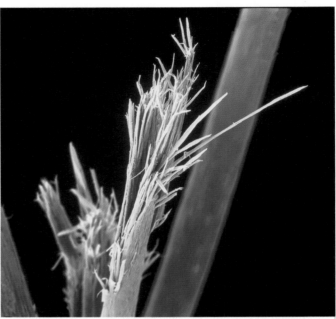

Hair in poor condition

Hair in good condition

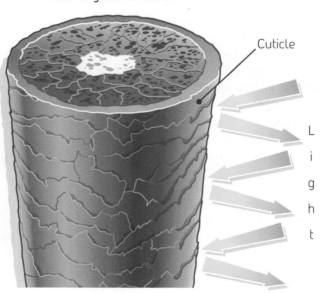

Cuticle

L i g h t

Hair in bad condition

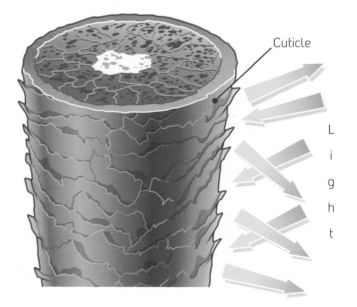

Cuticle

L i g h t

Healthy cuticle scales reflect the light to show shiny, healthy hair. Cuticle scales in poor condition bounce the light back in all directions giving the hair a flat, dull appearance

To keep the hair in optimum condition requires good health, a good diet, exercise and a skilled hairdresser who will provide excellent services and advise the client on a first-rate home-care routine. There are many things that may adversely affect the condition of the hair, such as:

- chemical damage caused by overuse of chemicals or poor application
- physical damage caused by over-brushing, blow-drying and overuse of heated styling appliances
- weather conditions, both very hot and very cold
- certain medication
- illness.

The factors above should be taken into consideration when carrying out consultations, as their effects will impact on the services and products that are suitable for the client.

When discussing the client's health and/or medication, both of which are personal and may be highly sensitive, you should always follow the salon's code of ethics and maintain confidentiality. Failure to do so may result in disciplinary action against you and loss of trust and goodwill on the part of the client.

Check it out

Does your salon have a policy of confidentiality towards clients? What should be covered within these rules?

Factors that may limit or affect services and products

There are several factors that may limit or affect the services and products you provide in the salon.

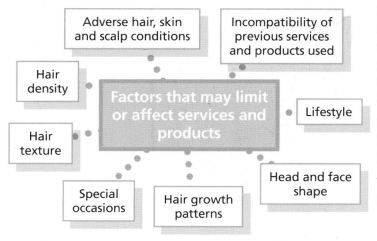

Adverse hair, skin and scalp conditions

It is essential that any adverse hair, skin and scalp conditions are identified and taken into consideration during the consultation. If the client has an infectious hair, skin or scalp condition, it needs to be recognised before the service commences to reduce the risk of cross-infection within the salon.

There are many different types of adverse hair, skin and scalp conditions and these usually fall into four main categories as follows:

- hair disorders
- infestations
- infectious or contagious skin or scalp conditions
- non-infectious skin or scalp conditions.

Hair disorders

Hair disorders are not usually infectious but may require special consideration when carrying out hairdressing services. The hair may be damaged or porous and be susceptible to breakage.

Infestations

Infestation is the name given to animal parasites that live on or in another living creature and have the potential to cause harm. The most common infestation seen by hairdressers is that of the head louse, although many hairdressers still do not recognise this condition or know how it should be treated. This infestation is becoming more prevalent and it is up to hairdressers to educate their clients as to the correct procedure to follow.

Most clients or parents are upset to discover they or their children have head lice and you must display tact and diplomacy when informing them. Salon services must not take place if a client has an infestation, but the client should be reassured that the problem is a common one and treatable. You should question the client/parent, as head lice are a common problem and are usually caught through close contact with children. You should refer the client to the pharmacist to purchase a suitable treatment and ensure the client checks through every member of the family, as they too will require treatment should they have head lice.

Once the client has left the salon, any tools and equipment that have been in contact with the client should be sterilised immediately to prevent the risk of cross-infection.

The table overleaf provides a quick reference to common infestations.

Name	Recognised by	Caused by	Referral to	Infectious/contagious
Scabies	A rash of red, raised spots and severe itching, especially at night. The burrows are sometimes visible, especially around the wrist	The sarcoptes scabiei mite, which burrows under the skin. The mite may be passed easily through close contact and commonly starts at the wrists (maybe through holding hands with an infected person	GP	Yes
Head lice (pediculosis capitis)	Intense itching and the presence of nits (the small eggs that are attached to the hair shaft, close to the scalp). On closer examination, there may be lice present	A parasitic infestation	Pharmacist or Trichologist, but treatment with conditioners is unsatisfactory and should be avoided	Yes

Infectious skin and scalp conditions

Infectious skin and scalp conditions will obviously cause problems if you fail to recognise them, or more importantly, the risk of cross-infection. An infection can usually be recognised by redness, swelling, excessive warmth to the touch or the presence of pus. The affected area will be sore to the touch and possibly itchy. Infectious conditions of the skin and scalp should always be referred to a Trichologist, as medical intervention is required.

The table below provides a quick reference to common infectious conditions.

Name	Recognised by	Caused by	Referral to	Infectious/contagious
Impetigo	Small blisters containing a pus-like substance that may break and form a flat, honey coloured crust. Most commonly seen on the face	Streptococcal or staphylococcal bacteria spread by fingers and towels, etc. Impetigo may be present as a secondary infection, associated with head lice. The skin is broken through scratching and the bacteria enters the skin	GP	Yes
Ringworm	First appears as small, round, red spots. As the spots enlarge, the centre begins to clear forming a ring with a raised border that is red and scaly. Hair will become brittle and fall out leaving bald patches	A fungal skin infection	Trichologist/GP	Yes

Name	Recognised by	Caused by	Referral to	Infectious/contagious
Folliculitis	Small yellow spots with a hair growing through, found in the follicle opening	A bacterial infection within the hair follicle, sometimes following scratching	Trichologist	Yes
Sycosis barbae (barber's itch)	A form of folliculitis. Small, red spots, often with a yellow pustule, around the follicle opening. Found in the beard area only	A bacterial infection. May be transmitted by infected shaving brushes, razors etc.	Trichologist/GP	Yes

Non-infectious skin and scalp conditions

Non-infectious skin or scalp conditions should pose no problem unless the skin is broken. If this is so, any products used may enter the skin and cause discomfort to the client. Clients with known scalp conditions should be informed if there is any deterioration in their condition. This will enable them to seek intervention before the problem worsens.

The table below provides a quick reference to common non-infectious conditions.

Name	Recognised by	Caused by	Referral to
Alopecia areata	A small round bald patch on the scalp, with surrounding hairs being short and appearing 'stubbly'. The skin in the patch is usually pale and glossy. The patch may appear overnight with the hairs being evident on the pillow the following morning	An auto-immune disorder where the cause is not fully understood, as there seem to be a number of possible reasons for it occurring. In some cases it is thought to be genetic; however, stress and shock are also thought to be contributory factors. In some instances there is no explanation at all	Trichologist / GP
Traction alopecia	Hair loss at the point of tension, for example, tight plaiting or braiding can result in hair loss at the base of the plait	The loosening of the hair in the follicle from constant pulling. Recommend all tension be removed until the hair grows back and then treat with extreme caution to prevent a recurrence	Trichologist

Name	Recognised by	Caused by	Referral to
Cicatrical alopecia	Loss of hair over an area of scarring	Baldness due to scarring. The follicles are absent in scar tissue. Take care when using chemical relaxers as they may burn and damage the skin, the same could apply to perm lotions	Trichologist, although there is little that may be done other than confirmation of the diagnosis
Diffuse alopecia	A gradual or more commonly sudden loss of hair without any itching or scaling present. Affects females for a variety of reasons	Following pregnancy (see hair growth cycle, page 39) changes in hormone levels, the contraceptive pill, thyroid problems, iron deficiency, illness or a side effect from certain medication	Trichologist
Androgenic alopecia (male pattern baldness)	Usually starts with a receding hairline, followed by loss at the crown area. Eventually the whole vertex is void of hair. The length of time the hair is in the anagen stage of the cycle reduces and the hair becomes gradually shorter and finer until the hairs do not re-grow	A genetic condition affecting some men from late teens through to old age	Trichologist
Trichotillomania	Areas of hair loss that are rarely complete patches and have irregular outlines. In right-handed people the hair loss is usually on the right-hand side	The twiddling of hair as a form of comfort or habit, or obsessive hair pulling is usually associated with some psychiatric disorders	Trichologist
Psoriasis	Well-defined, red, thickened areas of skin covered with large, silvery scales	An auto-immune disorder that is passed on in families, recurring in times of stress. Involves overactive production and shedding of the epidermal cells. It is not infectious and normal salon services may be carried out. It is not advisable to carry out chemical treatments if the skin is broken.	Trichologist

Name	Recognised by	Caused by	Referral to
Eczema	Patches of dry skin, which can itch, become sore, inflamed and weep. Usually found in the creases of the body, for example, behind the knees, but may affect large areas of the body and can affect the scalp alone	External or internal factors that give rise to an allergic response	Trichologist
Fragilitis crinium	Split ends	Harsh treatments, chemical over-processing or general weathering of the hair	The only real treatment for this is to cut them off, although 'end repair' products may give a temporary solution
Seborrhoeic dermatitis	Yellowish, greasy scales that flake, causing redness and itching. In severe cases this can extend into the eyebrows, around the nose and ears and onto the cheeks	Auto-immune disorder often associated with hormonal change	Trichologist (only after advising client to try appropriate salon products first)
Contact dermatitis	An allergic response to contact with for example shampoo, plants or rubber gloves	Over production of sebum in conjunction with dandruff and an inflamed scalp	Trichologist
Sebaceous cyst	A dome shaped lump under the skin. They are usually skin coloured unless infection is present. They may vary in size from 1–4 cm in diameter	The hair follicle has a small duct opening onto the surface of the skin. The sebaceous duct becomes plugged with sebum and the subsequent bacterial infection causes the cyst to gradually become larger. Many people with small cysts choose to ignore them. However, if they are unsightly or large, they may be removed by their GP	Trichologist/GP

Provide hairdressing consultation services **Unit G21**

Name	Recognised by	Caused by	Referral to
Keloid scarring	Scars that heal as a firm, smooth, hard growth. They have 'ridged' appearance. Keloids may be uncomfortable and itchy	An over-production of healthy tissue. It is seen more often in African type skin	Trichologist
Trichorrhexis nodosa	Small, split swellings appear on the hair shaft where the cortex has split	Harsh physical and/or chemical damage Incorrect use of heated electrical appliances Perm rubbers incorrectly placed or twisted Over-use of elastic bands to tie hair up	Trichologist
In-growing hair	A hard lump with a dark patch in the middle, underneath the surface of the skin	Short, curly hair that grows back on itself. It is quite often due to friction, for example, a shirt collar rubbing against the neck. Not infectious unless the in-growing hair has become infected	Trichologist (if it's become infected)
Monilethrix (beaded hair)	Along the hair shaft there are nodes and constrictions that make the hair look like a string of beads. This is caused by an uneven production of keratin. The hair must be handled with care, as it is liable to break where the hair constricts	A rare hereditary condition	Trichologist – this condition requires diagnosis as it cannot be seen with the naked eye. There is no cure for this.

Incompatibility of previous services or products used

Once you have identified your client's wishes and carried out an in-depth analysis of the client's hair and scalp, you may identify factors that will be incompatible with the requested service. For example, the client may have coloured their hair at home with a colourant that contains metallic salts and is therefore incompatible with any products that contain hydrogen peroxide.

Sometimes the condition of the client's hair means you will be unable to carry out the requested service, since the hair may become further damaged or break. This can prove to be very disappointing to the client, but the negative outcome that would undoubtedly occur could end up being far worse than any frustration felt by the client. When handling these situations, you must be sympathetic towards the client when you explain the problem but remain firm about your decision. This is the time when alternative services or products should be suggested and their outcomes explained to the client.

Honesty is the best policy

Mrs Smith went into the salon to book an appointment for a permanent wave. Sonia, one of the stylists, was sitting at the reception desk covering for the receptionist whilst she had lunch. Sonia looked at Mrs Smith's very fine, highly bleached hair and suggested a consultation before the appointment to be sure of the most suitable course of action to take. Mrs Smith agreed and returned to the salon later that day for her consultation appointment.

Sonia carried out a number of tests on cuttings from Mrs Smith's hair. The hair was porous and had very poor elasticity and it was obvious to Sonia that a perm was not advisable as it would cause severe damage to the hair and it would break. She explained the situation to Mrs Smith and then suggested a course of intensive conditioning treatments. She explained that when the hair condition had improved sufficiently, she would be able to carry out the perming service. Mrs Smith was not very happy with the outcome and said she would take her business elsewhere. Sonia was quite upset to have lost a client, but she still stood by her decision.

Four days later Mrs Smith returned to the salon, looking very uncomfortable. She was wearing a scarf around her head and asked to speak to Sonia. As Sonia walked over to see her, she removed her headscarf, which revealed hair that looked like cotton wool balls all over her head. She had taken her custom elsewhere and the result was disastrous. The hair had been over processed, which was not difficult given its condition to begin with, and there were random areas of breakage all over the scalp. Having realised her mistake, Mrs Smith went back to the hairdresser that she knew she could trust and asked for help to put it right. It was a long, slow process to repair the damage to the hair and Mrs Smith's confidence in hairdressers. However, Mrs Smith is still a regular client of Sonia's ten years later and has brought a lot of custom to the salon as a result of her experience.

- Was Sonia right to stand by her original decision?
- What would your professional opinion be of the hairdresser who carried out the perming service?

Head and face shape

Being able to carry out excellent hairdressing is only a part of what makes a successful hairdresser. You also need to be able to identify your client's head and face shape and ensure the service you provide will enhance it (or reduce the appearance of anything less than perfect). The illustrations below show a range of different face shapes. The oval face shape is considered to be the 'perfect' face shape and can support most hairstyles.

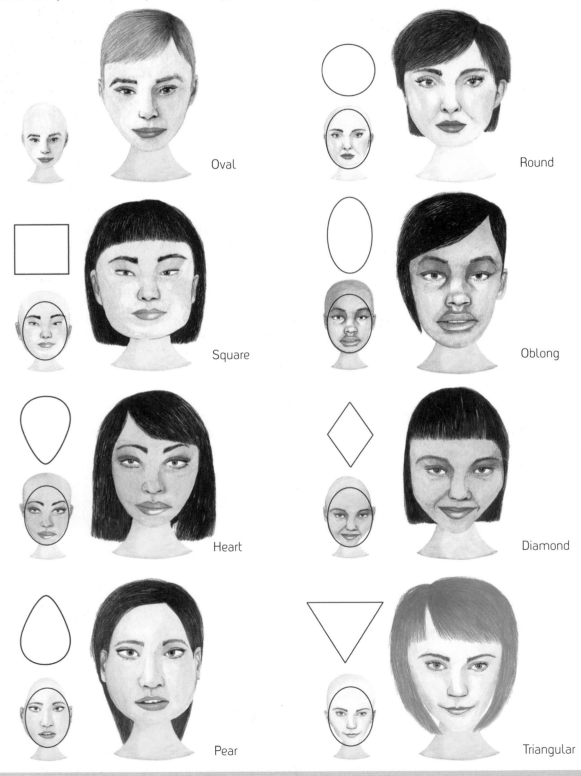

Oval

Round

Square

Oblong

Heart

Diamond

Pear

Triangular

The position of a parting can alter the shape of the face quite significantly. A client with a long face should avoid a centre parting, as this will lengthen the face; instead move the parting to the side and the face will appear shorter.

The position of the parting can lengthen or shorten the face:

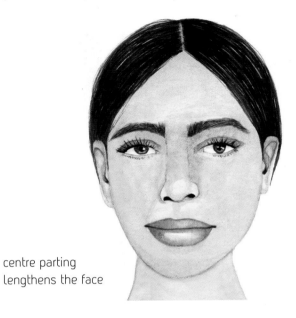

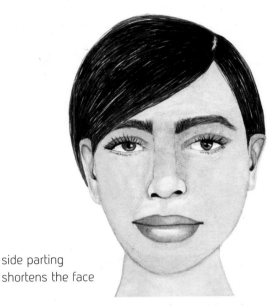

centre parting
lengthens the face

side parting
shortens the face

A side parting suits longer face shapes

A client with a small face should avoid a hairstyle that involves a lot of hair on the face, as the face will appear smaller still. This is also true for a client with glasses, as the face becomes hidden behind the hair and glasses. The addition of a fringe can camouflage a high forehead or lines and wrinkles that are best left hidden. It also softens the facial features of a more mature client.

You should always check the shape of your client's head before starting any salon service. Not every client will have a perfect head!

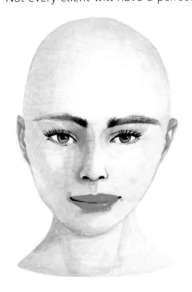

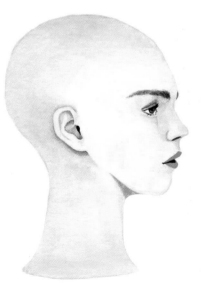

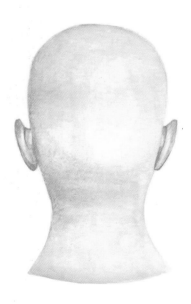

The ideal head shape

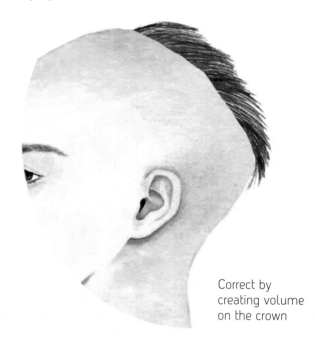

Correct by
creating volume
on the crown

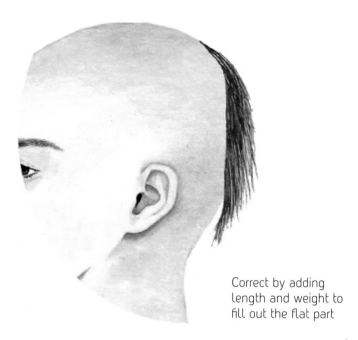

Correct by adding
length and weight to
fill out the flat part

Different head shapes and possible style solutions

Some salons now have a computer package that includes a digital camera that imposes different hairstyles and colours onto the client's face. This gives clients a visual impression of how they may look and removes the worry factor.

Lifestyle

Taking your client's lifestyle into consideration is vital. You must consider the following points:

- What amount of time does he or she have to spend on their hair each day?
- Can he or she commit to the upkeep?
- Does the proposed service complement his or her occupation?
- Is it suitable for any leisure activities he or she may pursue?

All of the above should be addressed during the consultation to ensure the client will be able to manage their hair between visits. The style you would recommend for a busy working person may differ greatly from a style for a client with a lot of leisure time on their hands.

You must ensure the client can commit to the upkeep of the style or colouring services you propose. A full head bleach would not be practical for a client who visits the salon every four months, as the re-growth would be unsightly. It may be advantageous to suggest highlights, as the re-growth would not be as noticeable. It is important that the client is aware of these implications, to ensure client satisfaction. Some occupations have quite stringent rules regarding the use of excessive styling and vibrant colours, and this must be considered.

You should find out whether your client pursues any leisure activities that could impact on your decision. A client with long, thick hair who swims every morning before work should not have their hair bleached as it may discolour if incorrectly treated. Your client may ride a motorbike and need to wear a crash helmet and so a low maintenance style may be more suitable.

Remember

You should ensure you have all the necessary facts to hand before you make your recommendations, as this will prevent an inappropriate service taking place.

Hair growth patterns

Hair growth patterns may limit or affect some services in the salon. These must be taken into consideration to ensure a satisfactory result. It is always better to work with the natural fall of the hair rather than 'fight it' so that the hair lies another way. The styling will be more durable and therefore easier for the client to maintain. A soft perm can add movement to some strong growth patterns and make them more versatile.

Double crown

You should be careful not to cut the hair too short, as it will not lie properly. You should leave the hair longer in this area as the hair will lie better. The addition of a few perm rods in this area will create some movement and help prevent the hair from lying awkwardly. You should always try to work with the client's hair growth patterns wherever possible, for example, if the client requires a style that is short and spiky, utilise the double crown to help you to achieve this look.

Widow's peak

A widow's peak is a very strong growth pattern. Consideration must be taken when cutting hair, especially around this area. It can prove difficult when cutting a fine fringe, as the hair will easily lift and split. Again, work with the natural growth pattern whenever possible to ensure the best results.

Cowlick

A cowlick makes it difficult to cut a straight fringe, as the hair tends to grow strongly to one side. However, styling the hair and utilising the natural movement will make the style more durable.

Nape whorl

Nape whorls must be considered when cutting hair and dressing long hair. The hair may not lie flat in the nape area if the hair is cut too short. Analyse the nape whorls and check the direction in which the hair grows to try to incorporate it into your cutting or styling.

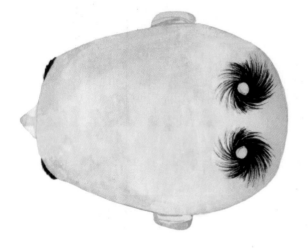

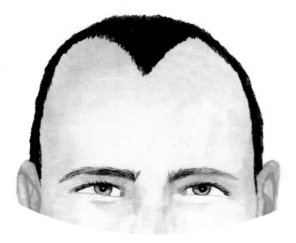

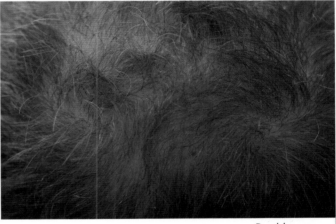

Double crown

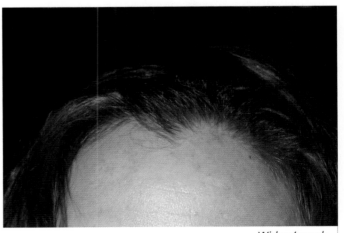

Widow's peak

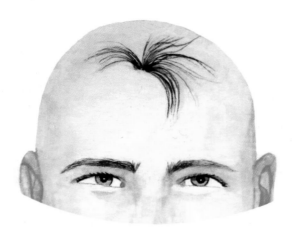

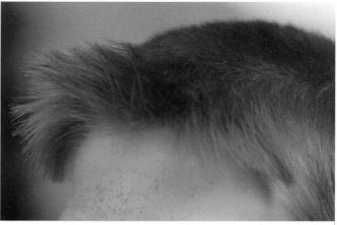

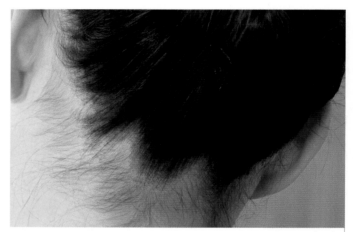

Cowlick

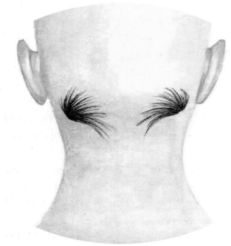

Nape whorl

Special occasions

If the client is having their hair styled for a special occasion, you must utilise the broad spectrum of skills you have and adapt them accordingly. For many clients, this type of occasion happens infrequently and therefore they will require something extraordinary. These occasions may include:

- bridal work
- fancy dress
- ball
- award ceremony
- milestone occasion (retirement, twenty-first birthday, and so on).

Your client may want a standout style for a special occasion

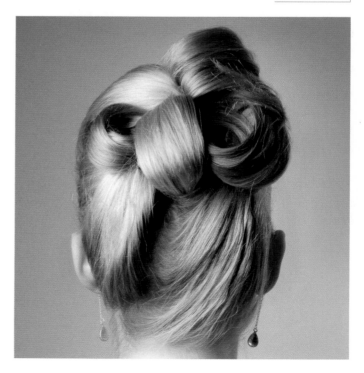

Once you become aware of the event the client will be attending, it should give you a clear indication of the type of service/styling the client may require. Remember to clarify the client's requirements as to whether they want something sexy and sophisticated, way out and funky, or modest but classy, but always ensure the service and styling will suit the occasion.

Some stylists like to carry out a trial run, as this helps to iron out any worries or anxieties the client may have. However, some stylists do not like to carry out trial runs as experience has taught them that it is not always possible to recreate the style so that it looks exactly as it did on the previous occasion. You should know your capabilities and use your own judgement as to whether the trial run is right for you.

> **Be professional ★★★**
>
> If carrying out trial runs, always take photographs of the final look the client decides on for the special occasion. This will help to refresh your memory on the day and ensure the client is satisfied.

Hair texture

The hair texture refers to the thickness of each individual hair. Fine hair is narrow in diameter, whereas coarse hair has a wider diameter. Fine hair is generally considered to be more receptive to perming and colouring services. However, you must remember there are exceptions to every rule, as some fine hair is known to be resistant to chemical processing. The hair may differ in texture across the head — it is usually finer at the front and this must be taken into consideration. It is essential that you know the texture of the client's hair prior to starting a service, as there are implications for most services carried out in the salon.

Hair density

The hair's density refers to the amount of hairs on the head. Many hairdressers confuse texture and density, as hair may be fine in texture but abundant in number. The average number of hairs on any head is said to be between 100,000–150,000, with blondes having the most and redheads having the least. However, blonde hair tends to be finer in texture than any of the other natural colours.

Providing analysis assistance to colleagues

There may be occasions in the salon when another member of staff is encountering difficulties with their own client analysis. This may be through lack of experience or lack of confidence. In either situation you should assist them promptly and effectively to enable them to continue with their work. This intervention should be carried out in an unthreatening manner to ensure you do not undermine their confidence.

> **Be professional ★★★**
>
> - You should have a thorough knowledge of all aspects of the hair, skin and scalp.
> - You should know how to gain information regarding the client's hair, skin and scalp.
> - You should be aware of the importance of pre-service testing and examination.
> - You should know about adverse hair, skin and scalp conditions and whether they may be treated in the salon.
> - You should recognise the importance of identifying the incompatibility of previous services and products used.
> - You should be able to identify head and face shapes and decide upon the most suitable style.
> - You should consider the effects of the client's lifestyle regarding the suitability of services and products.
> - You should be aware of hair growth patterns and how they affect your choice of styling.
> - You should recognise the importance of getting it right for a special occasion.

Unit G21 Provide hairdressing consultation services

Making recommendations to your client

Once your analysis is complete and you have identified your client's needs and wishes, you should then be able to make recommendations to your client as to the most suitable course of action. You must take into consideration the information you gained from your in-depth analysis, which includes the results of any tests you have undertaken. You must be aware of all the services and products that are available in the salon if you are to make an informed choice. This may include other parts of the salon that you are not familiar with. It would be advantageous for you to be aware of the beauty treatments that the salon offers so you can recommend a combined package to your client, for example, the bride or client about to take a holiday.

Remember

- Only when you are absolutely sure that you know what your client requires and you have carried out a full analysis of the hair and scalp, should you begin to make your own service recommendations.
- Under the Trade Descriptions Act 1968, any information you give to the client, including that of the **features** and **benefits** of a service or product, must be correct. You should be able to state the features and benefits of each service and product that is used or carried out in the salon. However, in reality, most clients are more interested in the benefits to themselves. Think about what the client has to gain from the service or product.

Check it out

Are you aware of all the services your salon offers to the clients? Can you list the features and benefits of each service and product used within the salon? You'll find this useful to refer back to when you are updating your knowledge of salon services.

 Key Skills Links: Level 2 Communication

Feature

what it does.

Benefit

how it helps the client.

Keep abreast of current trends

Your knowledge of current fashion trends should be up to date so you can offer the widest range of services and products available to your clients. There are numerous ways of updating your skills and knowledge, including:

- referring to trade magazines, such as the *International Hairdressers Journal*
- attending trade shows and exhibitions
- attending courses run by product manufacturers
- watching television, for example, programmes about fashion
- accessing hair and fashion websites.

You should be aware of current style icons and the impact they have on the general public and their concept of fashion. If you think back over the last few years, stars such as Kylie and David Beckham have re-invented themselves several times and on each occasion have helped to determine what becomes 'street fashion'. Agyness Deyn and Kelly Osbourne are also good examples of people in the public eye that change their look to reflect different situations.

You must keep abreast of these developments to ensure you can offer the requested service and know what the finished result should look like!

Some clients have aspirations regarding their hair that cannot be fulfilled. It is very disappointing for a client to be told the look they wish to achieve is not possible. There will always be a client with very fine, sparse hair who wants to look like Amy Winehouse! However, it is your job to explain the situation to the client using language the client can readily understand and offer alternatives. You may need to explore a number of different options until you find one that the client finds acceptable. You should display tact and diplomacy when dealing with this type of situation as the client's self-confidence may not withstand the brutal truth and you do not want to lose the client.

In some instances, the client's hair may not be able to withstand the preferred service and again you must explore all the options until you come up with a mutually agreeable alternative. You may wish to show the client evidence from any tests that you have carried out, especially those that clearly indicate deterioration in the hair's condition or unwanted colour. You should then make alternative suggestions regarding other services or products that may be used or given, which will give a positive outcome.

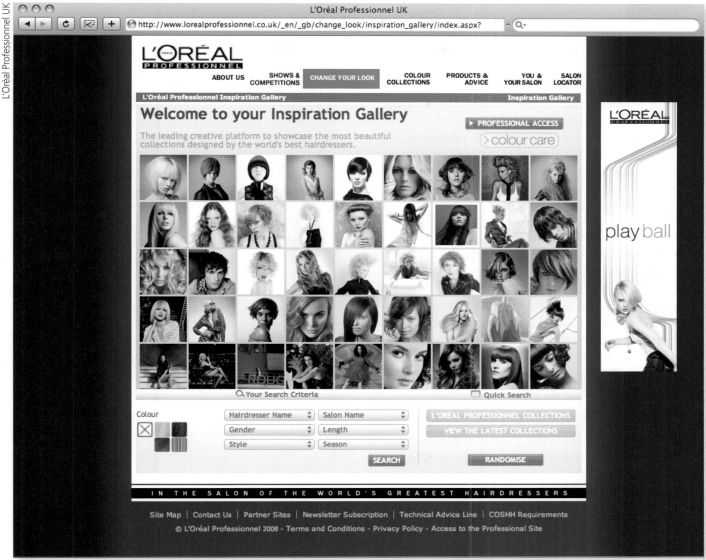

Keep abreast of current trends by visiting hair and fashion websites. This is the Inspiration Gallery from the L'Oréal Professionnel website

In the salon

To test or not to test, that is the question

A client comes into the salon for a re-growth application and has 25 per cent scattered white hair. However, since the last visit she has coloured her hair at home. An incompatibility test shows evidence of the presence of metallic salts, so you immediately know a permanent colour cannot be used. It may be possible to use a true semi-permanent colour (one that is not mixed with anything, but used directly from the bottle), as it does not contain hydrogen peroxide.

- What should you do next?

Referral

There are times when the client's preferred service is unavailable due to:

- the service not being offered in your salon
- adverse hair, skin and scalp conditions.

If a client requests a service that is not offered in your salon, rather than leave the client to find a salon that does offer the service, your salon should have a policy specifically for this purpose. If you refer the client to a specific salon, you must be sure the salon offers services to a good standard, as your reputation is at stake. If the service proves to be unsatis~~...~~ remember the client went there on your recommen~~...~~

09

Check it out

Does your salon have a policy for referring clients to other salons?

If your salon does not have a policy covering the referral of clients, but intends to put a policy in place, make sure you do your homework and find the best place for your clients, as this will reflect on your judgement as a professional hairdresser. If the number of requests for a specific service becomes substantial, it may be in the interest of the salon to train one of their existing staff to fulfil this opportunity, or employ somebody who can offer the service.

Referring clients to specialists

Some hair and scalp disorders are treatable in the salon, for example, using special products or treatments manufactured for treating dandruff. However, some disorders will need to be referred to a **trichologist** for more specialist treatment. In some instances, clients with hair and scalp problems will go to their stylist as a first point of call. Many clients are unaware of the role of the trichologist or are unsure of how to access one. You should be encouraging and supportive towards these clients as they may find the situation quite distressing.

Be professional ★★★

If you need to refer a client to see a registered trichologist and are not sure how to find one, the following website is very informative and user friendly: www.trichologists.org.uk

This website lists all the Institute's members from England, Scotland, Wales, the Channel Islands, Northern Ireland and the Republic of Ireland. Alternatively, you can call 08706 070602.

Trichologist

a hair and scalp doctor.

In the salon

A growing dilemma

Sally was a regular client. Every few months her mum Joan came to stay with her for a long weekend and as a treat she took her to the salon for a shampoo and blow-dry. Paul, the stylist, always did both Sally's and Joan's hair. One day, whilst blow-drying Joan's hair, Paul noticed a strange, dark brown, raised, unusual shape on the side of her face. He asked if it had been there long and Joan said she was not sure and asked him why it mattered. He made light of the situation but suggested she mention it to her GP when she was next there. During her next visit to the salon she told Paul that the doctor had 'burned the thing off her face'. He did not see Joan then for several months, but when she came to the salon, the brown, raised, unusual shape was back, but this time it was bigger. With each subsequent visit, Paul could see it getting bigger. He had no idea what it was, but felt it was not right and suggested again that she see her GP. He did not see Sally for ages and when she finally came into the salon she looked very worried. She told him that her mum had been in hospital having the sinister shape removed and this necessitated her having facial surgery. She was very poorly.

Paul knew he had done as much as he could for Joan. He was not a doctor and he was not sure what the lump was, but at least he had suggested the initial visit to the GP.

- Could Paul have done anything more?

In the types of situation described above, it is important not to diagnose specific conditions to the client. Medical practitioners are the experts and although you may be right in your diagnosis, there is always the possibility that you are not. Firstly, you must consider the stress and worry the client will have to endure, especially if they have to wait several days for an appointment. Secondly, if you wrongly diagnose a client's condition, they may endure unnecessary stress and worry and inevitably blame you (even if you were trying to help!).

It is more professional to say to the client, 'I'm not sure what the problem is, but I would suggest you see your GP before returning to the salon.' This may offend the client, but if the client has a contagious or potentially serious condition, your actions will cause the condition to be treated more quickly, reducing the risk of it worsening and preventing possible cross-infection.

When referring a client with a suspected infectious condition, you should say as little as possible to get your point across effectively. In the event of a client with head lice, they do not need to know how many lice you have actually seen, but you should tell them there is evidence of the condition and refer them to a pharmacist. If you elaborate in these situations, you may find you are giving the client information that is not really your responsibility to give. You should speak quietly or move your client to a private area of the salon to maintain discretion and show that you are complying with the salon rules of confidentiality.

You must not show disgust or repulsion towards the client, but empathise with them instead and try to make them understand that these things are common within the salon environment (even if they are not). You should maintain a relaxed manner so you do not cause alarm and the tone of your voice should be authoritative to ensure the client takes your referral seriously.

In all instances, you must ensure your clients realise that you are a professional person and your recommendations are in their best interest. This will help to promote trust and goodwill between you and your clients.

Be professional ★★★

- Check the availability of services and products within your salon.
- Know your responsibilities under the Trade Descriptions Act 1968.
- Keep abreast of current fashion trends and looks.
- Be aware of your salon's policy for client referrals.
- Understand the importance of using tact and diplomacy when referring clients.

Agreeing services with your client

When you are absolutely sure of your client's requirements, you should discuss what the service entails, the length of time the client can expect to be in the salon, and any special advice that may be necessary. For example, if you have a client having hair extensions, you must inform the client of the duration of the service, as they may not realise the length of time it takes, and the possibility that it may be uncomfortable. You must make sure the client has allowed sufficient time for the service to be carried out, as clients will quite often fit in a hairdressing appointment around other commitments.

It is frustrating for both the client and the stylist if the duration of the service takes longer than anticipated. This may involve the client having to leave the salon midway through the service or remaining in the salon but 'clock watching' the whole time. This leads to undue anxiety for the client and puts the stylist under unnecessary pressure. It shows a lack of professionalism and does not reflect well on the salon.

Check it out

How long does your salon allow for each service it offers? Make a comprehensive list.

 Key Skills Links: Level 2 Communication

Special requirements

Your clients should also be informed of any special requirements that may be needed for a specific service. It is very frustrating for a client to arrive at the salon for a service, only to be told the service cannot be carried out as something has been overlooked. Some examples of pre-service requirements include:

- the need for tests prior to the perming or colouring service – skin test, test cutting and so on
- special preparation requirements – a client having a relaxing service should not shampoo their hair for a least a week before the service as there should be a protective barrier on the scalp. They should be advised not to use excessive products on the hair during this time as it may prevent the relaxer from penetrating
- special clothing that needs to be worn – if you are preparing a client's hair for a special occasion, you must ensure they are wearing clothing that may be removed easily without disturbing the finished styling. You may suggest the client wears a top that buttons or zips up the front rather than a jumper that will be dragged over the head.

Establishing the cost of the service

Your clients should also be informed as to the outcome of the service, the products you will use and the cost of the service. To do this you must be able to calculate the likely charge for the salon service, which means that you must be familiar with the pricing structure within the salon.

If your salon has staff with varying levels of competence, they may be allowed extra time to complete certain services; however, you need to be aware of this if you are to pass this information on to the clients. In some salons, the prices for certain services start from a specific price, for example, highlights from £50, in which case you must inform the client if their highlights are likely to cost them £50 or more.

Check it out

To calculate the client's bill, you must ensure you have included all services the client has received, for example:

Cut	£17.50
Relaxing service and finish	£60.00
Semi-permanent colour	£19.95
Total	£97.45

Using your salon's price list, calculate the cost of:
1 a re-style, followed by a body perm and finish
2 colour polishing and cut and blow-dry
3 a man's re-style and re-design of facial hair.
You must include any additional products that may be used if these are charged separately.

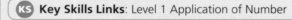 **Key Skills Links**: Level 1 Application of Number

Remember

Under the Sale and Supply of Goods Act 1994, there should be a reasonable charge for any service carried out unless a price was agreed prior to the service. As the client should be informed of the price prior to the service and their agreement sought, you should be fulfilling some of your responsibility under this piece of legislation.

Payment policies

Many salons have payment policies, which require clients to pay a deposit or, in some cases, pay for the whole service prior to their visit. Some salons maintain these policies at all times; others may implement the policies to cover:
- busy periods (for example, Christmas and New Year's Eve appointments)
- services that are time consuming (for example, extensions)
- clients who regularly default (do not turn up).

This is to ensure the salon receives an income even if the client has to cancel their appointment.

Record cards

Any information you have gained during your consultation that relates to the service your client will be having should be recorded on a client record card. Clients may not always have their requested service on the day of the consultation, therefore it is vital that you have the information to hand when the client comes in for the service.

To comply with the Data Protection Act 1998, all records should be accurate, up to date, legible and complete.

Once your client has agreed to the service, you are ready to commence. If the client has visited the salon for a consultation, you must ensure they make a suitable appointment prior to leaving the salon.

Be professional ★★★

- Inform clients of the cost, duration and any special requirements that may be necessary.
- Know your responsibilities under the Sale and Supply of Goods Act 1994.
- Know how client record cards should comply with the Data Protection Act 1998.

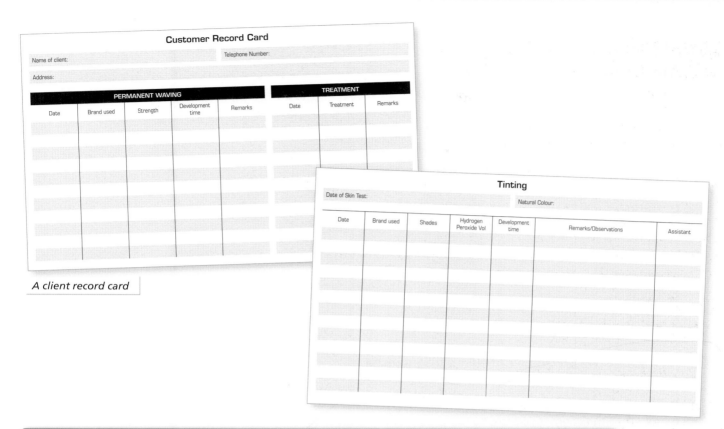

A client record card

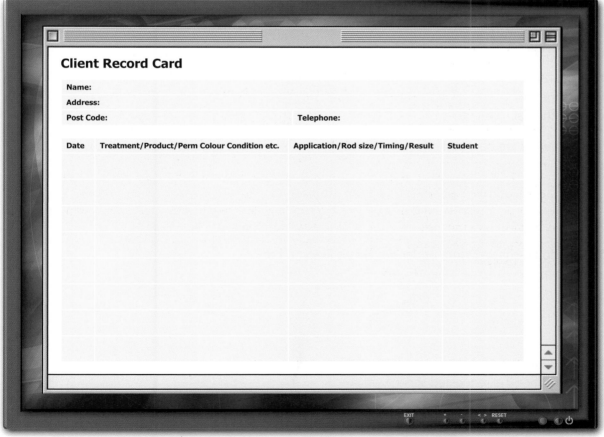

An electronic client record card

Check your knowledge

The following questions will help you to check your understanding of this unit. The answers can be found on page 417. Take care, as there may be more than one correct answer for some questions.

1   Which of the following are parts of the hair?
   a   Cortex
   b   Follicle
   c   Germinal matrix
   d   Cuticle

2   In which part of the hair growth cycle is the hair growing?
   a   Anagen
   b   Catagen
   c   Telogen
   d   Growgen

3   An elasticity test should be carried out to determine:
   a   the condition of the cuticles
   b   the presence of metallic salts
   c   whether the client is allergic to the products to be used
   d   the tensile strength of the cortex

4   A healthy hair can be recognised by:
   a   its dull appearance
   b   its shiny appearance
   c   the colour of the hair
   d   the texture of the hair

5   Which of the following are bacterial infections?
   a   Ringworm
   b   Trichotillomania
   c   Impetigo
   d   Folliculitis

6   A skin-coloured, dome-shaped lump under the skin is likely to be:
   a   keloid scarring
   b   an in-growing hair
   c   a sebaceous cyst
   d   ringworm

7   It's important to keep up with current trends and fashion to:
   a   ensure you can offer the requested service
   b   maintain satisfied clients
   c   ensure you wear the correct shoes for work
   d   keep your colleagues happy

8 Some salons have specific payment policies, including those that require the client to pay in advance. These may be:
  a services that are time consuming
  b the day the client is going on holiday
  c Christmas and/or New Year's Eve
  d clients that regularly default (don't turn up)

9 To comply with the Data Protection Act, all your records should be:
  a accessible to anyone who wishes to see them
  b accurate and up to date
  c legible
  d shredded every 4 months

10 You can update your hairdressing skills by:
  a reading trade magazines
  b attending hair shows and exhibitions
  c watching fashion-related programmes on TV
  d attending courses run by product manufacturers

Provide hairdressing consultation services **Unit G21**

Assessment guidance

You must demonstrate in your everyday work that you have met the standards for providing hairdressing consultation services.

You will be assessed on at least three different occasions and you will have to prove that you can competently carry out a thorough and effective consultation covering a minimum of three different technical units, for example, colouring, cutting and perming.

You must show that you have considered all the factors limiting or affecting services and used questioning, observation and testing during your consultations.

Although simulation may not be used during this unit, range three may be covered by knowledge evidence if performance evidence isn't available.

Unit G18

Promote additional services or products to clients

What you will learn:

- How to identify additional services or products that are available

- How to inform clients about, and gain client commitment to using, additional services or products and salon promotions.

Darren Ambrose

Introduction

The range of products and services available to promote within the salon is constantly changing, as you would expect from a fast-moving industry such as hairdressing. It is important for you to be aware of these changes in order to keep up with clients' needs and expectations. This unit is primarily concerned with how you promote products or services to clients in order to extend their use of your salon. The benefits to the salon are increased revenue and, for the client, the improved condition of their hair and a manageable style.

You the stylist

As a stylist working in the salon, your job will involve promoting services and products to your clients. You will be required to keep abreast of changes and developments in the range of services and products that are available in order to maximise what you can offer your client. Excellent communication skills are essential in order to fully respond to the needs of your clients and present the services and products of your salon. You will need to be aware of each person's role within the salon and ensure that you are working as part of the team in promoting services and products.

Depending on your job role within the salon, the part you play in promotion may differ. For example, if you are responsible for stock ordering, you will need to be aware of which services or products are on offer to ensure you have enough of the items in stock.

You may be responsible for organising the window display; therefore you need to be aware of what is on offer in order to change the window promotion. Staff meetings will play a vital role in ensuring that the correct information is shared, and chairing these meetings may be your responsibility. If you are a senior member of staff in your salon, you will probably have a larger part to play in ensuring that the promotion of services and products takes place, including monitoring and updating when it is necessary.

Remember

You may have productivity targets to reach on the promotion of additional products and services to clients. See pages 105–7 for information on productivity.

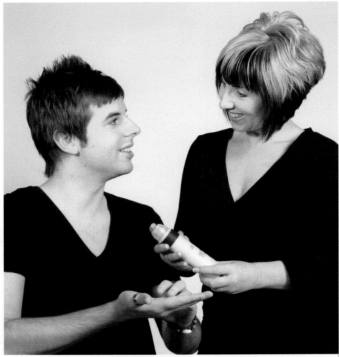

Keep abreast of the latest products so that you can advise your client on what is best for their hair

How to identify additional products or services that are available

In order to maximise the client's use of your salon, the whole team must play a role in making clients aware of what is available and encouraging them to return to the salon. There are many factors you should consider when promoting services or products. Both the salon and its employees have responsibilities to clients regarding legislation and regulations. The client also has rights as a consumer that you are legally bound to observe.

Products and services

The services that you offer in the salon are usually all the things that are listed on the salon's price list. However, there may be other services that on occasions you are asked for and will also provide, for example, special occasion styling or alternative colour techniques. The services you provide often change over time as your clients' expectations and requirements change.

The products that you use and offer in your salon may be supplied from several different companies. This is often the best way to operate in a salon. Using only one product supplier can inhibit the services you offer, for example, your supplier may not produce a hair straightener.

Wella

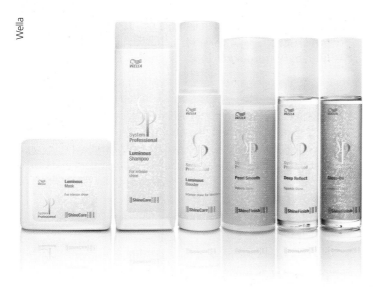

Products have features and benefits – make sure you know what they are

You must stay focused during discussion with your client in order to identify opportunities for offering your client additional services or products that will improve their client experience. For example, during consultation, if they are discussing hair condition and you know you have products to improve their hair, then this should be suggested. Or even something as basic as telling you that they are attending a special event soon, this again could be an opportunity to promote special occasion styling or beauty services.

Features and benefits

You will need to understand the features and benefits of the products and services before you can successfully promote them. Everything that you offer in the salon has a feature and a benefit. Features of a product or service are its attributes or characteristics, for example, using mousse will aid the styling process. The benefits of a product or service are the advantages that it will give to the client. For example, styling mousse provides hold and volume to the finished look.

The services and products that you provide in your salon will differ from that of another salon and will depend upon the hairdressing abilities of your staff. For example, you may have a long-hair expert working at your salon providing a lot of special occasion styles, or a nail technician, or even a trichologist with a specialist clinic. Whatever your salon set-up, it is essential that you remain aware of the changes and developments to the services and products that you provide. There are several ways in which you can update your knowledge of services and products and each one may hold possible advantages and disadvantages for you. These are summarised in the table below.

Method of updating knowledge	Advantages	Disadvantages
College courses	Not linked to any one manufacturer and can gain further qualifications / certificates	May have to take time off work to attend
Reading trade publications or researching on the Internet	Contains lots of information regarding numerous products and services	Two dimensional, can't try it for yourself. No one checks that information on websites is factually correct
Product manufacturer courses	Can gain further qualifications / certificates. Sometimes offer free courses as incentives	Can be the most expensive way of updating your knowledge
Trade events	Lots of companies to look at and can try them for yourself	May have to take time off work to attend

Informing clients about, and gaining client commitment to using, additional services and products

When supplying services and products to your clients you must also consider what you can promote outside of your salon. The term 'outside' does not have to mean exterior to the salon premises, it may just be a service that is outside of your hairdressing capabilities. Remember that you are trying to improve your clients' experience with you and this may require you to promote something that you do not necessarily provide yourself. There may be several other services that are linked to the salon, for example, a nail technician, beauty or holistic therapy services, or even a **trichology** clinic. It may even be something as remote as dog grooming or plumbing if the salon owner's partner also has a business. Through your communication with your client you will be able to determine their needs and advise accordingly, but take care to choose the most appropriate time to make recommendations as you can easily offend a client by being too pushy with your selling techniques — no one likes the feeling of being pounced on! You should also take care not to offer the client something that is out of your reach as they may become disheartened. Ensure that if you are offering to supply your client with a service or product that you can fulfil their requirements.

Trichology

the science of the hair and scalp.

In the salon

Special occasion hair

Joseph owns and works in a busy town centre salon. He has a varied client base but works predominantly as a colour technician in the salon. A regular client of his was going to a college ball and asked for her hair to be put up for this special occasion. Unfortunately, his long-hair technician was away on holiday. Not wanting to lose the client or disappoint her, he agreed to put up the client's hair himself and booked the appointment. When the client came into the salon, she brought a picture of how she wanted her hair to look. Joseph took one look at the style and knew in his heart that he would not be able to achieve it; however, he felt committed and did not want to let her down.

He tried to discourage her from the look and recommended something else but to no avail — the client had made her mind up. Joseph tried several times to achieve the look and the client was beginning to ask questions about whether he knew what he was doing. Eventually he admitted to the client that he could not achieve the look she wanted but could offer her an alternative style. The client had no choice but to agree in order to have her hair styled for the special occasion. However, she was very disappointed and, although a regular client at the salon, never returned again.

- Should Joseph have booked the appointment without letting her know that he was not a long-hair expert?
- Do you think he lacked professionalism in his judgement of the situation?
- How could he have handled this situation differently without losing a client?
- Why do you think the client never came back to the salon again?

Salon promotions

There are various types of promotions that you will be involved in whilst working in the salon, and you may even be responsible for running them. For example:

- promotional events at the salon
- advertising on radio or local newspapers
- using a website address
- advertising in trade magazines
- window display
- promotional leaflets or flyers.

Stages of a promotion

There are several stages to a promotion that must be considered. Initially, it should be well planned, looking at the budget and the resources available. The objectives must be set to ensure each individual is aware of their responsibilities and what is expected of them. Next, implement the promotion, monitoring its effectiveness as it progresses. Every promotion reaches a **saturation point** when it is no longer **commercially viable** and should be brought to a close. This will become evident through careful monitoring. Then, finally, evaluate its effectiveness, again involving the people who took part to ensure all accurate information is gathered. The evaluation will provide crucial information on its effectiveness and whether or not it has achieved its objectives. This information can be used to assess the benefits of further promotions.

Saturation point

the stage of a promotion where it no longer makes money and is not worth continuing with.

Commercially viable

generates enough money to make it worth doing.

You must be able to choose the most appropriate time and method of communication to introduce your client to additional services or products. Displaying the products for retail sale at reception is a subtle way of introducing your product range; you can then back this up by discussing their benefits whilst using them on your client. This type of promotion is commonly used; there are many ways of subtly bringing to your client's attention what you can offer, or alternatively, you may want to announce it in a loud and attention-grabbing way.

However you decide to carry it out, the timing and way you present a promotion is crucial. Clients can easily be put off by an attitude they find too brash. Alternatively, being quiet about it will not grab any attention. Think about what it is that you are trying to promote. If the product or service is new to the salon, then you may want to make a big statement as it may attract new clientele to the salon. For example, if a new member of staff begins working at the salon, they may provide different services than previously offered or may want to inform their client base of where they are now working.

Planning

Implementation

Evaluation

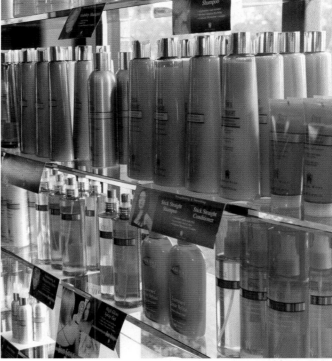

An attractive product display can catch the client's attention

Check it out

Look at your contract. Are there any restrictions as to where you can work on leaving the salon? If you are the salon owner, is this something that you may consider introducing to your contracts with staff? It could save you money in the long term if an employee was to set up a business nearby.

Be professional ★★★

If you are employing a member of staff that has worked locally, remember to check their contract from the previous salon; they may have a clause in their contract forbidding them from working within a specified area and you could end up being liable for poaching clients.

Promote additional services or products to clients **Unit G18**

Organise a launch party

If the salon is a new business, then you may want to organise a launch party. This could be as small or large as you want it to be. Consider inviting local people to attend to have a look around without any obligation and even offer them discount vouchers for their first treatment with you. You may want to use a variety of resources to promote the event, but you should not restrict yourself to just using the salon facilities.

> **Remember**
>
> The cost of promoting should never exceed the financial gain of the promotion.

Set up a website

Many salons now have websites that tempt clients into the salon without them having to physically enter. You can use the website to promote all the products and services of the salon, the arrival of new staff, download discount vouchers, buy products or even book appointments. One of the most important advantages of a website is that you can store lots of information about your salon and this should be as visually attractive as possible. You can also link to other websites, which is especially useful if the salon has a partner business, for example, a beauty salon. You can apply software in order to find out how visitors to the site found you, for example, what search criteria they used – this is particularly useful when updating your site and planning the content and key words. A salon website has many uses and you cannot afford to overlook its numerous advantages. However, it should never be used as the sole medium of promoting, as you would be excluding a vast number of clients who do not have Internet access. Using local newspapers or radio stations to promote the salon can be extremely effective, as they go out to a much wider audience. These methods can, however, be costly and this should be taken into consideration.

Window displays and retail stands

The cheapest and most cost-effective way of promoting is using the salon window. You do not necessarily need to employ a professional window dresser – just use your imagination, or there may be a member of staff with a flair for this. You can change the display according to the seasons, or when sales are down in order to target certain services. The only disadvantage is that it will only reach a limited audience, especially if your salon is not in a busy main road position. However, if used in conjunction with other promotional media, then it can be extremely cost effective. Retail stands and product display within the salon are just as cheap and cost effective in that you are utilising the space you have, but of course they are only seen by your current clients. It is important to keep these up to date and current and make sure they are cleaned regularly so they always look appealing.

> **Check it out**
>
> Do you have a returns policy in the salon? What is it and do you display this for clients to see?

Promotional leaflets and flyers

If you have a particular announcement to make about the salon, then promotional leaflets or flyers can be a successful way of getting the information across. You do, however, need to consider that they will have to be given out, which can take up a lot of working hours. Think about the amount of junk mail you receive yourself and what happens to it; this could be money spent being thrown in the bin.

> **Check it out**
>
> Design a promotional leaflet or flyer to be used in your salon offering a discount on the customer's first visit or a free sample product with a product purchase. Make it stylish and eye-catching and ensure it suits your **target audience**.
>
> **Key Skills Links**: Level 2 Communication

> **Target audience**
>
> the people you are aiming your promotion at, for example, teens, young professionals.

Magazine features

If you are a large salon with enough financial capital to spend, then you may want to consider promoting your salon via a trade magazine. If you have recently undergone a makeover, or are a newly opened salon, you could put yourself forward for a feature which would be a low-cost option for the salon.

Whichever method of promotion you decide to use, choose the right kind of promotion for you and always follow the three key stages.

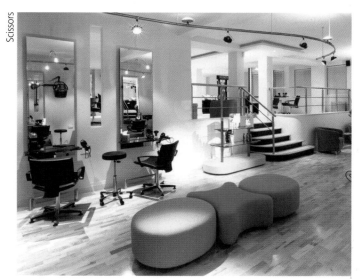

Promote your salon's makeover in a trade magazine feature

Communication

The way in which you communicate with your client will play a crucial role in the success of the promoting you do in the salon. Communication is the sending and receiving of information between persons by various methods. To make your communication effective you need to ensure that the information you are passing on is clear, legible (where necessary) and fully understood by the receiver. In the salon you will communicate with your clients and staff in many different ways. The art of communication has greatly advanced due to the development of technology at such a fast pace. However, the basic methods of communication remain the same, and these can be categorised into three areas: written, verbal and non-verbal.

Written communication

There are several forms of written communication that can be used effectively in the salon. Any written communication that takes place can be kept as proof of what has been said — for example, an invoice of outstanding payment or an enquiry about a product.

Possibly the two most important methods of written communication used in any salon are the appointment book and record cards. Firstly, the appointment book is essential in organising your working day. If the information stored in the appointment book is incorrect, this will lead to major disruption in the salon. It is therefore essential that all the staff be fully conversant with how the appointment system works. Secondly, the record cards are a necessary requirement in order to retain information about the client's hair, the treatment received and his or her personal details. The information stored on the card must be accurate, legible and up to date: this is a requirement of law under the Data Protection Act. For an example of a client's record card see page 31. Written communication for promotion may take the form of posters, flyers, salon websites or notices in the salon window or reception area. Whatever form you use, it should be clear, legible and stylish. This will also present a professional view of your salon.

Check it out

List all the types of written communication that are used in your salon and the advantages and disadvantages of each. This will help you to decide if you need to make any changes to the lines of communication that you are using.

Remember

A record card could be used as evidence in a court case if proceedings were to be brought against you. Therefore, it is crucial that the information stored on it is completely accurate.

Verbal communication

This type of communication applies to everything that is spoken in the salon. This includes both face-to-face and telephone conversations. In the salon you will have to deal with a variety of people, not all of them clients. Therefore, your communication skills will have to expand across many levels. You should pitch your conversation to the level of the client you are dealing with. Being versatile enough to recognise the level of language to use with different clients is essential. For example, the way you talk to a teenage client would be very different from the way you would talk to an elderly client. When speaking face to face and over the telephone, you need to be sure that you are clearly understood. The consultation process relies on good verbal communication, essentially to ensure you reach a positive end result for your client. Misunderstanding when communicating will lead to client dissatisfaction and lack

Unit G18

Promote additional services or products to clients

Scissors

of job satisfaction for you as a stylist. Therefore, maintain clear, concise and understandable communication at all times. When promoting verbally it is essential that you have a thorough and up-to-date knowledge of your services and products. You should be able to clearly explain the features and benefits of each service or product in order to sell it well.

Non-verbal communication

This type of communication covers everything that is expressed via your body language or facial expressions. It is the one type of communication that we often have little or no control over. It can be quite difficult to be continually aware of what we are saying with our body language and facial expressions. However, it can be used to your advantage, as the stylist, when communicating with your client to try to determine their requirements. For example, if you spot a client's attention drifting over to the retail display, or reading promotional materials, then this would be a good opportunity to introduce the benefits of what they are looking at, which could result in a sale.

Check it out

Ask someone you work with to look at your body language over a short period. Is it aggressive, intimidating or appropriate? Do you say one thing but convey something completely different with your body language?

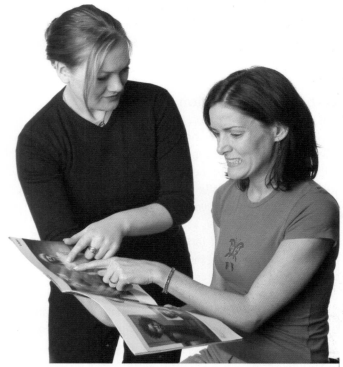

Observe your client's facial expressions when discussing the service – she may not like what you have in mind!

Be professional ★★★

When you are in the salon, mirrors surround you. Even if you think no one can see what you are doing, it is likely that someone will notice your facial expression. A client may easily take offence at a frown from you, even if it was not aimed at them. You should make a conscious effort to look at your non-verbal communication and ensure that it is appropriate.

Making eye contact

Positive eye contact is essential. Have you ever noticed how difficult it is to talk to a person without looking at them? You must be sure to look at the client you are dealing with, as offence can easily be taken if it appears that you are not paying attention. However, too much eye contact can be a negative. For example, if the client is shy, then trying to maintain eye contact can be an uncomfortable experience for him or her. The correct use of body language and facial expression can go a long way to impress the client, and this should never be forgotten.

Whichever way you communicate with your client, it should always be clear, polite and confident. This is important to ensure that there is no misunderstanding between you and the client and it will help to increase his or her confidence in your ability as a stylist. You should consider the manner with which you communicate – do you use a sympathetic tone or an empathetic tone? As an experienced hairdresser you will have come across many problems and crises that you have discussed with a client. Because of this vast experience it will be much easier to empathise with a client's needs based on the theory that you have dealt with this type of problem before. If you can only sympathise and not offer any real solutions, then your client may feel disheartened and lose confidence in your ability.

The communication skills that you use when promoting additional services or products need to be appropriate and balanced. It is of little use explaining to the client all the features and benefits of something if it is not what he or she is interested in. It is likely the client will become bored by you and may not return to the salon. Your knowledge of what you are promoting will help to increase your confidence in the way you communicate. If you have a strong and thorough service and product knowledge, and are able to relay all the features and benefits to the client, then this will be reflected in how you communicate with him or her.

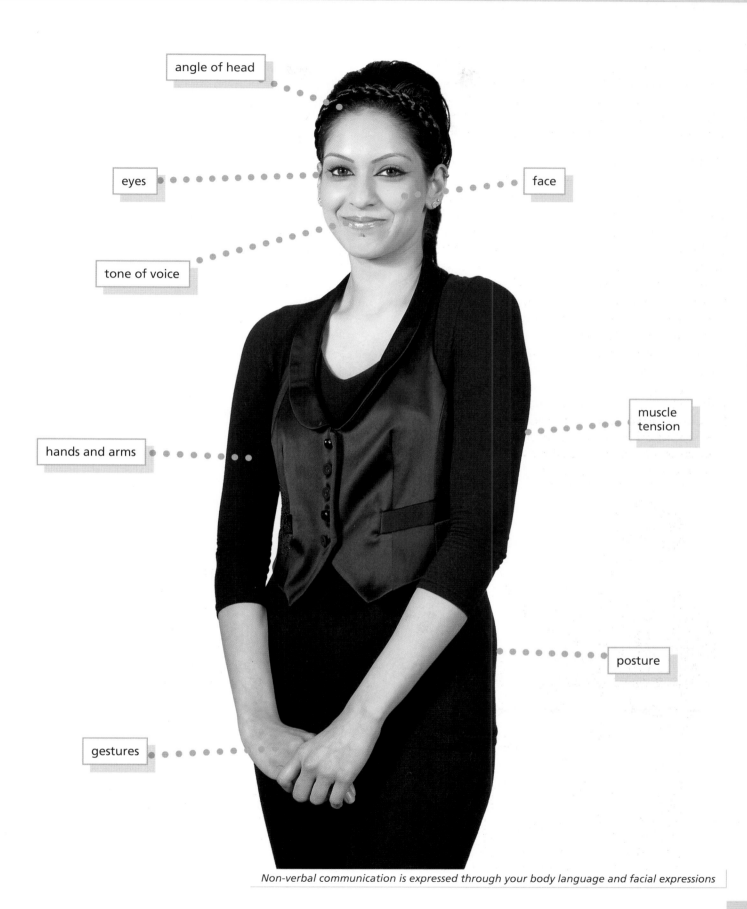

angle of head

eyes

face

tone of voice

muscle tension

hands and arms

posture

gestures

Non-verbal communication is expressed through your body language and facial expressions

In the salon

Effective promoting of services and products

Rosalyn had just started a new job at a local salon. Within the first few days she was looking at the product range to familiarise herself with the features and benefits. On her third day she had a client booked with her for a re-style and from starting the consultation it was obvious to her that the client was open to using additional products and trying out new services. Rosalyn recognised a good promotional opportunity but felt that she did not yet have a thorough knowledge of all the products and services available at the salon.

Not wanting to miss out on the opportunity, she asked the client if she would mind if she consulted with a senior member of staff about her requirements. Rosalyn took care to explain to the client that it was not due to the fact that she did not know what she was doing, but just felt that because she was new to the salon she may miss telling her about something that would be of benefit to her. This reassured the client of her ability as a stylist. After the client agreed, Rosalyn asked her colleague, who was a senior staff member, to lend a hand. The situation was resolved in a satisfactory way for both the client and the salon. No promotional opportunities were missed out on and the client received the best advice possible.

- Do you think that Rosalyn showed professionalism in her approach to the situation?
- What might have been the outcome if she had not brought in a colleague to assist?
- Have you ever been in this situation yourself and felt that you were out of your depth and, if so, would you have the confidence to ask for help?

If you give your client clear and detailed information regarding your salon's services and products, they can then reach an informed decision about what is right for them. Encourage them to ask questions on any points they wish to be clarified and check that you have fully answered their questions. Stay focused during the discussion and look for signals that your client is not interested; this will allow you to close the discussion at an appropriate point and prevent any awkwardness. Successfully promoting additional services or products to your clients will only serve to increase salon revenue and improve your salon's professional image.

Be professional ★★★

Always let your clients smell and feel the products you are promoting and clearly display prices so there is no embarrassment in having to ask.

76

Check your knowledge

The following questions will help you to check your understanding of this unit. The answers can be found on page 417. Take care, as there may be more than one correct answer for some questions.

1 What are the benefits, to both the salon and clients, of your salon promoting additional services and products?
   a It will make more money for the salon
   b The clients will have great hair
   c The staff can become competitive at selling
   d You can spend more on advertising

2 Why is clear and effective communication important in the salon?
   a To be sure that everyone enjoys conversation
   b So that staff and clients feel that they have a voice
   c To ensure there are no misunderstandings between anyone
   d So the client gets the best service possible

3 What type of questions elicits your client's feelings?
   a Closed questions
   b Open questions
   c Leading questions
   d Don't ask questions – it's rude

4 Which of the following are effective methods of promoting the salon?
   a Standing in the street talking loudly about how good the salon is
   b Advertising on local radio
   c Advertising in local papers
   d Word of mouth

5 What are the three stages of a promotion?
   a Planning, implementation, saturation
   b Preparation, implementation, evaluation
   c Planning, implementation, resting
   d Planning, implementation, evaluation

6 What essential information should be stored on a record card?
   a Client's name and address
   b Client's age
   c Client's email address
   d Client's service details

7 Why is it important to complete all written records clearly and legibly?

   a So that you don't have to do them again

   b In case they would have to be used in legal proceedings

   c So that you can read clearly and understand exactly what a client wants for next time

   d To waste time in the salon

8 What positive non-verbal communication should you be using in the salon?

   a Frowning at clients

   b Smiling at clients

   c Making positive eye contact

   d Staring constantly at a client

9 What should your verbal communication be like to ensure you are fully understood?

   a Clearly spoken at a normal pace

   b Speaking quickly

   c Talking with your hand over your mouth

   d Mumbling and talking quietly

10 Should a client be informed of the cost of a service and length of time prior to starting the service?

   a Only if they ask first

   b Yes, always

   c No, this might mislead them

   d Not if you don't like the client

Assessment guidance

For the practical element of this unit, evidence for your portfolio will be collected through observations of you promoting additional services or products to clients made by your assessor. To back this up you will also need to provide evidence showing that you know and understand:

- your salon's procedures and systems for encouraging the use of additional services or products

- thorough working knowledge of service and product promotion.

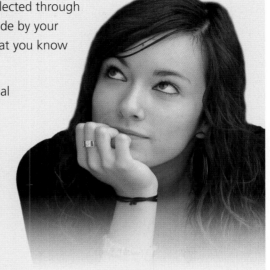

Unit G18 Promote additional services or products to clients

Unit G19

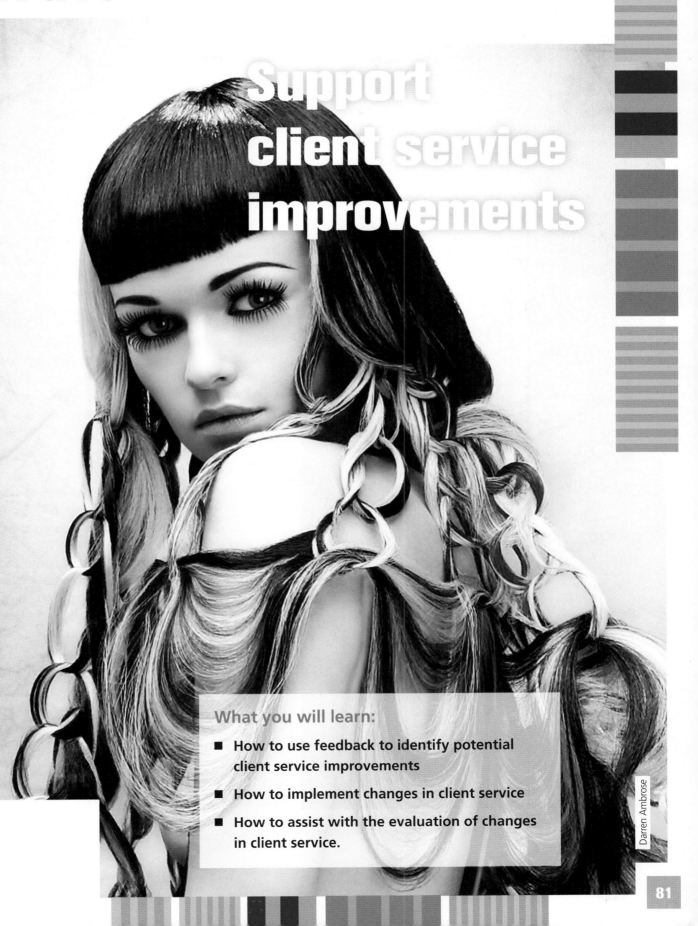

Support client service improvements

What you will learn:

- How to use feedback to identify potential client service improvements
- How to implement changes in client service
- How to assist with the evaluation of changes in client service.

Darren Ambrose

Introduction

This unit focuses on how you can improve the services you provide in the salon. Being aware of your clients' needs and making improvements that reflect those needs is essential. You should be prepared to keep an open mind and not allow yourself to be blinkered or narrow-minded in your decision making, as this can adversely affect your judgement about the right way for your salon to move forward. Throughout this unit, you will become familiar with ways of determining what your clients' needs are and how improvements can be made to the services your salon provides.

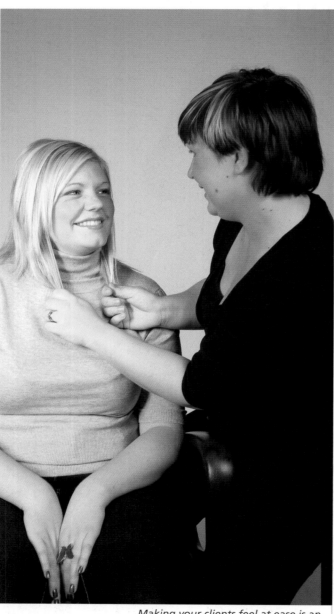

Making your clients feel at ease is an important part of running a successful salon

You the stylist

As a stylist, your job involves delivering a service to clients. It is important for you to be fully aware of your responsibilities regarding this and there are several factors that you must consider. You should:

- know the market you provide for
- have good knowledge of the products available for use
- have excellent communication skills
- maintain an awareness of fashion trends and changes
- regularly update your professional skills.

Salons change the way they deliver services to clients because clients demand change. You should, however, be aware that making changes for the sake of it will not always make good business sense. For example, if your client base is happy with the level of service you provide and your salon systems work well, why cause unnecessary disruption? You need to be aware of other salons and the services they provide in order to keep your eye on the competition. If your salon is implementing improvements, then you must support them and present them positively to your clients. Listening to clients' comments and putting your own views forward is an essential part of your job role. As a stylist in the salon, your opinions will matter to the salon owner. It will be the salon owner's responsibility to judge if your ideas have possibilities for change and improvement.

Communication

Understanding the importance of effective communication is an essential part of working in the salon. But what is meant by 'effective communication'? This is a common term that you will have come across many times whilst completing your hairdressing training, but do you fully understand it? Communication is the sending and receiving of information between people using various methods. In the salon there are three methods that are relevant to you as a hairdresser. These are written, verbal and non-verbal communication. Refer to Unit G21 (pages 29–32) and Unit G18 (pages 73–5) for information on and examples of methods of communication.

Services and products

The services and products that you offer in your salon will be similar to those of other salons but not exactly the same. The services you offer will be dependent on the ability of the staff that work in your salon and the needs of your clients. If your salon is located in an area where there is a large ethnic community, then you will be looking to provide specialist hairdressing services in order to service your local community.

If your salon is located in a rural village, you will not necessarily have the same demands for updating the services that you offer. You need to target the services you provide in relation to the client base you are providing for.

The services that you provide are enhanced by the products you offer. Again, your product range needs to be relevant to your clients' needs. It does not make good financial sense to buy products that your clients will never require or they would consider too expensive. Enhancing the services you provide with small but important features, for example, free refreshments or a discount for loyalty, will ensure your clients' satisfaction.

Check it out

Discuss with your clients if they are aware of your responsibility for implementing service improvements. Check that you are fulfilling your job role in this area – it is easy to become indifferent about what the salon has to offer.

KS **Key Skills Links**: Level 2 Communication

Check it out

Think about the lines of communication that you use in the salon. It is easy to forget their importance when you are using them on a daily basis in your working life. List them all and then as you progress through this unit, check to see if there are any that you have forgotten.

Remember

Word-of-mouth advertising is completely free to you. If a client leaves the salon with a fantastic hairstyle and feels you have treated them well, they are sure to tell their friends. However, you must not forget that clients will also be quick to tell their friends if the service was poor and this will harm the salon's reputation.

Using feedback to identify potential client service improvement

You need to look at ways of finding out how clients feel about the services you provide in the salon. There are various methods you can use to identify your clients' needs, which can be labelled as either formal or informal.

Informal methods

Informal methods are probably the most commonly used. Each day, whilst dealing with your clients, you will question them and extract information about the services and products that you offer. Most of this information will never actually be recorded anywhere for future reference. Non-verbal communication is another form of informal feedback. For example, if a client is not happy with the service provision, although they may not say it directly, the look on their face can tell a different story. Perception of non-verbal communication, such as body language and facial expression, is crucial in order for it to be used as a means of identifying feedback. You may occasionally write a comment on a client record card regarding a service or product used, especially if a client had an allergy or dislike. At staff meetings, management may ask for client feedback, particularly if there have been any changes at the salon. This will be an opportunity to discuss and formalise (via the minutes of meetings) client feedback gained on a day-to-day basis.

Image provided by label.m professional haircare

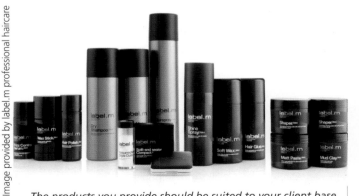

The products you provide should be suited to your client base

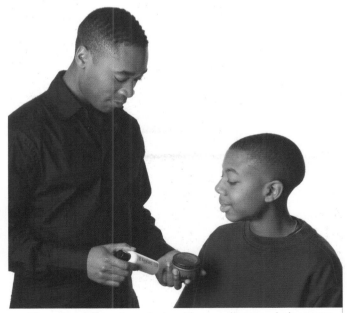

Discussing different products with your client can help you to identify his needs

Formal methods

It may, from time to time, be necessary to carry out a formal client feedback procedure to ensure that you are maintaining a high level of service provision for your clientele. The need to develop and enhance your service provision may have been highlighted by informal feedback given by clients. For example, if, during a discussion at a staff meeting, you uncover the same negative comments from several clients, then this should be recognised and acted upon.

There are a variety of methods that you can adopt in order to gain formal feedback from your client base including:

- a written survey
- a telephone survey
- an interview
- client suggestion box
- via the salon website.

Written client survey

In order to improve services that you provide in the salon, you may consider using a client survey. This will be more effectively carried out in written form to enable you to collate all the information given. It is a valuable tool if used correctly. Consider keeping it anonymous to try to extract your client's true feelings. If not, then think of the implications of storing information under the Data Protection Act. You need to be clear about what you are trying to gain from the survey before you start. This will ensure you retrieve the information you require in order to make your improvements. You could post it on the website, allowing clients to complete it in this way.

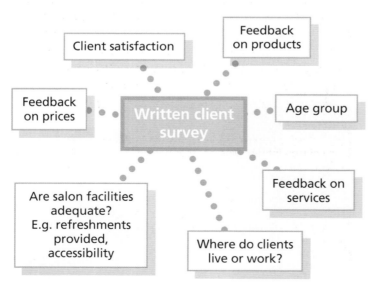

These are just a few of the many different facts and figures you may want to look at. How you deliver the survey is also an important factor. You also need to consider whether the survey caters for the needs of all your clients, for example, both men and women. If your client base is mainly one sex, then you must ensure that if the survey is to be given out to both, that it will be fair. It would be beneficial to discuss this with all the staff and decide among yourselves how you will deliver it in the salon. This will ensure fairness and you will know that everyone is informed of his or her exact role.

You need to develop a plan for completion of the survey from start to finish, ensuring start and end dates are included. You will need to consider:

- where the survey is to be carried out — for example, in the salon or will clients take it home
- at what time during the service the client will complete the survey — for example, whilst waiting at reception, during chemical processes or paying at the end
- how the survey is to be carried out — for example, client completes it anonymously or staff ask the questions
- who is responsible for ensuring its completion — for example, the receptionist or the stylist.

Types of questions

In the survey, there are specific ways in which you can question clients to determine the information you require.

Closed/open questions

Closed questions are more commonly used, as they make a survey quick and easy for a client to complete. You will ask a question and the client will only have to give a yes or no answer. This type of information is much easier to collate and analyse. However, you should consider that this could limit the amount of feedback you will gain. To overcome this, you may want to follow it with an open question. This type of question is much more difficult to collate and analyse, as it requires the client to put down their own thoughts and feelings. Open questions will generate a wider response and are particularly useful if you are not sure of the likely replies.

Leading questions

Leading questions are easy to devise, especially if you have a strong opinion on the questions you are asking. Be careful of using a leading question — if you are prompting a particular response to the question, would you be receiving the client's true feelings?

Unit G19 support client service improvements

Personal information

A client may be put off completing the survey if you are asking personal questions, so only put them in if it is absolutely necessary. Make sure they are aware of why you are asking them to give reassurance, and put these types of questions towards the end, so as not to put them off. If you are trying to extract information from a client that is personal, such as age or income, then do not ask for specifics. It is much more likely that they will reply if they are offered a range. Look at the client survey below for an example of this. When you have decided on the types of questions you are going to ask, devise the survey in a logical order, for example, grouping the questions in sequential order so that one question leads to another.

Client Survey

As part of our ongoing commitment to the services we provide in the salon for you, we ask you to take a small amount of time to complete this short questionnaire. It is necessary to assist us with our improvements that we ask for a small amount of personal information. May all the staff at the salon thank you in anticipation of your completion of this survey, as it will greatly assist us to improve the services we offer you.

1. Do you feel the reception/waiting area is welcoming and comfortable?

   Yes/No

2. When you entered the salon were you greeted immediately and in a friendly manner?

   Yes/No

3. Do you feel the retail display looks inviting and attractive?

   Yes/No

4. How do you think the retail product range could be changed to encompass your needs?

   _____
   _____
   _____

5. Which age category do you fall into?

   Under 18   19–28   29–38   39–48   49–65   over 65

6. Are there any other comments that you would wish to make about the services, facilities or products used at the salon? If so, please write your comments on the next page.

   Many Thanks

Telephone survey

This type of survey can take up a lot of working hours, as staff will actually have to take the time to read out the questions and write out the client's response. The advantage is the immediate response you get from it. You would have to go through the same process of devising the questionnaire as you would for a written survey, looking at the types of questions and how it should be collated.

Interview

Interviewing a client to get responses will allow you to focus on an issue in more depth. As it involves speaking to the interviewee directly, it captures in greater detail personal views and experiences. Interviews can draw out feelings and reasons in a way that a questionnaire cannot. However, you should bear in mind that the interviewer may influence the answers given. Normal gestures shown by the **interviewer**, such as nodding or smiling, can lead the **interviewee** to give a false response. Recording the interview will allow you to replay the interview many times and extract the correct information.

Interviewer

any person interviewing another person.

Interviewee

any person being interviewed by another person.

Client suggestion box

Consider how many times you have taken the time to write down how good a product or service was compared with the amount of times you have taken the time to complain. Receiving constructive feedback from a suggestion box is unlikely, and it also limits the type and amount of information you can get. However, if you actively encourage all clients to regularly complete the suggestion slips and use it as a tool to make improvements or stay up to date with your clients' needs, it can prove to be a useful resource.

Salon website

Using the salon website as a means of obtaining feedback is a good method. There are many uses of the website; in fact, all of the methods listed can be used successfully (with the exception of an interview). If a client is looking at your website, they are more likely to take a minute or two more to complete a questionnaire or comment box. You can ask as much or as little as you like without the client feeling embarrassed or uncomfortable at not having enough time or not being interested.

Identifying the improvements to be made

When the survey has been successfully completed, you must collate the information and decide how you will use it. It may be beneficial to share this information with staff and decide amongst you all what the best options for your salon would be. You will need to decide if the information gained from the survey should be made public to the staff. Sometimes it can contain comments that are not entirely complementary. You will need to deal with this as you see fit. For example, if a comment made about a receptionist states that his or her telephone manner is poor, then you will need to raise this on an individual basis. An important question that you must ask is: did it achieve the objectives set? If not, do you need to revisit the survey and look at ways in which you can alter it to meet your requirements? The client survey should provide you with an opportunity to look at any improvements you need to make. It is important that, following its completion, you act upon this and implement the necessary changes.

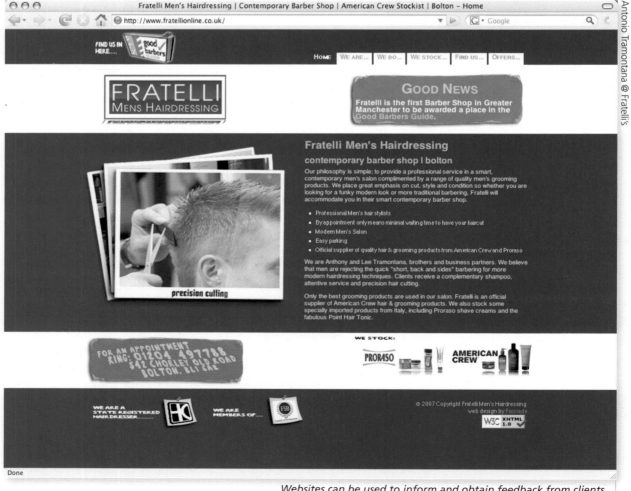

Antonio Tramontana @ Fratelli's

Websites can be used to inform and obtain feedback from clients

These changes may take many different forms. For example:

- re-pricing the product range
- re-pricing the service charges
- changing the product range
- introducing special offers
- staff training
- enhancements to the services offered
- updating facilities
- organising social events
- introducing new products and services.

If you show the clients that you have acted on the information given in the survey, you will be showing that you value their opinion.

> **Remember**
>
> Listening to your clients' needs is important in order to sustain a healthy business. There is a lot of competition waiting to steal your clients away from your salon. You need to stay ahead by listening to and acting upon your clients' needs.

Implementing changes in client service

When working in the salon as part of a team, you will have to implement changes in the services you provide. It is important to work as a team and stay positive and focused whilst implementing any changes. Ensure that you all communicate and check the progress of the changes as you go along. This section covers:

- recognising the need for change
- presenting your ideas for change
- how to implement changes
- working as a team to implement changes.

Recognising the need for change

How will you know when your salon needs to implement changes? You are now familiar with the ways in which you can gain client feedback to help determine any changes required. You also have a responsibility to be alert to the changes that need to be made yourself. If you work in the same environment day-in and day-out, it is easy to become indifferent to your surroundings.

Updating the salon can be a small task or a major overhaul depending on your financial situation. A new coat of paint can dramatically change the appearance of your surroundings without costing a lot of money. If, however, you are in a position to redesign the salon, then this would be a good time to ask your clients' opinions. Check if your clients have any particular requirements that you may have overlooked. They may provide you with a wealth of good ideas. The changes that you feel need to be implemented may not even be on so grand a scale. For example, you may feel that the stock ordering system needs updating or a new method of distributing the tips given by clients is needed.

> **Check it out**
>
> Take the time to look around your salon at the décor and all the fixtures and fittings. Is the salon in good decorative order? Is it ready for a change? Are the fixtures and fittings in need of repair or updating? Take some time to research what changes you could make and work out the expenditure.
>
> **Key Skills Links**: Level 2 Communication & Level 2 Application of Number

> **Remember**
>
> If you are redesigning or making any physical changes to the salon, check that these changes comply with the Disability Discrimination Act.

Presenting your ideas for change

Regardless of how trivial or crucial the change you feel is needed, it is important to bring it to the attention of the appropriate staff before implementing the change within the salon. How you do this is vital as to whether or not your suggestions are taken seriously. You need to be sure that you can justify why the changes are necessary, especially if you have to present your ideas to a manager or salon owner. Decide if you may need the other staff to support your idea and, if so, discuss it with them first. This option could be particularly useful if you need help on deciding how you will present your ideas. Alternatively, it may be a suggestion that you would like to discuss with management without the other staff knowing, for example, if you felt certain staff need more training in a particular area. You will need to judge the delicacy of the situation and how others might feel about the proposed changes.

In the salon

Ali's salon improvement plans

Following a recent client survey, Ali, the salon owner, decided to redecorate and modernise the salon. After a brief meeting with the staff, during which he informed them of his intentions, he set to work planning the improvements. Ali was very busy over the next few weeks with research and planning. Finally, he called another meeting to inform the staff of his ideas. The staff were already feeling concerned at not being involved in any of the planning and on seeing their boss' intentions they became alarmed at the changes he was proposing.

Firstly, the salon had a large storeroom upstairs that the staff also used as a staff room. Ali was proposing to change this into salon floor space and for all the chemical work to take place upstairs. The staff pointed out that not only would it limit access for clients with disabilities but that they would lose their recreational area. Secondly, the layout of the salon and the choice of decor would be very restrictive. The staff felt that putting in more salon stations would reduce each other's workspace and again limit access for clients with disabilities. They also felt that the blue colour scheme Ali was planning for the salon would adversely affect the colours reflected on clients' hair.

At first, Ali was hurt that all his hard work was being dismissed in this way, though he soon realised that he would have to listen to what his staff felt about the improvements. After much discussion, which at times became heated, Ali and the staff managed to make several compromises. He understood that the changes to the upper floor would be depriving the staff of their recreational area and decided to scale down the changes, allowing them to keep an area for themselves, but placing a couple of work stations upstairs for training purposes or when the salon was extremely busy. He allowed the staff to have input into the new colour scheme for the salon and to show him different ways of how it could be laid out, utilising the space available to its best advantage. When all the staff had agreed as a team on the way to go forward with the improvements, Ali began to put them into place. Once finished, the team and clients were extremely happy with the outcome, feeling the improvements to the salon's surroundings and facilities were beneficial.

- Did Ali initially consider the needs of all his staff on making plans for improvements?
- Why do you think the staff were concerned when he did not involve them?
- Would you feel upset at not being consulted about major changes that affected your working conditions?
- Do you think his staff were justified in pointing out his discrimination to disabled clients?

Be professional ★★★

To keep a successful and happy team, you must communicate openly and discuss ideas and changes freely.

How to implement changes

When you have decided what changes need to be implemented, you must then look at how this will be done. You need to be sure that all staff are made aware of how the improvements are to be carried out and that clients are also kept informed. You can use various methods to inform clients of the changes; however, you need to be sure you choose the right one and that all clients are fully updated throughout to prevent them from feeling undervalued. The table below indicates a few methods, with the advantages and disadvantages of each listed alongside.

Method	Advantage	Disadvantage
Poster	Good way to inform clients about specific information e.g. prices, dates or times	Clients will still ask and you will have to discuss with each
Inform each client on an individual basis	You can be sure you have told them exactly and explained the benefits fully	You may forget to tell someone and it could be particularly important
Leaflet distribution	A leaflet can contain lots of information about the salon, e.g. special offers, location	Time consuming and easily dismissed as junk mail
Media advertising	Will reach a wider audience	Can be very expensive and not all your clients may see it
Internet via website	Can reach a much wider audience	Not all clients have access to the Internet

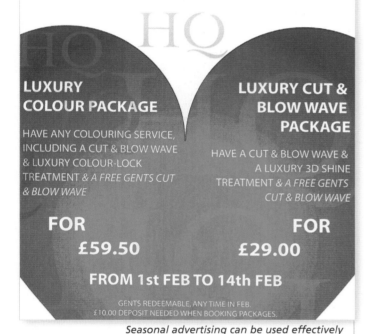

HQ Professional Hairdressing

HQ VALENTINES PAMPER PACKAGES

ANY LENGTH, ANY DAY, ANY STYLIST: NO HIDDEN EXTRAS!

LUXURY COLOUR PACKAGE

HAVE ANY COLOURING SERVICE, INCLUDING A CUT & BLOW WAVE & LUXURY COLOUR-LOCK TREATMENT *& A FREE GENTS CUT & BLOW WAVE*

LUXURY CUT & BLOW WAVE PACKAGE

HAVE A CUT & BLOW WAVE & A LUXURY 3D SHINE TREATMENT *& A FREE GENTS CUT & BLOW WAVE*

FOR **£59.50**

FOR **£29.00**

FROM 1st FEB TO 14th FEB

GENTS REDEEMABLE, ANY TIME IN FEB.
£10.00 DEPOSIT NEEDED WHEN BOOKING PACKAGES.

Seasonal advertising can be used effectively

Working as a team to implement changes

As a team, all the staff need to present a positive approach to the improvements being made. If you or anyone else has any doubts about the changes, then it will become difficult to remain enthusiastic. This will be reflected in your approach to the improvements and clients will become aware of it. If you display concerns, then clients will lack confidence in the improvements being implemented and this can result in disaster for the salon. Alternatively, if you present a positive, united campaign, then clients cannot fail to be impressed by the improvements made.

Be professional ★★★

You have a duty within the salon to promote equal opportunities for people with disabilities. Your salon should be promoting good practice by widening its service provisions depending on the needs of each individual.

Assisting with the evaluation of changes in client service

Evaluating the changes

Staff meetings are crucial at this stage to evaluate the improvements you have made. As a team, you will need to work flexibly. Ensure that each individual is fully aware of their responsibilities and is working towards achieving them. If problems do occur, then they need to be addressed. A group discussion will help to formulate a plan of action, and this is where flexibility is paramount. It may be that job roles have to change and as an individual you will have to adapt. You may also have to support other staff with this task, again showing your flexibility. Client feedback is very important at this stage. Each member of the team will have different comments to make and it is important that they are considered no matter how trivial they appear.

Check it out

If you are involved in any team meetings, make sure that minutes are taken and you keep copies to refer back to so that any discrepancies can be clarified.

 Key Skills Links: Level 2 Communication

Support client service improvements **Unit G19**

Dealing with negative effects of changes

One problem that you may encounter is how to present negative feedback to staff, especially if the changes were their ideas. Any negativity needs to be handled with caution. It is easy to upset a person's feelings with a flippant comment and you need to be tactful in your approach. Be sure to deliver it with a positive comment, then the negative, and finish with a positive. This is sometimes called a 'feedback sandwich'. This will show that you have considered their feelings and that you are not totally disregarding their ideas. Alternatively, it may be your idea that is being presented with some negative feedback. You must be able to look at it with maturity and not take it personally, especially if the feedback is constructive. Constructive criticism should be used as a learning tool. However, blatant criticism can be both demoralising and demotivating. Most importantly, take steps as soon as possible to correct any negative effects from changes. Being able to evaluate ideas and correct any problems as they occur will ensure continued success for the salon.

Supporting client service improvements can prove to be a motivating factor within your job role. It is essential that you see it as a necessity in order to maintain a healthy salon. Any support that you give must be positive and assured. This will promote a healthy working environment in the salon and help to increase the financial effectiveness of the business.

Check your knowledge

The following questions will help you to check your understanding of this unit. The answers can be found on page 417. Take care, as there may be more than one correct answer for some questions.

1 Look at the factors below and decide which ones, if any, are important when providing good customer service.
  a The salon has no refreshments provision
  b Staff have good knowledge of the products that they use
  c There is no parking close to the salon
  d The staff are highly trained with excellent communication skills

2 What is communication?
  a Good driving skills
  b Excellent braiding skills
  c Sending and receiving of information between people using various methods
  d Always paying bills on time

3 Why should the services and products you provide be suited to your client base?
  a To prevent your clients from becoming bored
  b To make sure that your clients enjoy their holidays
  c To be able to boast to your friends
  d To ensure that you provide for your market, which will increase revenue

4 Why is it important to use client feedback to make customer service improvements?
  a To ensure you are providing a service that suits the needs of your clients
  b To show to your accountant
  c To keep staff busy
  d To show your clients that you value their opinion of the service you provide

5 What is the difference between formal and informal methods of feedback?
  a Formal means you don't record it, e.g. just a chat with a client, and informal means something recorded, e.g. on a customer survey
  b Informal means you don't record it, e.g. just a chat with a client, and formal means something recorded, e.g. on a customer survey
  c Formal is more important than informal
  d Informal is more important than formal

6 Which of the following are formal methods of feedback?
  a Client suggestion box
  b Discussion at reception
  c Feedback via the salon website
  d Facial expressions

7 Which of the following would be suitable to ask questions about on a client survey carried out in the salon?

   a Client age group

   b Whether clients have any pets

   c Where clients live or work

   d Whether clients use/like the salon products

8 Why should all the team be involved in evaluating feedback and making improvements?

   a To allow them to spend time off the salon floor

   b To ensure you present a positive, united campaign to clients

   c So that all staff feel valued and important

   d So that the salon can be closed over the lunch hour

9 Why must you present a positive impression of changes that have been made?

   a To impress your boss

   b To show clients that you feel these are of benefit to the salon and them

   c Because you are told to

   d To see if you can get a higher tip

10 How can you avoid negative effects of any changes made?

   a By believing in and staying focused on the positives of the changes made

   b By encouraging staff and clients to see the benefits of the changes

   c By ignoring the changes as much as possible

   d By avoiding discussion about the changes with staff and clients

Assessment guidance

All the practical assessments for this unit must be from work carried out with clients in the salon. You will be expected to gain feedback from your client and use this to implement any changes found to be necessary, for example, completing a client questionnaire. Within the practical element of this unit you must also show that you have supported improvements over a period of time by both individual efforts and working as part of a team. The evidence will come from changes that have been implemented, and these can be things such as:

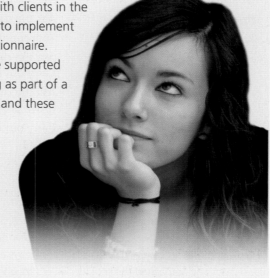

- changes to products or services offered, for example, a new product range
- changes in how they are supplied, for example, new retail displays
- changes in conduct when delivering products or services to clients, for example, issuing a 'Hair prescription' to ensure maximum selling opportunities.

You will also have to show in your practical work that you took part in evaluating the changes made with both clients and the staff of the salon.

Unit G11

Contribute to the financial effectiveness of the business

What you will learn:

- Salon and legal requirements relating to the use of resources

- How to contribute to the effective use and monitoring of resources

- How to meet productivity and development targets.

JFK

Introduction

The main aim of any business is to make a profit and the hairdressing business is no exception. However, this should not be at the expense of health and safety, client comfort, or staff welfare and career progression. In this unit, you will learn about the ways you can help the business become more profitable by monitoring the effective use of resources, and the impact of productivity and development targets as a means of generating income. You will also need to ensure that any other staff for whom you have responsibility are working effectively.

You the stylist

As a stylist, you need to understand the implications of using resources effectively. This is to ensure maximum profitability and minimise waste. You will need to monitor members of staff whose job role is to assist you in your work to ensure that they comply with the above aims.

Throughout your working life in the hairdressing industry, you will be required to meet monetary targets; this is to ensure the salon owner's business remains viable. Hairdressing is a fast-moving fashion industry with new products and services being introduced all the time. You need to keep abreast of these changes if you are to remain a productive member of the staff; therefore, further training and development will be necessary to achieve this.

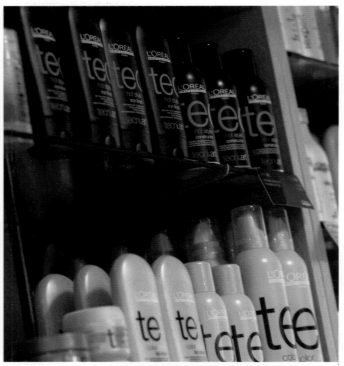

Ensure that stock levels of all products are monitored effectively

Salon and legal requirements relating to the use of resources

There are numerous legal requirements relating to the use of resources that are relevant to the hairdressing business, many of which have been covered in Unit G18 (page 68) and G22 (HSS3) (pages 5–11). These include:

- the Health and Safety at Work Act 1974
- the Manual Handling Operations Regulations 1992
- the Reporting of Injuries, Diseases and Dangerous Occurrences Regulations (RIDDOR) 1995
- the Electricity at Work Regulations 1989
- the Cosmetic Products (Safety) Regulations 2008
- the Control of Substances Hazardous to Health (COSHH) Regulations 2002.

However, there is additional legislation you should be aware of to enable you to contribute to the financial effectiveness of the business.

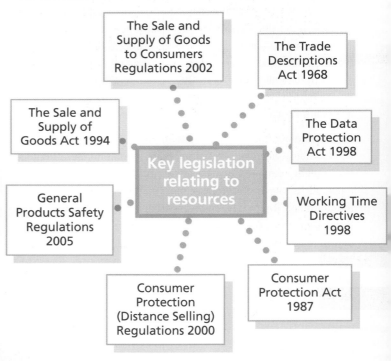

The Sale and Supply of Goods to Consumers Regulations 2002

The Trade Descriptions Act 1968

The Sale and Supply of Goods Act 1994

The Data Protection Act 1998

Key legislation relating to resources

General Products Safety Regulations 2005

Working Time Directives 1998

Consumer Protection (Distance Selling) Regulations 2000

Consumer Protection Act 1987

Much of this legislation is there to protect the salon from possible litigation. Any litigation against the business can prove to be costly in both time and money, and the negative publicity will undoubtedly have an impact on the salon's financial security. Other pieces of legislation exist to ensure all members of staff are treated fairly and their working conditions are considered acceptable. Staff who consider their working conditions to be up to standard are more likely to cooperate with their employers and therefore the working environment will be conducive to good productivity.

Legislation and consumer rights

Sale of Goods

The Sale of Goods Act 1979 has been amended by the Sale and Supply of Goods Act 1994 and The Sale and Supply of Goods to Consumer Regulations 2002.

When you sell goods or a service to your clients, you are entering into a legally binding contract. The contract may be written or verbal. The Sale and Supply of Goods to Consumer Regulations states that goods must be:

- of satisfactory quality — this covers minor and cosmetic defects, as well as substantial problems. It also means that the products must last a reasonable length of time. It does not give the consumer any rights if a fault was obvious or pointed out at the time of purchase
- sold as described — this refers to any verbal or written description made by the seller
- fit for purpose — this means not only the obvious function of the item but any queries that were made on its function and given assurance on.

Anything that is bought is protected under this law and clients are entitled to their money back under certain circumstances. Faulty goods must be returned immediately and as the supplier you must seek compensation from the manufacturer. If the client feels the goods are not of a satisfactory quality, they have the right to return the goods and you must refund their money. In this instance, the client must return the goods within a reasonable time scale. Your salon should have a returns policy to ensure compliance with this Act.

Remember

Since the introduction of the Sale and Supply of Goods to Consumers Regulations, if a product was faulty when purchased, then returned to the retailer, then the consumer is entitled to:
- a full refund
- a reasonable amount of compensation (or 'damages')
- a repair or replacement.

The Sale and Supply of Goods Act 1994

This Act applies to the hairdressing industry, as it is a service provider. It has implications for both labour and the materials used during the service. The Act states that you must:

- carry out the service with reasonable skill and care
- complete the service within a reasonable time (unless a prior agreement was made specifying the time)
- make a reasonable charge for the service (unless a price was agreed prior to the service)
- use materials that are of a satisfactory quality and fit for the purpose.

It is also becoming a more recognised procedure within the hairdressing industry to make clients aware of the cost of the service beforehand. In the past, the hairdressing industry has gained a bad reputation for adding items onto a client's bill without their knowledge. This type of practice caused clients to mistrust hairdressers. With the heightened awareness of consumer rights, this type of poor practice will no longer be tolerated.

Check it out

Have you received sufficient training for the services you carry out in the salon, thus covering the 'reasonable skill' issue within this Act?

The Trade Descriptions Act 1968

This Act ensures that the description of goods, services and prices is accurate and not misleading in any way. The trade description may be given verbally, in writing, by photo or by inference, but whichever way it is made, if the information is incorrect, it is an offence, even if it was made unintentionally. Therefore, it is important to think carefully before you unwittingly give out incorrect information, as you can still be penalised if you have acted without due diligence. Failure to comply with these regulations could result in lack of client confidence, negative publicity, and/or loss of clientele, not to mention the cost of litigation.

Consumer Protection Act 1987 and General Products Safety Regulations 2005

The Consumer Protection Act is the main piece of legislation dealing with consumer safety. It is there to protect the consumer from defective products, that is, products that do not reach a reasonable level of safety. The Consumer Protection Act gives consumers the right to sue for damages if they have been injured or suffered damage to property (over a certain value).

The General Product Safety Regulations 2005 also deal with product safety and, in part, replaces the Consumer

Protection Act 1987. It is the responsibility of all businesses to ensure that their products are safe. The responsibilities included within this piece of legislation are to provide relevant information to consumers regarding the risks of the products they are supplying.

Consumer Protection (Distance Selling) Regulations 2000

These regulations were introduced to increase consumer confidence. They will apply to you if the salon where you work sells goods or services via the Internet, by phone, by fax, or mail order. The key points of the regulations are:

- the consumer must be given clear information about the goods or services on offer — this information includes the price, delivery costs, arrangements for payment and delivery, and so on
- the consumer must be sent confirmation after making a purchase
- the consumer must have a seven-day cooling off period (this supposedly equates to the time the consumer would spend in the salon deciding whether to purchase).

It is likely that this regulation does not apply to your salon if you do not usually supply clients in this way, but perhaps you agree to as a one-off request. However, if the business regularly handles one-off requests, it is likely the salon should comply with these regulations. If this is the case, the salon should also ensure it has registered with and is fulfilling the requirements of the Data Protection Act 1998.

Data Protection Act 1998

The Data Protection Act is in place to protect the personal information you hold on individuals. You are required to ensure appropriate security measures are in place to prevent any unlawful or unauthorised access to data, although it's also worth remembering that your clients must have access to their own information if and when requested. If your salon is holding personal data, you must be registered with the Information Commissioner. It is worth checking to find out if you should be registered, as failure to do so may result in prosecution.

All information held must be accurate, up to date and relevant.

> **Remember**
>
> It is not only client record cards that are covered by this Act. If your salon carries out distance selling, any information held on the client requires the salon to be registered. The salon may hold staff details, for example, salary, commission paid, working times, and so on, and these are covered by this Act. Some paper-based data is also included.

Working Time Directive 1998

Up until the Working Time Directive was introduced in 1998, employers were free to set working times and holiday entitlements. Although many employers and employees negotiated terms and conditions, some employees were still treated badly by their employers. The general rule, which has been applicable since the introduction of this law, is that an employer must take reasonable steps that are in keeping with the need to protect the health and safety of their employees.

The main provisions of the Working Time Directive relating to hairdressing salons include:

- a limit on the average working week
- minimum daily and weekly rest breaks
- rest breaks at work
- paid holiday entitlement.

The law applies to full-time, part-time and casual workers, which is anyone with a contract of employment (whether written or not). These regulations do not cover the self-employed.

Key points of the Working Time Directive

- You should not be asked to work more than 48 hours a week, averaged over a seventeen-week period.
- You are entitled to a rest period of eleven consecutive hours between each working day.
- You are also entitled to a minimum of one day off per week.
- You are entitled to an uninterrupted break of 20 minutes if you work more than six hours per day. It should be a break in working time, not taken at the start or end of the working day.
- You are allowed at least four weeks paid holiday per year. This is calculated on your right to take a twelfth of your holiday entitlement for each month worked (rounded up to the nearest half day). One week's holiday is the equivalent to the time you would normally work per week, for example, if you work three days per week, your annual holiday entitlement would be twelve days. If your contract of employment is terminated before you have taken your leave entitlement, you have the right to payment in lieu.
- For staff aged over sixteen but under eighteen, the law is slightly different. The entitled rest period is increased to twelve consecutive hours rest in every 24 hours, and they are entitled to an uninterrupted break of 30 minutes if they have worked for more than four-and-a-half hours.

Your employer must keep records to show they are complying with this directive and they must keep them for two years from the date on which they were started.

Contribute to the effective use and monitoring of resources

The resources covered within this part of the unit are:

- stock
- tools and equipment
- human resources (people)
- time.

Stock

Stock is a valuable commodity within any salon. A business may have large amounts of money tied up in stock and it is essential that the stock is used appropriately as misuse may cost the salon owner money.

Stock control

Stock control is an important aspect in any salon, as it is essential to the smooth running of the salon. If the salon were to run out of a specific item, it could lead to a disappointed client and give an unprofessional image of the salon, both of which may lead to negative publicity. There may also be seasonal changes that need to be considered, for example, more clients request blonde highlights during the summer months and warm/red colours in the winter. The salon may stock holiday hair products to retail during the summer and this should be well thought out when ordering stock. If the salon is running any promotional offers, it is essential that the stock be available.

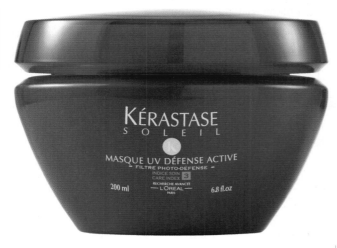

Kérastase Soleil

Ensure that you stock holiday hair products during the summer

Stock includes items such as:

- products used for salon services
- retail items
- equipment used in the salon, for example, hairdryer, climazone, and so on
- consumable items, such as cotton wool and tissue
- semi-consumable items, for example, protective gloves and aprons.

Stock should be monitored following the procedures laid down by your employer, who should set minimum stock levels for products used in the salon and for retail products. They should also set the frequency of the stocktaking. Minimum stock levels are set to ensure the stock on the shelves does not exceed its shelf life. Items of stock that are used frequently or a good retail line may have a higher minimum stock level set than items that are seldom used. For example, you may retail more shampoos and conditioners for colour-treated hair than dandruff-control shampoo. Therefore, the minimum stock levels for the range of products for colour-treated hair would be greater as you will use or sell more.

Stocktaking should be carried out on a regular basis and may be done in several different ways. Your salon may stocktake manually, that is, count each individual product and record your findings. You should then compare this against the minimum stock level set and this will tell you if the product needs re-ordering. Manufacturers will often provide stock sheets to record your stocktaking.

Many salons have computerised systems, which deduct the specific stock used during each transaction. The system is then able to identify products that need to be re-ordered. This will only work if accurate records are made of the products used within each service. This method readily shows any discrepancies in the stock and highlights, for example, any shortfalls in the stock.

In the salon there should be one person responsible for stock control. Their responsibilities include:

- carrying out regular stock checks
- ordering stock
- checking the stock on arrival at the salon
- dealing with any discrepancies
- storing the stock, including stock rotation
- monitoring stock usage
- keeping the necessary records relating to the above.

Check it out

- Does your salon have an appropriate system for stock control?
- Who is responsible for ordering stock in your salon?

Clynol

Styling Range

		STOCK LEVEL		DATE																						
		MIN	MAX	UNIT	Stock	Order	Stock	Order	Stock	Order	Stock	Order	Stock	Order	Stock	Order	Stock	Order	Stock	Order	Stock	Order	Stock	Order	Stock	Order
862206	Lift Mousse 250ml			6																						
862207	Lift Mousse 500ml			1																						
862209	Move Mousse 250ml			6																						
862210	Move Mousse 500ml			1																						
862215	Stay 300ml Hairspray			6																						
862216	Stay 750ml Hairspray			1																						
862202	Freeflow 300ml Hairspray			6																						
862203	Freeflow 750ml Hairspray			1																						
862220	Upgrade Rootboost 250ml			6																						
862156	Create Styling Creme 200ml			6																						
1053700	Massive Volume Spray 200ml			6																						
1053695	Animator Finishing Spray 200ml			6																						
862159	Fibreform Shaping Gum 130ml			6																						
862160	Fix Wax Spray 150ml			6																						
862212	Construct Moulding Clay 75ml			6																						
862213	Shape Gel Wax 100ml			6																						
862219	Titanium Extra Hold Gel 200ml			6																						
862158	Hot CurlCurl Protection Spray 200ml			6																						
862157	Swirl Curl Cream 150ml			6																						
862201	Flatter Iron Spray 200ml			6																						
862204	Gloss Shine Spray 150ml			6																						
862214	Frizz Free Shine Serum 50ml			6																						
862217	Stretch Flattening Balm 100ml			6																						
862218	Tame Smoothing Lotion 100ml			6																						
968983	Wrap Up 150ml			6																						

An example of a manufacturer's stock sheet

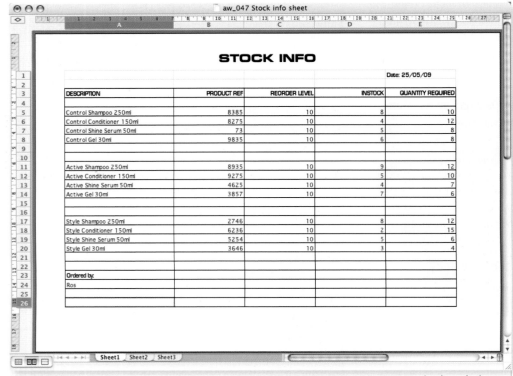

A computerised stock sheet

Unit G11 contribute to the financial effectiveness of the business

Ideally, stocktaking is carried out at a set time each week and the subsequent order placed with the supplier. In a busy salon this is not always possible and stock control may become haphazard, which may lead to problems, as low levels of stock may not be noticed until it is too late. You should be aware of your salon's ordering system, as this will allow salon staff plenty of time to inform the person responsible for ordering stock if there are any shortages that may have been overlooked, or if they become aware that a large amount of a specific product is required the following week. The table below offers solutions to a common stock problem.

Resource problem	Possible cause	Outcome	Solution
No base colours	Poor stock control	Client dissatisfaction	Implement a good stock control system
	Unexpected usage over a short period of time		Inform staff of the procedures if and when they notice low levels of stock
	Poor service from the supplier		Try to come to an agreement with the supplier or shop around for a more reliable one

Ordering stock

There are several different methods that may be used when ordering stock. Whichever method your salon employs, records must be kept to show this. This is to make sure the order is correct on its arrival.

Stock may be ordered by:
- sending your order by post
- telephone
- fax
- email / on line
- in person.

The method your salon uses should be reliable, ensuring the required stock arrives on time. Your employer may need to shop around to find the most competitive prices and a supplier who can guarantee efficient service.

Checking the stock on arrival

When the stock arrives, it should be accompanied by a delivery note that states the contents of the package. This should be checked against the original order to make sure the delivery matches and the correct goods have been received. The delivery should then be checked to make sure the order is complete and undamaged.

Dealing with any discrepancies

Any shortfalls, discrepancies or breakages should be reported to the salon owner (if applicable) and the supplier immediately. Damaged, substandard or unrequested goods should be returned to the supplier with a returns note, stating the problem.

Storing the stock, including stock rotation

All stock should be stored in the correct place in the stock room. Large or heavy items should be stored at ground level; this is to safeguard against them falling and injuring someone. Frequently used stock should be stored at eye level to ensure it is easily accessible. All products covered by COSHH should be stored according to the regulations. This is to maintain health and safety within the salon and to prolong the shelf life of the products. For example, aerosols should be stored in a cool place away from direct sunlight and other sources of heat.

Stock rotation is an integral part of the stock control system. All new stock should be placed at the back of the shelf and the old stock brought forward. This will ensure that the stock is used in the order in which it was purchased and should guarantee it is in optimum condition. Some salons find it advantageous to date all stock as it arrives, allowing them immediate information regarding the age of the product.

Check it out

How do the Manual Handling Operations Regulations relate to your work role and that of others when receiving and storing stock?

Monitoring stock usage

You are responsible for estimating the amount of stock you require for each service. Although you must make sure you are using sufficient products to carry out the service effectively, you should also try to eliminate any waste. Any leftover products that have to be disposed of equate to money down the drain for your employer. You should be able to estimate the quantities of each product you will use and prepare them accordingly to minimise wastage.

Be professional ★★★

If you find it difficult to estimate the quantity of product to mix, it is more cost effective to mix more as and when it is needed.

If you are responsible for other members of staff, for example, juniors, you are also accountable for their product usage. It may be that you are required to train your staff to use all resources effectively to minimise waste. This may include turning off the taps whilst shampooing to save money on heating the water or using the telephone for business calls only, as using the telephone for personal calls will run up unnecessary phone bills and also prevent clients getting through to make appointments. If it is not within your job specification to deal with resource problems such as this, then you should notify the person responsible as soon as possible. Your salon should actively encourage you to put forward any recommendations for improving the use of resources.

When making recommendations, you must be able to justify them and state the reasons why they will benefit the salon. In the instance above, you may suggest a pay phone is installed for staff to use, reducing the telephone bill and not tying up the line for incoming calls. If the salon is to carry out training in the effective use of resources, it is more cost effective to carry out this type of training with several staff members at a time. This will also ensure that the information they receive is identical, which will ensure consistency within the staff.

In the salon

Less is more

Shabir was a colour technician in a busy salon. To save time he always asked the junior stylists to mix the tint for him, as they had been trained to mix colour products and knew which ratios of colour to oxidant to use. Some of Shabir's clients had up to four different colours on their hair. He always noticed that when Michael mixed the colour there seemed to be a lot left in the tint bowl at the end of the service. After several weeks, Shabir asked Michael how much tint he was mixing. Michael replied, 'Oh, a whole tube. It's easier to work out how much oxidant to use.'

- How do you think this affected the salon's finances?
- What should Shabir do now he has identified a problem?

Keeping the necessary records

All records or documentary evidence relating to the salon's stock control systems must be accurate and up to date. There are two main reasons for this.

1　To check the stock levels are accurate at any given time.
2　These records will also be used by the salon's accountant when drawing up the end-of-year accounts.

Consumable and **semi-consumable** items should be checked and ordered following the same procedure. It would not be safe, practical or professional for the salon to run out of essential items such as cotton wool or protective gloves.

Consumable

things that are used once, e.g. cotton wool.

Semi-consumable

things that may be used more than once, but won't necessarily last for a long time, e.g. protective gloves.

Be professional ★★★

If items such as cotton wool and protective gloves do not appear on your stock sheet, suggest to the member of staff responsible for stock to add them on at the bottom to ensure they are not overlooked.

Check it out

To whom would you go when suggesting recommendations for improving the use of salon resources? Why don't you devise a proforma to be used as a written record of recommendations that you put forward, e.g. a salon memo sheet?

 Key Skills Links: Level 2 Communication

Tools and equipment

Salon tools and equipment are monitored in the same way as salon and retail products; the main difference is that stocktaking of tools and equipment is carried out more infrequently, as tools and equipment should last longer provided they are properly maintained and only used for business purposes. To ensure the optimum life expectancy of electrical equipment, you should make sure you are complying with the Electricity at Work Regulations (refer to page 6 if you are unsure).

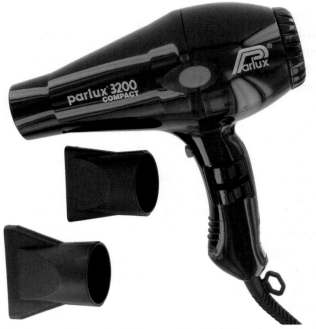

All salon equipment should be regularly checked and maintained

It is important to monitor the levels of tools and equipment in the salon for several reasons, which are:
- to ensure the correct number of working items that are needed for the smooth running of the salon (some may be out of use, either broken or awaiting repair)
- to calculate if the levels need to be increased to meet the demands of the salon (if there are more stylists employed, more equipment will be needed)
- to make sure the end-of-year audit is correct with regard to items that may be offset against tax due from the business.

If you are aware of any shortages of tools and equipment, you should report them immediately to the designated person within your salon. This will ensure the smooth running of the salon, avoiding unnecessary problems such as clients being kept waiting whilst another stylist finishes their client. The following table shows a common resource problem and solution.

Resource problem	Possible cause	Outcome	Solution
Five hairdryers broken within the last few weeks	Misuse	Clients kept waiting until resources become available	Ensure resources are repaired or replaced in sufficient time to ensure smooth running of the salon
	Accidental damage		
	Unauthorised use for out of salon work	Client dissatisfaction	

Human resources

The people that work in the salon should be a valuable asset to any business. However, for the salon to remain profitable, this should mean employing the right people for the right job, for example, your colour technician should have received proper training in this area and have the expertise to carry out the role. If they do not, this may lead to client dissatisfaction, resulting in loss of clientele, negative publicity and/or litigation (see the Sale and Supply of Goods Act 1994, page 97). A stylist carrying out the duties of a junior (on a stylist's pay) would not be cost effective, as the stylist would not be bringing sufficient revenue into the salon to cover their wages.

Remember

If you employ a 'Saturday junior' you need to check your local by-laws. Do you need a licence to employ people under 16?

The table below shows a common resource problem and solutions.

Resource problem	Outcome	Solution
Stylist phones in sick	A whole column of clients have no stylist	Try to share out the work amongst the other staff (with similar levels of competency)
		Telephone clients, explain the situation, then reschedule where possible
		Cancelling appointments should be a last resort

All staff should have good working conditions as laid down in law, examples of which are the Working Time Directive and the Health and Safety at Work Act.

Time

Time is another valuable resource in the salon environment. It is essential that all staff make good use of their time at work, as time is money! All the services carried out in the salon are priced to include the cost of materials (products, electricity, water, etc.) and the time it takes to complete the service. It is essential that you are able to carry out all salon services in a commercially viable time and, by doing so, you are fulfilling part of your obligations under the Sale and Supply of Goods Act 1994.

Some services allow time for other services to be carried out whilst the stylist is not needed, for example, the stylist

should be able to carry out an additional client while another client's hair colour is developing. All appointments should be booked in this way to allow optimum use of time. This will benefit both the business and the stylist, as it will bring more money into the salon and increase the amount of commission the stylist earns each week.

Check it out

Your awarding body has set timings for technical services that are deemed commercially viable. Are you aware of these timings? If you are not, you should speak to your tutor or assessor and ask them for this information.

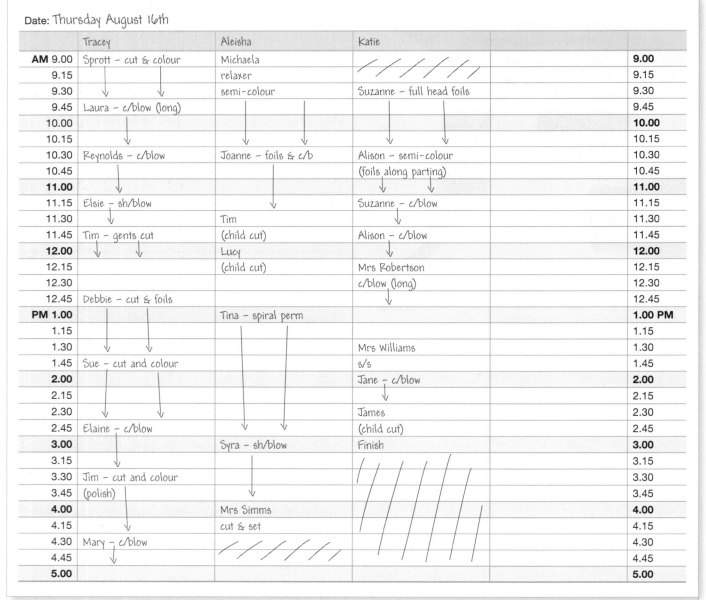

Date: Thursday August 16th

	Tracey	Aleisha	Katie		
AM 9.00	Sprott – cut & colour	Michaela	/////		9.00
9.15		relaxer			9.15
9.30		semi-colour	Suzanne – full head foils		9.30
9.45	Laura – c/blow (long)				9.45
10.00					10.00
10.15					10.15
10.30	Reynolds – c/blow	Joanne – foils & c/b	Alison – semi-colour		10.30
10.45			(foils along parting)		10.45
11.00					11.00
11.15	Elsie – sh/blow		Suzanne – c/blow		11.15
11.30		Tim			11.30
11.45	Tim – gents cut	(child cut)	Alison – c/blow		11.45
12.00		Lucy			12.00
12.15		(child cut)	Mrs Robertson		12.15
12.30			c/blow (long)		12.30
12.45	Debbie – cut & foils				12.45
PM 1.00		Tina – spiral perm			1.00 PM
1.15					1.15
1.30			Mrs Williams		1.30
1.45	Sue – cut and colour		s/s		1.45
2.00			Jane – c/blow		2.00
2.15					2.15
2.30			James		2.30
2.45	Elaine – c/blow		(child cut)		2.45
3.00		Syra – sh/blow	Finish		3.00
3.15			/////		3.15
3.30	Jim – cut and colour				3.30
3.45	(polish)				3.45
4.00		Mrs Simms			4.00
4.15		cut & set			4.15
4.30	Mary – c/blow	/////			4.30
4.45					4.45
5.00					5.00

A salon appointments book

In the salon

Time is money

Sylvie worked as a stylist in a busy salon. Each Friday she carried out a full column of cut and blow-dries. The salon allocated 45 minutes per cut and blow-dry client. Despite the amount of work she carried out, she still needed to earn more commission each week (as her expenses were more than her income). On looking through the appointment book, she noticed that the way her appointments had been booked, she sometimes had an hour to complete each client. She then realised that if her clients were rescheduled, she could actually do another three clients each Friday and still have a lunch break! Sylvie explained this to the salon receptionist and asked her to reschedule all her clients (as far as she was able) and to then make sure she booked all her cut and blow-dry clients at 45-minute intervals so she could maximise her opportunities to meet her targets and increase her commission.

- Was this Sylvie's responsibility?
- Whose responsibility is it to ensure that all working time is utilised to the full?

The table below shows a common time problem and solutions.

Resource problem	Possible causes	Outcome	Solution
Stylist is continually running behind schedule	Stylist is not up to speed	All other clients kept waiting, leading to client dissatisfaction	Enlist the help of other members of staff to either take over one of the clients or assist the stylist in order to help to catch up
	Junior member of staff is not fulfilling their own job role effectively, causing unnecessary problems for the salon	May cause unnecessary friction between the stylist and the junior	Junior needs retraining
	Instructions from the stylist are unclear or poorly timed	Stylist may not meet productivity targets	Stylist needs to improve communication skills

In some instances, it may be necessary to allow the stylist more time per client when booking appointments depending on the speed and experience of each individual. It may also be that the stylist needs some retraining in certain areas to enable them to get up to speed.

Meeting productivity and development targets

Hairdressing is a fast-moving industry. In order to keep abreast or ahead of any competitors, it is essential that you continually update your existing skills and learn new ones. To maintain your client base and generate income for the salon, it is important that you do not allow yourself to stagnate professionally. Change can sometimes be viewed as threatening; however, if it enables you to remain in employment it must be looked upon in a positive manner. To enable you to fulfil the requirements of this outcome, you should have regular meetings with your employer or salon owner to discuss, negotiate and review your productivity and development targets.

Your employer should have quite clear objectives regarding the salon's business and ways of keeping up with or ahead of the competition. This is a necessary skill for any employer who wishes to maximise the potential of their business. You may also be able to identify gaps in the market or areas you feel could be developed within the salon. You may get ideas from reading trade journals such as *International Hairdressers Journal*, as these contain information relating to all areas of the industry. You should also be expected to analyse your own performance in the salon and identify any areas of weakness you may have that you can then work to improve. This will have a positive impact on the salon and your productivity levels should improve accordingly.

Productivity

Within a business context, the salon's income comes from your ability to produce work of a good standard (in other words, you continue to bring money into the salon). Your employer needs to make sure you are able to maintain the required level of productivity to ensure both his/her and your income. If your wages cost your employer more than you bring into the salon, the business may not remain viable. Many employers offer incentive schemes or productivity bonuses to ensure their staff remain motivated and enthusiastic. You may already work in a salon that offers commission or other bonus schemes if you meet or exceed your targets.

Productivity targets cover retail sales and technical services. Retail sales are an excellent source of income for a salon, as any profit made does not need to be offset against the service. All members of staff may have productivity targets for retailing. To succeed in selling retail products, you must have excellent product knowledge to ensure you are selling the correct product for the client's requirements.

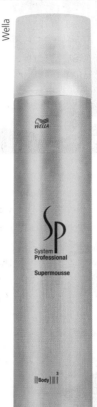

Wella

Knowing your product range well will help you to achieve your productivity targets

Any productivity targets should be negotiated and agreed by both you and your manager then recorded for future reference. The information may be recorded manually or the data may be entered onto the computer (if this is the case, the information held is covered by the Data Protection Act). Any targets set should be short term, for example, four to six weeks, and reviewed on a regular basis. The monetary targets that are set will vary depending on your capabilities and the prices charged in your salon. Any targets that are set should be achievable; there is nothing more demotivating and demoralising than failing to achieve your targets week after week. If you meet your targets easily, your employer may increase them to make sure you are working to full capacity and maintaining the challenge. However, if you fail to meet your targets, it may identify areas of weakness, for example, poor knowledge of retail products and their uses. This will necessitate additional training to improve your knowledge.

There are many different types of opportunities within the salon that you may use to help you achieve your productivity targets.

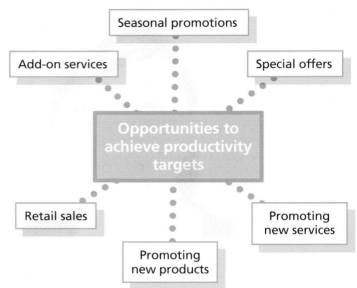

However, to carry these out effectively, you must have excellent product knowledge and a good awareness of other services that are offered within the salon.

Developing targets for personal learning and improvement

In addition to your productivity targets, you should also be encouraged to develop new skills and improve your existing skills. In this way you will continue to be an asset to the salon.

Before meeting with your employer to negotiate targets for your personal learning and development, it is a good idea to analyse your own performance in the salon and identify any areas of weakness you may have. You may also find it useful to gain feedback on your work from other members of staff. This information will enable you to put forward your own suggestions at the meeting. This should be looked upon in a positive way, as it shows you are able to be objective about your capabilities and limitations.

You may have your own thoughts regarding ways in which the salon can improve its financial effectiveness, for example, by introducing new services or products. However, when presenting this information, you must make sure you have given adequate thought to your suggestions, any potential problems that may arise, and how the problems may be overcome. This should enable you to present the benefits of your recommendations in a positive way. The way should then be open for you and your employer to discuss your suggestions objectively.

Any developmental targets set by your employer should have been negotiated and agreed by you both, with the necessary documentation completed. If you do not feel the targets your employer suggests are achievable, you should discuss this with them, using sound reasoning. Your targets may then be adjusted accordingly. Your employer may want to introduce new services into the salon, in which case you may be required to undergo training. It can be very difficult for a salon to progress if the staff are resistant to change and the atmosphere in the salon becomes tense. This does not reflect well on the salon, as the clients will pick up on the negativity. This will have an adverse effect on the business, therefore you should take up the challenge to progress and help the business and yourself whilst doing so. You may also be required to develop and improve your existing skills, as this may improve your productivity within the salon.

The timescale for developing new skills should be longer (than for productivity) and reflect the amount of time needed to perfect the skill. However, it is important that you meet your targets within the allocated timescale, as your employer may have included the potential income in the salon's business plan.

If you become aware that you are not going to achieve your developmental targets, you must inform your employer as soon as possible and give reasons as to why this is so. It is better if your employer hears this from you, rather than from another member of staff, as this can cause friction between the staff and create an unpleasant working environment. Your employer may ask you to explain the reasons why you are unable to meet your targets and if your reasons are justifiable, your employer may reconsider the original timescale, providing it is within the salon's budget.

Communication

Communication is an all-important part of salon life. Effective communication ensures total understanding between all the people involved. It will promote a professional image to both clients and junior members of staff (remember, they learn by example). It also sends out a good message to the clients, which will gain their trust and goodwill. Refer to Unit G21 (pages 29–32) and Unit G18 (pages 73–5) for more information on and examples of methods of communication.

In the salon

Good manners cost nothing

Salman was a junior in a busy salon assisting several of the stylists with their work. Mercedes, one of the stylists, had a habit of barking orders at Salman, whereas Natalie, another stylist, always asked him nicely if she required assistance. Salman liked to work with Natalie, as she did not make him feel insignificant or stupid in front of the clients. Salman began to hate working with Mercedes and avoided her whenever he could. Consequently, Mercedes found it difficult at work, as she did not receive the support she ought to. This had an impact on her ability to achieve her productivity targets.

- What should Mercedes do to improve the situation?
- If you were a junior member of staff, which of the stylists would you want to work with?

You may be required to order stock by telephone, in which case you must make sure your requirements are made quite clear. It is good practice to have your order repeated back to you. This way you can check there have been no misunderstandings. You will also need to communicate effectively with your employer during reviews or appraisals to negotiate productivity levels or development targets.

Be professional ★★★

'Actions speak louder than words.' Your body language can tell someone far more about how you are feeling than what you may actually say. You may think you can cover up feeling hurt or angry, but those who can read body language will know exactly what you are saying without words.

Written communication

Although the majority of your job role involves verbal and non-verbal communication, there are certain times when written communication needs to be used. This may be when compiling an order form for stock purchasing, completing stock records or filling in target sheets with your employer.

It may be necessary to use written communication on the staff notice board when notifying staff of your intention to send an order for stock and asking if they have any suggestions. This is especially effective if the salon has part-time staff and you do not always see them. It allows these staff to feel that they are valued members of the team. Client record cards must be completed accurately, as the information contained on a client record card communicates to other members of staff the exact nature of the service.

A badly filled in record card may be misinterpreted by another member of staff and cause client dissatisfaction if the end result is not as expected. It will also cost the salon money to fix the client's hair in terms of time and products.

Receiving and dealing with negative feedback

It is not always easy to deal with criticism or negative feedback; however, providing the criticism is constructive, you should use this as a tool for improvement. When responding to suggestions made for your self-improvement, these should be seen in a positive way and any constructive criticism accepted readily and acted upon. It is not always easy to respond in a positive manner, especially when you have received negative feedback and your immediate instinct is to feel hurt. However, it is important that you try to remain positive and look upon this as a learning tool, that is, something that is there to help you. This will lead to a more pleasant working environment for all the staff, which will be reflected in the salon atmosphere.

When receiving negative feedback, you must also remember your non-verbal communication skills are sending a message back to the sender and, although you may be saying all the right things, your non-verbal communication may be sending out a different message.

Check your knowledge

The following questions will help you to check your understanding of this unit. The answers can be found on page 418. Take care, as there may be more than one correct answer for some questions.

1 Why is it important to have an effective stock control system?
  a So each staff member has responsibility for a specific job in the salon
  b So all stock can be monitored and recorded
  c To make sure there is always sufficient stock
  d To make sure that junior staff have training

2 What are the potential consequences of stock levels falling below functional levels?
  a The salon may lose money
  b Client dissatisfaction
  c More money in the bank
  d More space in the stockroom

3 Which legislation do you need to consider when retailing products to the clients?
  a Working Time Directive
  b The Trade Descriptions Act
  c COSHH
  d The Sale and Supply of Goods to Consumers Regulations

4 Why is it important to adhere to consumer legislation when selling retail products?
  a To prevent litigation
  b To maintain a professional image
  c To ensure maximum profits
  d To ensure all products are sold before they become discontinued stock items

5 Why is it essential to your employer that you utilise all your working time effectively?
  a To maximise profits
  b To reduce waste
  c To set a good example to the other staff members
  d To ensure the receptionist is doing their job correctly

6 Why is it important to continually update your skills and learn new ones?
  a To prevent boredom
  b To set a good example to other staff members
  c To maximise your own earning potential
  d To maximise the salon's profits

7 What kinds of opportunities are there in the salon to help you achieve your productivity targets?
  a Seasonal promotions
  b Promoting new products and services
  c Excellent assistants
  d Using a suggestions box

8 What are the benefits of regular target reviews?

   a To ensure the stylist remains focused

   b To ensure the manager is kept busy

   c To allow regular contact with the manager

   d To help with the development of reflective skills

9 What are the potential consequences of poor communication skills during discussions with clients?

   a The clients may not understand the information they have been given

   b The wrong products may be used

   c Clients may decide to go to another salon

   d Clients may be offended

10 A shortage of resources may result in:

   a clients being kept waiting until resources become available

   b staff redundancies

   c client dissatisfaction

   d the salon running smoothly

Assessment guidance

You must demonstrate in your everyday work that you have met the standards for contributing to the financial effectiveness of the business.

You will have to prove that you can competently:
- monitor and effectively use all the resources listed in the range
- set and achieve your own productivity targets for technical services and retail sales.

You will be assessed once while carrying out your contribution to the monitoring and effective use of resources in the salon. The rest of your evidence will most likely be documentary evidence that you have gathered during a specified period of time. You may not use simulated activities at all.

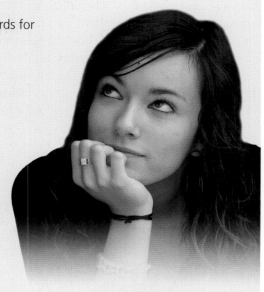

Unit G11 Contribute to the financial effectiveness of the business

2

Professional skills – hairdressing

Creatively cut hair using a combination of techniques

What you will learn:

- How to prepare the client
- How to create the look
- How to proceed after the service.

Goldwell

Introduction

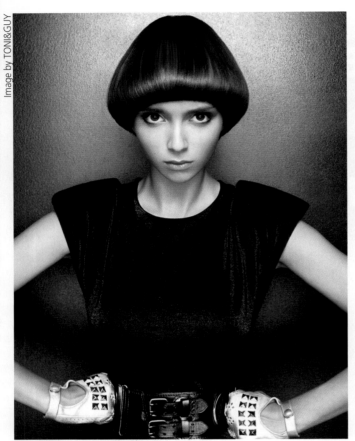

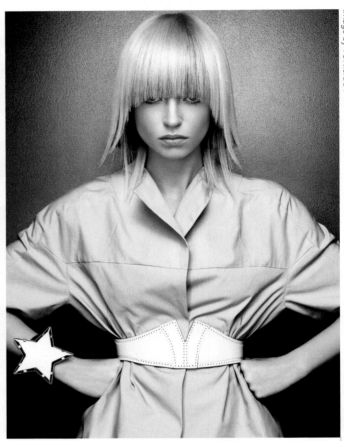

Cutting techniques can be used to create varied and contrasting looks

Throughout this unit, we will be looking at how to use a variety of cutting techniques to creatively re-style women's hair. You will see step-by-step examples of re-styled looks using creative cutting. There are many different techniques involved in cutting, all of which can be developed and applied in innovative and creative ways to produce varied and contrasting looks. You will use all of the basic principles that you learnt whilst completing your initial hairdressing training, but will now need to develop and apply those skills with greater accuracy and invention. The demands that a client will put on you for a total re-style will require you to have a higher skill level and a broader use of imagination.

You the stylist

This is the point at which you will need to have self-belief in your ability and commitment in the work you produce. Free your mind, find your creative flair and, most importantly, enjoy it.

Preparing the client

This section highlights all the things that are important when preparing your client for the cutting service, for example, using the correct personal protective equipment and ensuring you have ready the relevant tools that are appropriate for the task. As always, there are several health and safety regulations that you need to be fully aware of before you begin the cutting service.

Check it out

Reread Unit G22 (pages 3–25) and make a list of all the acts and regulations that you think might be relevant to cutting a client's hair. Then, as you progress through this unit, check that you have remembered them all.

Thorough consultation

When a client comes into the salon for a cut, it is important for you, the stylist, to conduct a thorough consultation with them. You must note what the client is wearing (ensure your assistant does not put a gown on until you have seen them). Ask about their job and lifestyle, for example, do they go to the gym regularly? Look at the client's hair as they enter the salon and before it is shampooed, just in case he or she asks for it to be styled in the same way. At this stage, find out as much background information as you can, as this will help you make an informed decision on the choices available to your client. Do not skimp on the detail and take the time to find out about them now, so that you can be sure to advise them on the best possible options that are available to them.

Use of visual aids

You will need to use sound communication skills to extract the right information from your client (see pages 29–32 in Unit G21 and pages 73–5 in Unit G18 for more information on communication skills). Your aim is to build up a picture in your mind of what exactly the client requires of you and you need to make sure that you are both thinking along the same lines. You must ensure that you fully understand your client's requirements; one method of doing this is to use stylebooks or magazines to illustrate the proposed look. It will be much easier for both you and your client if you have a firm idea of the look she is seeking to achieve.

An important factor that you must consider during a consultation is whether the client's hair has the potential to achieve the look that you both may want. A ten-minute consultation will be wasted time if the hair texture, length or amount of movement is not suitable to achieve or maintain the look. During the consultation, it is good practice to push the client's hair back off the face so that you can look at their head and face shape. Keep a close eye on your client's facial expressions as these can reveal whether she is happy with your suggestions or not.

Checking for contra-indications

When you are looking at your client's hair, remember to check the scalp for infections and infestations. You should also be checking the hair's texture and density, as this can be a **critical factor** in determining the right style for the client. For example, if the hair is very coarse and abundant, and the client has chosen a look that is best suited to finer hair, you may have to advise them against it or adapt your cutting technique to take this into account. It may be necessary to use a razor or thinning scissors to remove some bulk.

Critical factor

something which must be considered to ensure the best outcome.

You may need to ask your client when they last had their hair cut, as this will give you a good indication of how much to cut off, bearing in mind that most people's hair grows about one centimetre a month. Another good indicator is the demarcation line of a colour growing out, as this gives you an idea of your client's hair growth rate.

Once your client has been shampooed and has returned to you, look at the hair again and check the growth patterns. The client may have disguised these by styling the hair but shampooing the hair will allow it to lie back in its natural fall. Also, while the hair is wet, it is important to check the hair's elasticity; if it is poor and stretches considerably, this must be taken into account during cutting to prevent taking off too much.

Personal hygiene

During the time you spend with your client, you must consider your own personal hygiene. You will be in close contact with your client as you talk to them and lean over them. You should have fresh breath and a clean smell about you. Strong smells such as nicotine can be very off-putting for the client, particularly if they are a non-smoker. For this reason, it is good practice to appoint a rule of no smoking in the salon. Not only are there the risks associated with passive smoking, but there is also the risk associated with smoking near flammable products. You should ensure that your hands and fingernails are clean and presentable – this will instil confidence in both you and your client regarding your personal standards and professionalism.

Salon life

Poor consultation

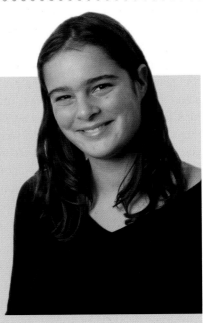

Simone's story

Today I had a new client come into the salon that I hadn't met before. I had a quick chat with her about how she wanted her hair to look before she went off to be shampooed by my assistant. Although I hadn't met her before we were happily chatting away about her job and as I came to cut the sides of her hair I asked her, 'Would you like your hair cutting over your ear?' and she just said, 'yes'. Then she gasped and looked horrified so I asked her what was wrong and she was really upset saying that I had cut her hair too short over her ear and that she wanted her hair to come over her ears so that she could keep them covered. She was quite distressed and said that she always thought her ears were too big and that she was really conscious of them. I couldn't apologise enough. I felt terrible as I had already cut it now and would have to continue the cut knowing how much I had upset her. I know that what I did was really unprofessional and the client said she will not come back to the salon again!

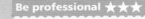

Be professional ★★★

- Never skip over detail during consultation – really listen and take the time to fully understand your client's requirements and to ensure they understand what is achievable and the likely outcome.
- Build the time for a thorough consultation into your pricing structure – if you have to charge slightly more because of the time taken, it will be worth it in the long term to ensure your professionalism is maintained.
- Use as many visual aids as possible during consultation – if your client cannot find a photo of a style they like, then try sketching a look for them. Alternatively invest in a computerised system that allows you to show the client how their new style will look on them before taking the plunge with a re-style.

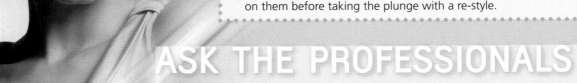

ASK THE PROFESSIONALS

Q *What is the key to an effective consultation?*

A You must have excellent communication skills, both verbal and non-verbal. If you are able to get your point across accurately and really listen to your client's requirements, also noticing facial expressions during the discussion, then you can ensure an effective consultation.

Q *What will good consultation techniques do for your salon image?*

A If a client is more than happy with their look then they will tell their friends; any discussion outside the salon about you is important to build a good and professional image of your salon and your ability as a hairdresser.

Personal protective equipment

Once you have fully explored every option with your client and you have agreed on the end result, you must prepare the hair for cutting. Gowning the client and using the correct protective equipment is essential. For example, a cutting collar or towel will not only prevent hair from falling onto the client's clothing, which causes uncomfortable itching, but it is also cleaner and creates a professional appearance. Attention to little details like this is what raises you from being a 'run-of-the-mill' hairdresser to being a specialist. Using a good shampoo and conditioner relevant to your client's hair type is essential. The hair must be thoroughly cleansed to aid with combing during cutting and also to prevent damage to your cutting tools. You will find the hair easier to handle if it is thoroughly clean and detangled; this will ensure you take clean sectioning lines and keep good tension during cutting.

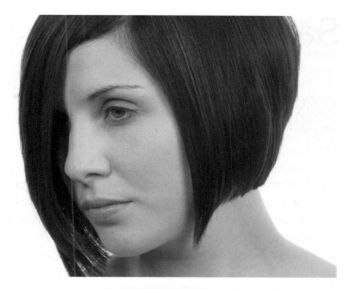

Preparing your work area

While your assistant is shampooing your client, you have a few minutes to prepare your work area. Utilise this time wisely to ensure that you get all the tools and equipment ready that you think you will need. Once you get into the routine of doing this, it will become natural good practice. You cannot always rely on your assistant to know which tools you are planning to use. However, you should be able to rely on the junior staff to ensure that all tools and equipment are clean and sterilised (see Unit G22, pages 13–14). This will prevent any risk of cross-infection, infestation, or damage to tools due to them being unclean or unfit for purpose. Scissors and combs can be sterilised by placing them in an ultra-violet cabinet, but remember, they must be turned over to ensure both sides have been done. It is also good practice to keep combs in a chemical jar and replace the solution frequently to ensure its effectiveness.

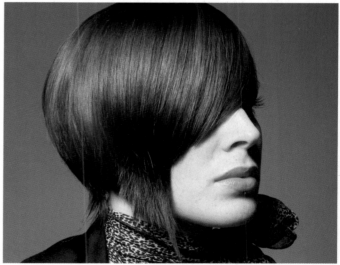

Creating the look

You need to be able to use advanced cutting skills to enhance your clients overall look and to give the hair a completely new re-style. You will have to find the confidence to build upon the basic cutting skills that you already have and use them to create individual re-styled looks.

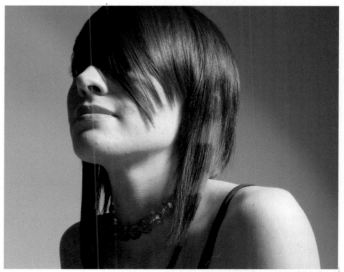

Some examples of re-styled looks using creative cutting techniques

Cutting tools and their uses

There are many cutting tools available for use. You need to be familiar with each one and the effects you can achieve by using them.

Scissors

Scissors come in many different designs and several lengths of blades. They are used for a variety of cutting techniques such as club cutting, slicing, texturising or thinning. It is very important to find the right pair; remember that they need to feel comfortable to use, as they are really just an extension to your hand. Be familiar with all the working parts of your scissors. It will help you to use them if you know how they work. Below is a diagram of a pair of scissors with all the parts labelled.

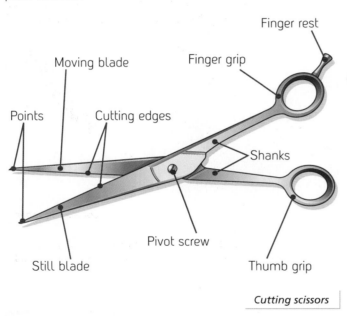

Cutting scissors

Thinning scissors

As well as straight-edged scissors, there are also thinning scissors with serrated edges. These can also be called **aesculap** or texturising scissors. They have one or more edges with serration. It is also possible to buy scissors with varying degrees of serration, which allow the stylist to produce much more imaginative styles. Thinning scissors are used to remove bulk, not length, and must be used only on dry hair.

Aesculap

initially a brand name of a company that developed thinning scissors; because of their popularity it became the most common name used for this type of scissor.

Remember

Your scissors must be handled with care and well maintained in order to prolong their working life and to ensure they give you the best possible results with each cut. Blunt scissors can cause damage to the hair ends by splitting them. Each time you use your scissors, wipe them when you have finished the cut to clean them. Use light oil on the hinge regularly, as this will prevent them from rusting or seizing up. You must sterilise them to prevent the passing on of infection or infestation. Because you are using them so close to the hair and skin, it is inevitable that they pick up bacteria from one client that could easily be passed on to another.

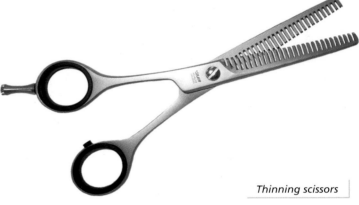

Thinning scissors

Clippers

Clippers are used for club cutting and are extremely good to use on very short styles. Clippers have two blades with serrated edges, one of which moves and the other stays still. Because of the type of edge, it is essential that you have them sharpened by the manufacturer or a specialist sharpening service. You can use small clippers for tapering and outlining as they cut much closer and finer. They are especially good for removing any hair outside of the hairline after cutting. Outlining is particularly important when providing a very short cut close to the skin as it can be used to neaten off a finished style. However, even when outlining, you can use ordinary-size clippers, but be sure to close the blades by using the lever on the sides, as this will give a much closer cut.

Remember

Clippers are electrical and you must use them in line with the Electricity at Work Regulations. Look back at Unit G22 (page 6) for a quick reminder.

> **Check it out**
>
> Look at the clippers that you use in your salon. Find out how they should be maintained and stored following the manufacturer's instructions.

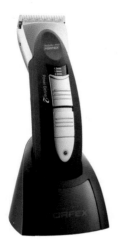

Clippers

Although clippers are mainly used for club cutting, if you are confident in their use, then they can be used to create various effects, such as scooping out at the root area to thin the hair (texturising). Clippers must be maintained by removing the hair around the blades with a clipper brush with stiff bristles, often provided by the manufacturer. Use clipper oil on the blades regularly but ensure they do not have oil on them whilst cutting or else this will hinder their performance during the cut. In recent years, cordless clippers have become more popular and this type of clipper has the advantage of causing less of a hazard due to trailing wires. They are recharged when placed back in the base unit after use.

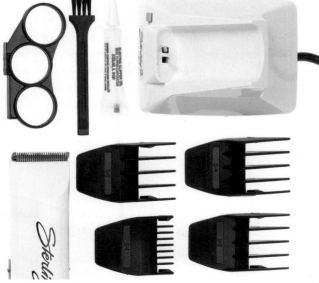

Cordless clippers with attachments, cleaning brush and oil

> **Remember**
>
> Whilst completing your Hairdressing Level 3 qualification, the use of a clipper attachment is not allowed.

Clippers are now available with a pivot head, which makes them easier to use as the head of the clipper is more flexible. They also come in various colours, which appeals to our fashion-conscious industry. Hairdressers are often nervous of using clippers, as they are afraid that they might cut the skin, when in fact they are safer to use than scissors as the blades are always parallel to the skin.

Razors

Razors can be used when cutting the hair to remove bulk or to thin out the ends. They are especially good for creating textured looks. You have the choice when using a razor for cutting hair of an open razor, a safety razor, or a shaper as shown below.

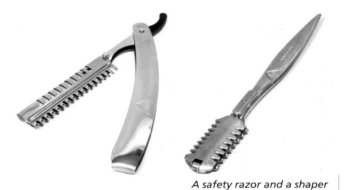

A safety razor and a shaper

It is essential that you hold and use a razor correctly, not only for your own and the client's safety, but also to prevent damage to the hair.

> **Check it out**
>
> In the photograph below, study how to hold the razor correctly when cutting and practise holding the razor this way.

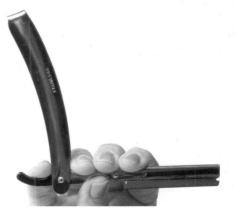

The safety guard must be facing you as you work

You must keep the hair wet at all times when cutting with a razor, as this will allow the razor to slice into the hair and cut precisely. You should also ensure that your blade is extremely sharp. The advantage of modern razors is that you can change the blades frequently, especially if you are using them to shave excess hair from below the outline. For instance, in the nape area of a short cut, if you shave the hair away, you must replace the blade following your salon policy for disposal of sharps. This is to prevent the risk of cross-infection. Care must be taken as it is very easy to slice the skin when using a razor, especially when you are working around the eye or ear area.

An important point that you must make to your client is that there is a risk of in-growing hairs after close razor or even clipper work. This can happen if the hair curls as it is growing and starts to grow back into the skin. It would be evident from a small lump in the skin that can become infected. They are, however, usually easy to remove by piercing the skin with a sterile surgical needle, allowing the hair to be freed. In-growing hairs are more likely to happen to a client with curly or African type hair. A client with dark skin will need to be advised about the changes that can happen to the skin with repeated use of close clipper or razor work. The area of skin that has been clippered or razored may start to thicken or darken, causing discoloration of the skin that will be very noticeable below the hairline. This is known as 'shadowing'.

Cutting techniques and effects

Now that you are aware of cutting tools and their uses, we can begin to look at the various cutting techniques in more detail.

Club cutting

This technique removes the hair length only. It gives the hair ends a very blunt look and is the most commonly used technique. Clubbing or blunt cutting allows you to cut very straight and precise lines, for example, in the cutting of a one-length bob. When club cutting, it is the angle at which you hold the hair that determines the finished effect. You have to hold the hair firmly between the fingers with even tension and ensure each section is thoroughly combed to produce even cutting. You can club cut on wet or dry hair, but it is more precise on wet. When you clipper cut the hair, you are also club cutting.

Thinning

This method of cutting is used to remove bulk from the hair but not length. It is more commonly carried out with thinning scissors; however, there are scissor-thinning techniques that you can use. For instance, chipping into the hair at the root area will remove bulk and the shorter hairs will help to provide style support to the longer lengths.

Be professional ★★★

- Thinning scissors should be used only on dry hair to prevent too much hair from being removed. They should not be used on partings or around hairlines as short hairs can be seen protruding once the hair has been styled.
- Thinning scissors are not suitable for use on fine or thinning hair, but they are good for very thick or coarse hair. You can use the thinning scissors at any point along the hair length depending on the amount of hair you wish to remove and the effect you want to create.
- If you have cut hair very short and there are 'steps' in the haircut that you cannot remove, a good tip is to use thinning scissors to go over the hair ends to remove them.

Razoring

This technique has become very popular again as very textured looks are currently fashionable. Razors should only ever be used on wet hair as the hair ends can be easily damaged by using a razor on dry hair. It will also be uncomfortable for the client as it drags along the hair shaft, giving the feeling of hair being ripped out of the head. You must also make sure that your razor's edge is always sharp, again to prevent damage or discomfort. Razor cutting can be done anywhere in a haircut and removes bulk and/or length, depending on where you use the technique.

With razor cutting, the hair is held between the fingers and can be cut either on top or below the section, with the razor held at a slight angle to the hair shaft. The amount of pressure you apply will determine the amount of hair removed, so take care — it is much safer to remove a little at a time than to take off too much. Razor cutting is especially good for creating very textured looks or for blending short layers into very long layers.

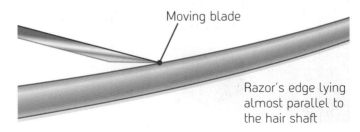

Moving blade

Razor's edge lying almost parallel to the hair shaft

Free hand

This technique can be done on wet or dry hair and is carried out by cutting the hair without holding it between the fingers. The hair is just combed into place and the ends cut to allow it to fall in its natural lie. It is especially good when cutting the hair around unusual growth patterns. For example, if a client has a cowlick at the front hairline and you were to cut the fringe between the fingers, when you let go it would jump up and look uneven in length. Similarly, if you were cutting around nape whorls, it would look much better for the client if you cut it to its natural lie.

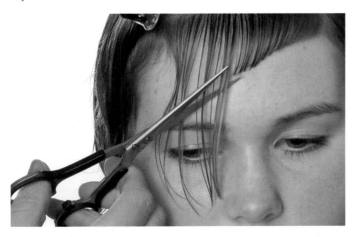

Texturising/point cutting

This can also be called chipping or point thinning. It can be carried out on wet or dry hair and is used to remove either length or bulk. The ends of the scissors are used to cut into the hair anywhere along the hair shaft from mid-lengths to ends, depending on the effect you are trying to create. It will give a look a much more choppy uneven finish, with softer broken edges. It can be incorporated into many different styles; for instance, a client with a very straight-edged look can require a softer fringe that has been point cut.

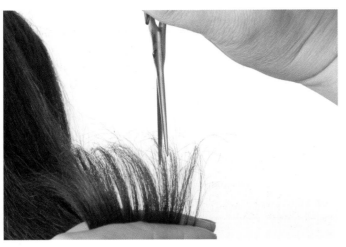

Tapering/slicing

This technique is used when you want to remove bulk or join together short layers with long layers. It can be done on wet hair if using a razor and dry if using scissors. The scissors are allowed to slide into the hair, as you slightly open and close the blades, in a backcombing type of movement. With the razor method, you scoop into the hair sections and apply pressure according to the amount of hair you want to remove. This method requires a great deal of accuracy and skill so as not to cut off too much hair.

Scissor-over-comb

Although more commonly used in men's hairdressing, it is inevitable that you will have to cut a short tapered neckline on a woman's haircut. It can be carried out on wet or dry hair. Care must be taken not to cut 'steps' into the hair. For this technique, you place the comb into the hair at the root area and pull out the comb away from the scalp up to the desired length. You cut the hair that protrudes through the teeth of the comb while maintaining a flowing movement; the scissors must open and close to cut at the same pace up the haircut or else lines will develop. Again, this type of cutting requires accuracy and a great deal of practice. Clipper-over-comb is done in exactly the same way, except the clipper blades are run over the hair protruding through the teeth of the comb.

Check it out

You can practise the movement of scissor-over-comb in the work-station mirror. Make sure that the comb follows the movement of the opening and closing scissor action and that you hold your comb in a way so that you can flip it over to comb down each section that you have just cut.

Bevelling

The bevelling technique is used when you want to introduce graduation into your cutting line. The hair is held between the fingers but the fingers are turned over to allow the hair to wrap slightly around. This small amount of drag will provide slight graduation. It can be done on wet or dry hair but, as with most haircuts, it will be more precise if carried out on wet hair. This technique would never be used for precision cutting where neat cutting lines are required.

Disconnecting

This technique is used when you want to achieve a look that contains shorter and longer sections within the haircut. Instead of blending the shorter lengths to the longer lengths they are left disconnected, which gives a more dramatic effect and has become increasingly popular. It is also useful for taking bulk out of a cut and cutting shorter layers underneath for style support.

Creatively cut hair using a combination of techniques **Unit GH16**

Cutting angles, baselines and guidelines

Now that you have looked at all the cutting techniques, you need to familiarise yourself with the effects you will be creating by cutting angles. They fall into two main types: layering and graduation. You will no doubt be familiar with the terminology, but do you fully understand the difference between the two? Firstly, you will layer most haircuts, except for one-length cuts. The most common layering technique is the uniform layer — this is where the hair is cut at a 90-degree angle to the scalp and is cut to the same length all over the head, as shown in the illustration below.

Cutting angle

the angle at which the hair is cut.

Baseline

the initial cutting that you will follow throughout the haircut.

Guideline

the line of the hair cut that you follow as you progress through the cut.

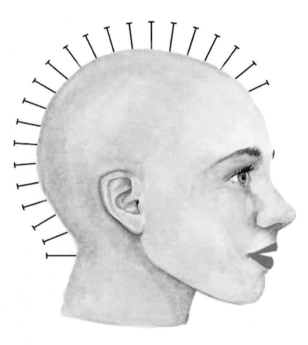
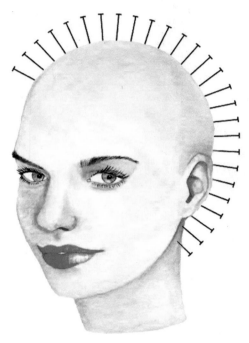

Hair cut in a uniform layer

Graduation is when the hair is cut to varying lengths throughout the haircut. For example, the layers on top may be quite short but through the back they are substantially longer; this is known as increased graduation. To achieve increased graduation you need to over direct the layers through the back and sides, pulling them all over to the shorter length guidelines at the top. The cutting angle will fall anywhere between 90 to 180 degrees depending on the amount of graduation. Alternatively, when the layers through the top are much longer than the underneath layers, this is known as reverse graduation. For this type of graduation, the cutting angle will fall anywhere between 45 to 90 degrees, again, depending on the amount of graduation. Examples of these are shown in the illustrations opposite.

Remember

It is extremely important that throughout the cut you are aware of the cutting angles you are using, as they will affect the finished shape and balance of the hair. Not only is this important, but you must be accurate in the way that you section the haircut. It is not always necessary to start at the back, but be sure to section off the hair and follow neat and even sections throughout the cut. Good sectioning will allow you to follow your guideline and ensure that no areas are missed. This also looks professional to the client. It is also important to take clean sections to ensure you achieve the desired effect.

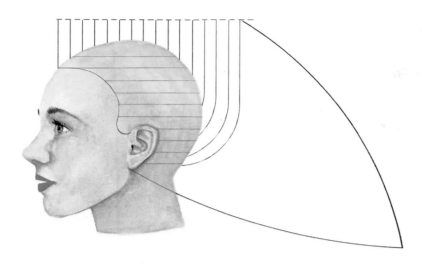

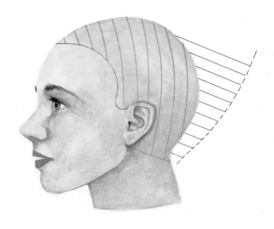

Increased and reverse graduation

The initial guideline or baseline you cut will be important in determining the overall length, shape and balance of the cut. Sometimes you will cut the outer line of the hair first, as in a one-length cut, or you may cut the inner length of the hair first, as in a uniform layer cut. Either way, you will always have to cut both the outer and the inner lengths. Guide or baselines can be cut in a variety of shapes, each of which is detailed below.

- Symmetric: the haircut is evenly balanced over both sides, as in a hairstyle with a centre parting of equal lengths on both sides of the head.
- Asymmetric: the hair is unevenly balanced over both sides, for instance, if the hair has a side parting and more hair is distributed to one side of the head.
- Straight: the hair is cut to a straight baseline as in one-length looks.
- Concave: the baseline will be cut curving inwards or downward; think of a concave bob where the hair curves downwards towards the sides.
- Convex: the baseline is cut longer from the sides into the middle section, which gives a curve of longer in the back to shorter towards the front.

Look at each of the illustrations on the right to help you visualise them all.

You may, however, cut a client's hair and not have to follow a guideline — some cutting, if it is freehand or texturising, relies on your feel for the hair and knowing how to create balance within a cut without following a guide line. This will only come with practice and the more cutting you do, the more of a feel you will have for what is right!

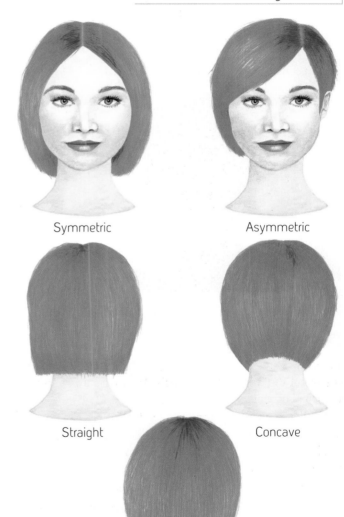

Symmetric

Asymmetric

Straight

Concave

Convex

Unit GH16

Creatively cut hair using a combination of techniques

Re-styling the hair using creative cutting techniques – step by step

1 Having cleansed the hair, remove the bulk by cutting off the ponytail.

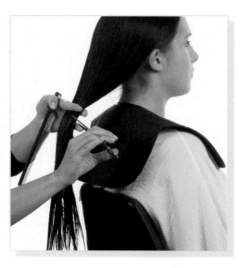

2 Create the first section as an off triangle at the front hairline. Draw a second triangle section asymmetrically across the top of the head. Proceed to the side area and create a third smaller triangle section above the ear. Draw a fourth triangle the same as the third on the opposite side of the head.

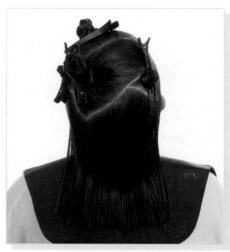

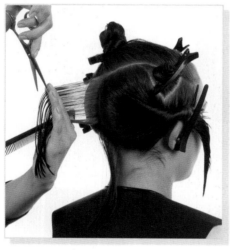

3 The remaining hair is now cut starting at the centre back. Draw a vertical section, elevate parallel to head shape and blunt cut.

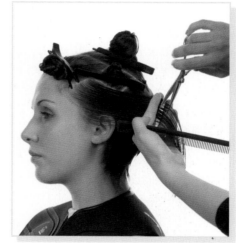

4 Over direct the hair in front of the ear area to behind the ear area by taking diagonal angles. Use a blunt cutting technique to retain length.

5 Cut the side sections by holding the hair between the fingers with minimum tension on a diagonal angle. Use a blunt cutting technique.

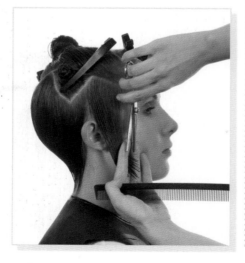

6 Cut the perimeter shape to the desired length using a point cutting technique.

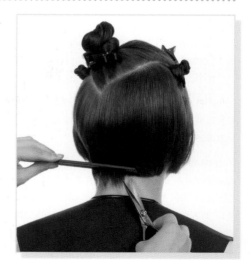

7 Cut the triangle at the front of the head using a blunt cutting technique. Elevate the hair vertically and cut on a diagonal angle creating a short to long effect, retaining length on the front hair line.

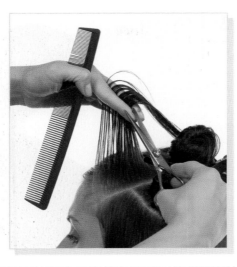

8 Continue to cut this section by pivoting from the shortest point until complete. This will give an asymmetric effect.

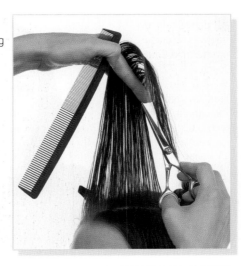

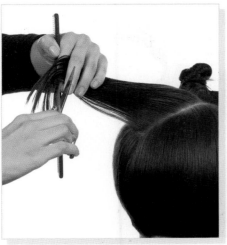

9 Continue working sections by pivoting and over directing each section back to the original guideline. This will retain length around the front/side area.

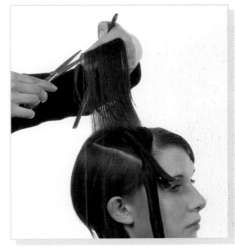

10 Cut the remaining triangle shape by elevating sections to a diagonal angle and blunt cutting.

11 Continue by pivoting from the shortest point and over direct each section to the original guideline.

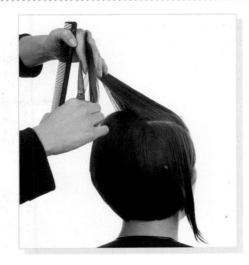

12 The finished look.

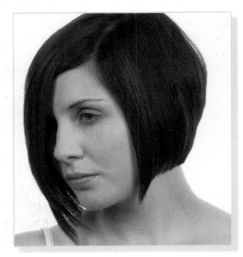

Re-styling the hair using creative cutting techniques 2 — step-by-step

1 Before cutting, hair was coloured using Wella Colour Touch ¼ — 77.45, ¾ —7.0, plus a teardrop section through the fringe with 5.0.

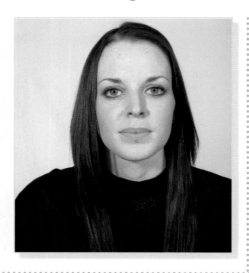

2 Cut off the pony tail to remove the bulk of the length.

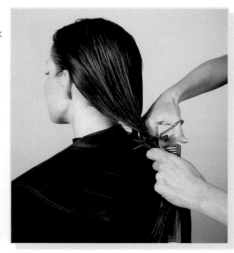

3 Take the first section from the temple to the ear at an offset angle.

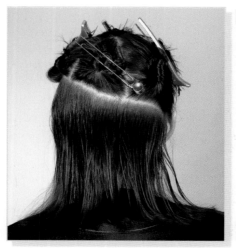

4 Cut this section using a graduated cutting line from shorter in the nape to longer at the crown.

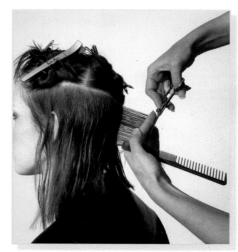

5 Cut the right-hand sections with less graduation to take this side shorter.

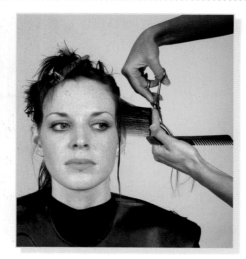

6 Tidy the neckline using both freehand and point cut techniques.

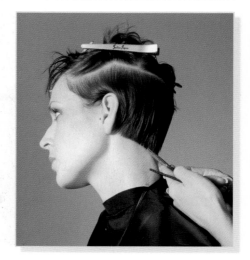

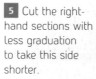

7 Disconnect the top sections and razor cut following the head shape to leave an overhang over the graduated under layers.

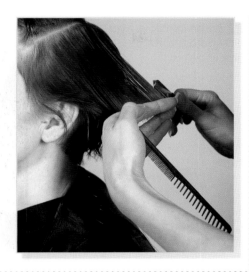

8 Carve into the front hairline using a razor.

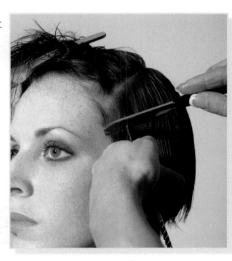

9 Overdirect the right-hand side to where the head rounds and carve into using the razor.

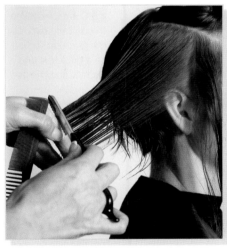

10 Razor the longer layers through the right-hand side from temple to earlobe to create softness and feathering.

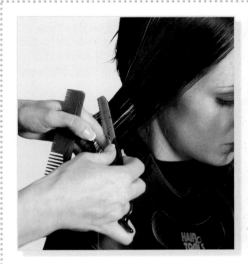

11 Point cut the edges to add final definition to the cut.

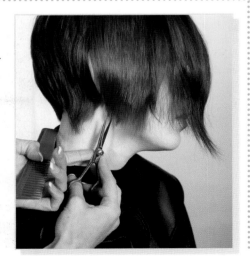

12 The finished look.

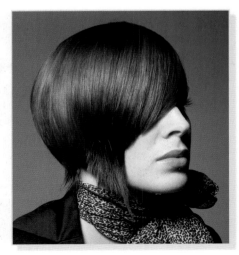

Creatively cut hair using a combination of techniques **Unit GH16**

127

Re-styling the hair using creative cutting techniques 3 — step-by-step

1 Before cutting, hair was coloured using Wella Koleston Perfect 55/65 and two triangular sections at the sides using 33/0.

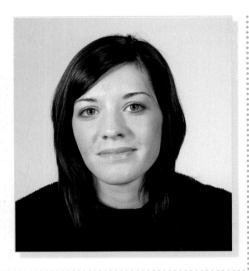

2 Section the hair in a heart shape at the back of the head.

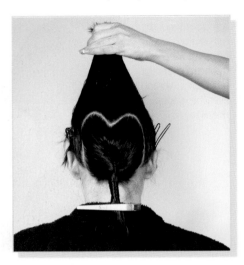

3 Take a vertical section down the back of the head and cut with some graduation.

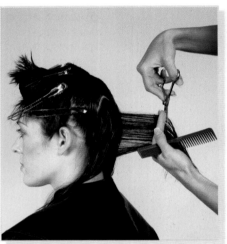

4 Cut each section through the back using the previous section as a guideline and slightly overdirected, leaving the heart shape disconnected through the centre.

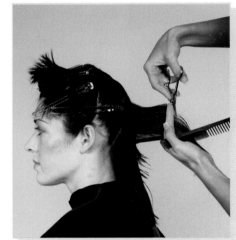

5 Cut the neckline to the required length leaving the hair longer at the sides.

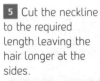
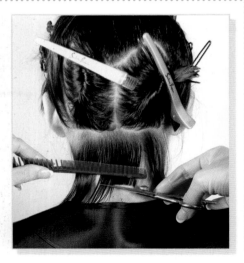

6 Hold up the centre section and cut on a plateau leaving the hair longer to the front.

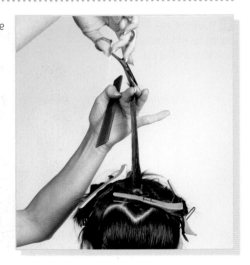

7 Take diamond-shaped sections to cut through to the front and point cut the ends — irregular sectioning adds definition.

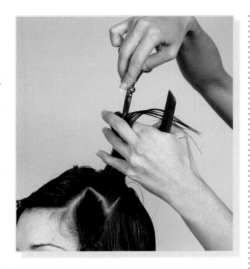

8 Slither cut the hair to retain length and disconnect. The hair will be cut again when dry to personalise.

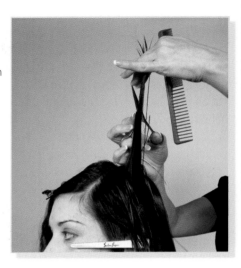

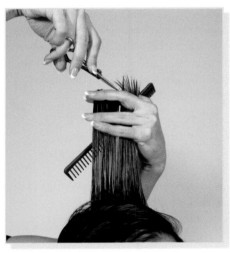

9 Plateau point cut across the top section and overdirect towards the front.

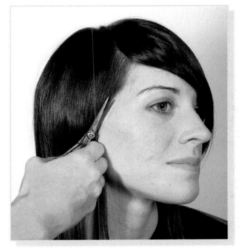

10 Comb hair flat onto the face and carve through the cheekbone area freehand.

11 Slice into the back and sides to personalise the cut.

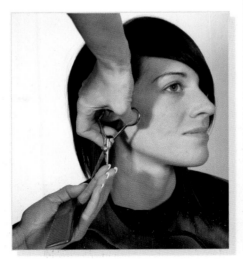

12 The finished look — a clip-in extension has been placed in the hair to add dramatic colour.

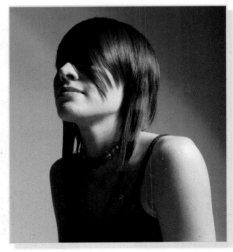

Creatively cut hair using a combination of techniques **Unit GH16**

Cross-checking

While you are carrying out the cut, you must maintain the consultation throughout. You will find that as the cut builds up, you may have different ideas about where it is going and you need to check this out with the client before making those changes yourself. It is also vital to cross-check the cut and check the balance throughout to ensure you have not made any mistakes. When cross-checking, look at it the opposite way to how it was first cut. For instance, if you took vertical sections, then take horizontal ones. Remove any hair only if you find it out of line. The point of cross-checking is to look for mistakes, not to re-cut the hair and take it another centimetre shorter. The client will not thank you for this and it is a waste of your time. Also, look at the length of the hair all over the head and make sure that you have not missed any areas.

Correct positioning of self and client

The positioning of yourself and your client during the cut is something that you must be aware of at all times. If the client is sitting awkwardly or slouching with his or her legs crossed, then this could affect your finished cut. If the client is slouching to one side, then you could end up with the hair longer on that side. It is much easier to cut hair if you position the head correctly. For instance, in the difficult-to-reach areas, such as the nape of the neck, you must ensure the head is placed down as far as is comfortable for the client. Not only is the client's position an **influencing factor**, but also your own body stance is very important. If you are stooped over clients all day and not keeping your back straight, you will soon feel discomfort in your back. It is essential to prevent long-term

injury or damage by ensuring that your own posture is good. Think about balancing the weight over your body when you stand and not leaning to one side for long periods. It is far too easy to put unnecessary strain on muscles and ligaments by over-reaching or stretching. However, this can be avoided by taking the time to adopt good posture while working. Eventually it will become habit to stand in the correct position and you will do it without realising.

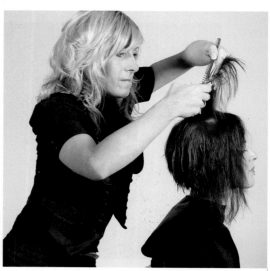

Do not strain your back by leaning over your client

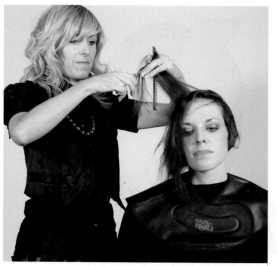

Keep your back straight and balance your weight correctly

Influencing factor

a point which must be considered as it will affect the outcome.

Timing

Timing is very important while you are training. You should be checking the length of time it takes you to carry out services in the salon. As a guide, a cut and finish should take no longer than 45 minutes on short hair, and a re-style or long-hair cut and finish should take about one hour. However, this may vary depending on the type of salon that you work in.

Check it out

> Think about the timings allowed in the salon for all the cutting services that you offer. Do senior members of staff have a different time allowed to them from the junior staff?

Solving cutting problems

There are various types of problems that you may come across during the cut and you need to feel you can deal with these as they arise. Usually, they are because your consultation was not accurate. For instance, you begin to cut and then find that there is a conflicting hair growth pattern that is preventing you from getting the look you require. You will have to deal with problems such as these whenever they occur, but remember to keep the client informed, use your professional judgement, and be tactful in explaining the situation. If you have a confident manner then your client will feel confident in your ability, whereas if you are floundering and unsure, they will realise this and may begin to panic. This type of situation will get you nowhere; it will look totally unprofessional and could harm your reputation. Even if you are not fully confident, do not panic but just keep talking to the client while you plan your course of action.

Below is a table showing common cutting problems with possible remedies.

Cutting problem	Possible remedy
Sides are not even on finished cut	Cross-check, use the mirror and remove the longer length to even up
Can't get close enough into the nape to cut to required length	Adjust the way you hold the hair for cutting, or use a different cutting technique
Hair won't lie correctly around hairline	Adjust the finished style to incorporate the hairlines natural lie
Cut the client's or own skin	Stop immediately and clean the wound so it's free from hair and apply pressure to stop bleeding. Use a band-aid if continuing
During the cut you notice head lice	Advise client to go and treat the hair as soon as possible

One problem that can easily be avoided is getting cut hair on the client's clothing. When you use a cutting gown, make sure it fits over all the client's clothing and that it is correctly fastened. You can use either a towel or a cutting collar around the shoulders. The benefit of a cutting collar is that it fits well over the shoulders and does not get in the way when cutting around the shoulder or neck area as a towel might. It is also a good idea and looks professional if, at regular intervals throughout the cut, you remove any hair that has fallen onto the skin or shoulders. This will also help to prevent any hair going down the neck area and causing discomfort to the client.

Remember

> A good tip if the cut hair is wet and sticking to the skin, is to use a little talcum powder on your neck brush to help to remove it.

Be professional ★★★

- Remain aware of critical influencing factors, such as growth patterns, at all times.
- If cutting wet hair, keep it wet throughout, especially if using a razor.
- Always take neat, even sections.
- Ensure that your tension is good and even throughout the cut.
- Make sure you can see your guideline before you cut.
- Never cut shorter than your guideline.
- Check regularly throughout the cut that it is level.
- Always cross-check your cut.
- Do not cut off too much hair when cross-checking, only the hair you have missed.
- Maintain the consultation throughout with the client to check what you are doing is to their requirements.
- If things go wrong, do not let the client see that you are panicking.
- Remember, if you cut the hair too short, there is nothing you can do about it!

If you cut hair using these rules, you will not go far wrong. Make them your cutting commandments and you will have many happy clients!

Cutting techniques and effects: a quick reference guide

Technique	Effect	Cut on wet, dry or either	Best suited on straight or curly hair
Clubbing	Gives a blunt, straight edge to the hair ends	Either, but more precise on wet hair	Either, but will help to reduce curl
Clippering	Gives a blunt straight edge to the hair ends	Dry	Can be used on either, but open the blades slightly to aid cutting on curly hair
Thinning	Removes bulk but not length	Dry	Either, but will encourage curl
Razoring	Removes bulk and length, good for texturising	Wet	Either, but will encourage curl
Freehand	Removes length and bulk	Either	Either
Point cutting / Texturising	Produces softer, broken edges	Either	Either
Slicing / Tapering	Removes bulk, gives texture	Wet with razor and dry with scissors	Either
Scissor over comb	Club cutting on short hair	Either	Either
Bevelling	Creates graduation at the ends of the hair	Either	Either
Disconnecting	Creates long and short lengths that do not blend together	Either	Either

After the service

Once you have finished the client's hair, just sending them out of the salon is not enough. You need to discuss with them how to maintain the look and book them another appointment for the next service that you recommend. Include in your discussion any after-care advice or recommendations that you feel are relevant.

Disposal of waste, including sharps

On immediately finishing the cut and checking with the client that it is what they require, it is most important that you remove any loose hair cuttings from the client's gown and skin so as to prevent any discomfort. If you brushed off the hair cuttings as you went along, then this will be a small task. You can use the hairdryer to blast away any hair from the chair or skin that you cannot brush off. The more hair you remove from the client and surrounding area, the more professional it will look and there will be less chance of them feeling itchy.

At this point, you must also sweep up all the hair from the floor and dispose of it following your salon policy. Hair cuttings left on the floor can cause a slippery surface and this then becomes a hazard in the salon, both to you and to the client when they stand up. Salons will dispose of hair cuttings in different ways, but generally it is more hygienic to ensure that they are placed in a covered bin and put in the outside bin in a tied-up bag to prevent hair spilling out. At the end of the cutting service, you may need to dispose of sharps and again this must be done in line with salon policy. However, it is a strict health and safety rule that used sharps are disposed of in a sharps bin. This has to be a sealed container clearly labelled with its purpose.

> **Check it out**
>
> Visit your council offices and look up the local bylaws for the disposal of used sharps and waste to see if there are written codes of practice. You will usually find that they have them and you should be observing and following these.
>
> **Key Skills Links**: Level 2 Communication

Using styling products to finish

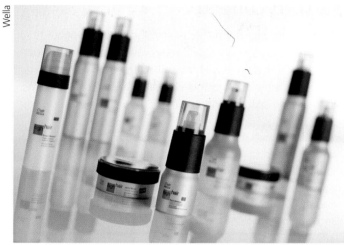

Wella

Let clients try different finishing products – it could encourage them to buy!

When you are styling the client's hair, you must select the correct styling products to complete the desired effect. It is also a great opportunity for recommending the products you use to sell to the client. Remember that it will be harder for them to style and maintain the look without the professional products that you are using in the salon. Let the client look at and feel the products and put a little in their hand for them to smell and feel. This will let them know that you have every confidence in the products that you are using and that you are proud to show off their quality. It is impossible to achieve a good finish using styling products of poor quality.

Know your styling products well – if you have thorough product knowledge, it will show your professionalism and will allow you to recommend with confidence. This is especially important if you work in a salon that pays you commission on your sales. This can be a good boost to your income. There are often other perks thrown in for the best salesperson, such as free products.

Check it out

When you have a spare few minutes in the salon, look at the products for sale and read the manufacturer's information to see if you have forgotten any of the benefits that they offer. Make yourself an easy reference guide to use in your work in the salon. Do this regularly, as it is easy to forget how good a product is when you use it day in and day out. It will help you sell to your client if you are fully conversant with what the products can do for their hair.

KS **Key Skills Links**: Level 2 Communication

Look at the table below. It lists several of the styling products available for use and the effects they will help you to achieve.

Styling product	Effect
Gel / Gel spray	Firm to ultra hold
Mousse	Volume, natural to extra firm hold
Wax	Texture, defines curl
Hairspray	Natural to ultra firm hold
Dressing / Styling cream	Adds shine, reduces static, defines curl
Gloss / shine spray	Adds shine, reduces static
Blow dry lotion	Volume, natural to firm hold
Straightening creme	Helps hair to stay straight, defies humidity

Any styling product that you use will need to be applied following the manufacturer's instructions. Take time out to read these on first use, as it will ensure that you get the maximum effect and best results from whatever you are using. If it says use a pea-sized amount, then you should just use that much; however, you will need to judge if the hair is thick and abundant and requires more of the product, or if it is fine and requires less of the product.

Remember

All of the styling products that you are using are likely to be flammable. You must take care that you do not use them near a naked flame, for example, near a cigarette lighter.

Any products that you use in the salon must be stored, handled, used and disposed of following COSHH regulations (refer to Unit G22, page 7, for more detailed information). Following COSHH regulations will show professionalism, ensure that safety is of the utmost importance to you and sets a good example to other staff.

Remember

A good tip is to ask the wholesalers or company representative to let you try the products for free before you buy them for the salon. You need to judge for yourself if the styling products will deliver what they say they offer and who better to try them than you!

Unit GH16

Creatively cut hair using a combination of techniques

Keeping up to date

There are many different manufacturers and types of product available to aid styling. Usually you find products that you can rely on and trust and you will tend to stick to this particular manufacturer. However, new products are being developed all the time and you need to keep up to date on the latest developments by taking regular trips to the wholesalers or receiving visits from the company representative.

Confirmation of the finished look

When you have finished styling the hair, you will need to check the balance of the finished look and confirm with the client that he or she likes the end result. Always look in the mirror and check the overall balance from every angle around the head, as this is what everyone will see of your client's look. Show the client the back, making sure that he or she can actually see through the back mirror. A good rule of thumb is if you can see the back or sides through the mirrors then your client will also.

Sometimes the cut will need a little adjusting after drying. Explain this to the client and keep them informed at all times of where and how much you are cutting off. You may find that the feathering is finer on one side; this is sometimes visible only on dry hair. You may find that a small piece of hair, when wet, was stuck behind the ear and you missed it. Do not be afraid to tell the client that you have spotted something that needs correcting. They will thank you in the long run and be happier with the style once they have left if it is corrected now instead of on the next cut.

Removing the client's protective clothing correctly

Once you have applied the styling products and are about to start styling, you (or your client) may want to remove the gown, especially if it is a hot day in the salon. It is, however, important not to remove the gown before applying styling products so as to prevent any spillage onto the client's own clothes.

> **Be professional ★★★**
>
> If you do need to remove the gown at this stage, explain to the client that cut hair may still fall off the head during styling and onto the clothing, causing discomfort later. They may reconsider if they have to go to work or go shopping and are unable to change soon.

When removing the gown, always take care to take it off properly. Unfasten it correctly and ensure that any cut hair is thrown from the gown onto the floor and not over the client's clothing. If you do find there is some on their clothes, offer them a clothes brush to remove it – never let them leave the salon with hair on their clothes. This looks messy and does not give a good impression of the salon. Remember that a client is looking for an all-round excellent service; they may think that although you have given them a fabulous haircut your customer service skills leave a lot to be desired. It is likely that it will stick in their mind and be what they tell their friends about your salon.

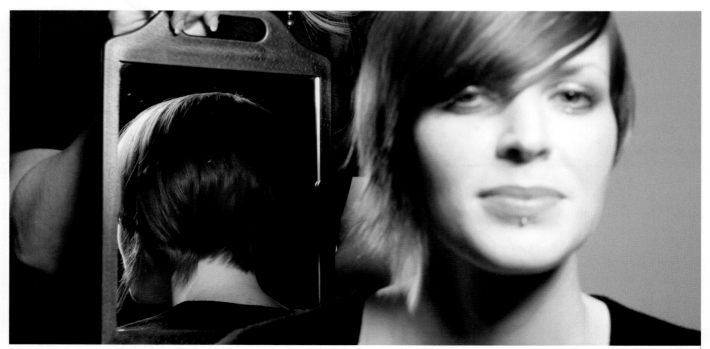

Make sure your client can see through the back mirror

Recommendations

Finishing off the style can be a very relaxing experience for clients and they often tell you that the final styling is the best part of the service. If it is a regular client that trusts you, then they may just want to close their eyes and relax. Alternatively, they may want you to explain how you are drying it so they can re-create the look at home. As you are styling the hair, you can discuss with your client the techniques you are using and why and how the products are helping you to achieve the final look. Ensure you have a selection of brushes and equipment available for retail sale. A client may find it easier to style at home using the tools that you use and it is another good selling opportunity. Never shy away from giving clients advice on styling — it is a reflection of your salon's good name if their hair always looks good. They are, after all, a walking advertisement for you out on the streets.

> **Check it out**
>
> Using a selection of pictures or photographs of your own work, describe how you achieved the overall look and incorporated different cutting techniques. In your descriptions, indicate the cutting angles and list the tools and equipment you used. State which products you used to create the looks.
>
> **Key Skills Links**: Level 2 Communication

Intervals between cuts

Remember to advise the client on when they will need to return to the salon for their next appointment. This may be for a service other than cutting, but generally, clients have their haircut maintained between every four to six weeks, unless they are growing their hair in which case they may want to leave a longer gap. Usually, no longer than ten weeks between cuts is advised. If it is left any longer, the ends of the hair become more susceptible to splitting (**fragilitis crinium** — see page 49 Unit G21) and the style will begin to look messy, causing the client to have difficulty with it at home. Always ask the client to book their next appointment before they leave; do not miss the opportunity while you still have the client in the salon. This will make sure they return to you and do not have the chance to go elsewhere in the meantime. It will also make them think that you care about keeping their hair in good condition and, if you work in a busy salon, they may need to book early to avoid the disappointment of you not being able to fit them in.

> **Fragiltis crinium**
>
> commonly known as split ends: the ends of the hair have become damaged and split open.

Unit GH16 creatively cut hair using a combination of techniques

Check your knowledge

The following questions will help you to check your understanding of this unit. The answers can be found on page 418. Take care, as there may be more than one correct answer for some questions.

1 What is the name of the act governing safe use of electrical equipment?
  a Data Protection Act 1998
  b Electricity at Work Regulations 1989
  c Gas Safety (Installation and Use) Regulations 1994
  d Health and Safety at Work Act 1974

2 Why is it important to protect the client's clothing from loose hair cuttings?
  a To prevent discomfort
  b It looks professional
  c It may add decoration
  d The client may like it

3 Why should you position your cutting tools for ease of use?
  a To save time
  b To show the client you don't care
  c To prevent them from being stolen
  d To prevent accidents

4 Why must you continue your consultation throughout the cutting service?
  a So you can annoy the client
  b To be able to tell your friends what the client has said
  c So you can ignore the client
  d To ensure you fully understand the client's requirements

5 What may happen to curly hair if you continually cut it close to the skin?
  a Nothing – it has no effect whatsoever
  b Skin can become itchy
  c Scarring of the skin
  d Hair may start to in-grow

6 Why must hair products be removed from the hair prior to hair cutting?
  a To prevent damage to your cutting tools
  b To prevent products coming into contact with your skin
  c To prevent the risk of cross-infection
  d So the hair is clean which aids the cutting process

7 Is razor cutting carried out on wet or dry hair?
  a Dry only
  b Wet only
  c Both
  d None of the above

8 Why should you cross-check the haircut?
  a Because it takes up more time
  b To make the client think you are not sure of what you are doing
  c To highlight any mistakes that need to be corrected
  d It helps to provide a professional service

9 Half way through cutting a client's hair you notice head lice and eggs. Should you:
  a shriek and throw down your scissors and comb
  b quietly inform the client
  c clean and sterilise all tools and equipment immediately when finished
  d refuse to continue with the haircut

10 When carrying out a haircut, why is it important to give advice on maintaining the look at home?
  a To keep the client for longer
  b To ensure the client can look after her hair at home
  c To open up a retail sale opportunity
  d To show professionalism in your work

Assessment guidance

In order to prove your competence in this unit you must demonstrate advanced cutting skills that will improve your clients' overall image. All the practical assessments for this unit must be from work carried out with clients in the salon using a combination of cutting techniques, and no simulation is allowed for any performance evidence. You will be assessed cutting at least six creative re-styles on different clients and at least one must include precision cutting. There are ten cutting techniques but only seven out of the ten must be witnessed by your assessor. In order to prove competence in the other three you must provide other evidence, for example, photos or videos of you using the cutting techniques or written statements from a witness that you have used the techniques.

Unit GH16 creatively cut hair using a combination of techniques

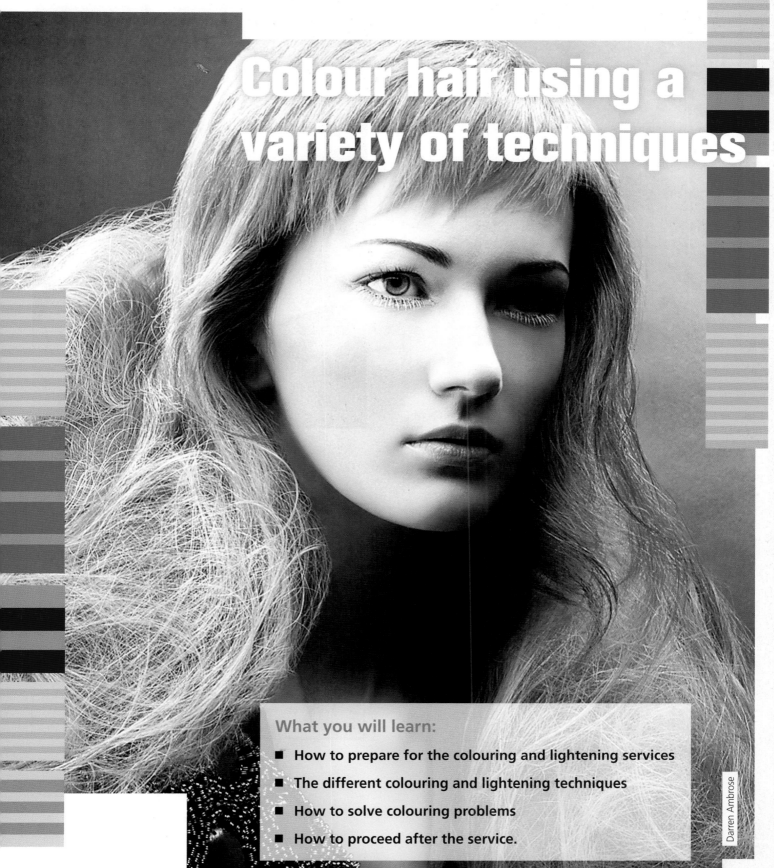

Unit GH17

Colour hair using a variety of techniques

What you will learn:

- How to prepare for the colouring and lightening services
- The different colouring and lightening techniques
- How to solve colouring problems
- How to proceed after the service.

Darren Ambrose

Introduction

This unit is concerned with combining, adapting and personalising colouring techniques. You will need to be able to produce a variety of fashion effects in a way that complements the style you are creating. You will also be required to restore depth and tone of colour and neutralise unwanted colour tones. Colouring the hair will allow you to use your artistic flair and represent the looks you are creating in an innovative way. In terms of chemical treatments, colouring the hair has become substantially more popular than perming over the last decade and, with this in mind, product manufacturers have developed many more interesting and expansive colour ranges and treatments. This gives you, the stylist, a broader spectrum of choice when colouring a client's hair, allowing you more versatility in the work you produce.

You should consider all the reasons why a client may come to the salon for a colour. This will help you to realise the importance of colouring in the salon.

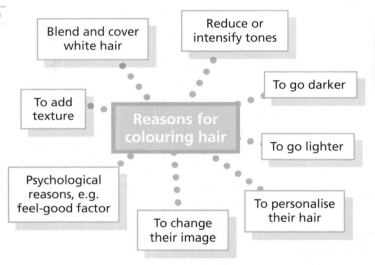

Blend and cover white hair

Reduce or intensify tones

To add texture

Reasons for colouring hair

To go darker

To go lighter

Psychological reasons, e.g. feel-good factor

To personalise their hair

To change their image

You the stylist

While carrying out your initial training, you will have learnt the importance of the shade chart and the international colouring system. In building on this foundation of knowledge, you must now move forward and develop your colouring skills further to allow you vision and diversity in your colouring work. The more confidence you build in your ability, the more inspirational your work will become.

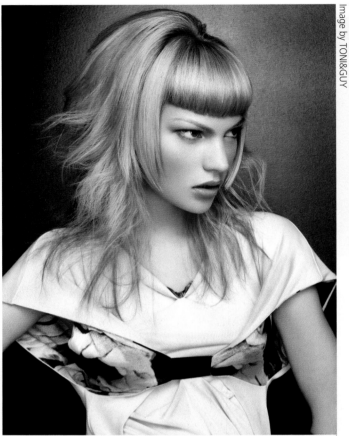

Image by TONI&GUY

Colour allows you to create more innovative looks

Preparing for the colouring and lightening service

Preparation is the key to success when colouring and lightening. Thorough preparation will prevent problems arising, such as running out of a colouring product or incompatibility of the product you are using with the client's hair. Ensuring you are fully prepared and ready for the service will not only present a professional image, but also allow you to work within the expected service times for your salon.

Check it out

What are your salon's expected service times for colouring and lightening work?

Thorough consultation

Before providing colouring services to your clients, the consultation you carry out is essential to extract the correct information, allowing you to proceed with the correct colour choice and techniques. Remember, the use of visual aids, such as shade charts, is very useful in helping the client choose a colour. In addition, you may wish to utilise other sources or creative inspiration, such as historical or cultural trends. You must ensure you keep up to date with what is currently fashionable; this may be carried out via the Internet, trade and fashion magazines etc. You will have to rely on your excellent communication skills, as clients are not always aware of the consequences of misinforming the stylist regarding any previous colour treatments they have had. To ensure your success, you should complete a consultation sheet with your client. This will not only prevent you from forgetting to ask an important question, but will serve as a written record of the discussion you have had. This could prove to be extremely useful if you are faced with legal action as a result of a colouring service.

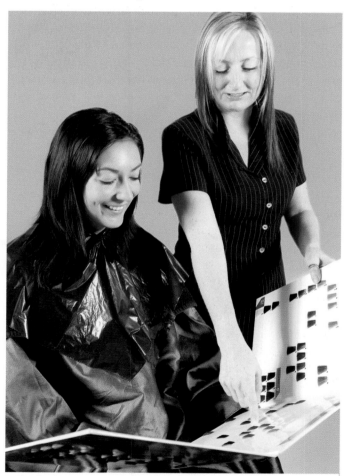

Shade charts or samples can help your client to choose a colour

Be professional ★★★

If a client wants a particular colour service and you suspect there is something on the hair that may cause a problem, you cannot always trust a client to tell you the truth, even if you have explained the consequences. Therefore, any written record of the consultation will prove useful if the client challenges you later.

During the consultation you will need to assess how the client's hair needs to be prepared for the service. If you are unsure, always check the manufacturer's instructions, as it may be a requirement that the colour is applied to clean, freshly shampooed hair. The way the hair is prepared for the service will play a vital role in the colour result and, if you prepare the hair incorrectly, the results may not be as you or the client expected. This would cause both yourself and your client to feel unhappy and dissatisfied and you may lose the client, along with your confidence in your ability to colour hair.

Contra-indications and influencing factors

Although these two can be very similar, they are not exactly the same. A contra-indication would prevent you from continuing with the service; whereas influencing factors may not necessarily prevent you, but must be considered in all the decisions you make while the colouring service is taking place. Influencing factors can sometimes prove to be contra-indications. For example, if a client is suffering from an adverse skin condition and it proves to be infectious, this would present you with a contra-indication that would prevent you from continuing.

Contra-indications

It is important that you question your client to ascertain whether they have any contra-indications to the colouring service, as sometimes they may not be apparent by observation alone. A few minutes spent questioning your client may save hours of time and possibly money should there be problems (which could have been avoided) during or after the service.

Contra-indications should always be carefully considered. Never overlook their presence, as this could present you with problems that you did not foresee. The table overleaf shows contra-indications and methods that may be used to assess the problem.

Unit GH17 Colour hair using a variety of techniques

Contra-indications	How to assess the problem
Skin sensitivities	Carry out a skin test prior to the service
Previous history of allergic reaction to permanent colouring services	Ask the client during consultation and look at previous record card or consultation sheet information
Other known allergies	Ask the client during consultation and record any known allergies
Skin disorders	Thoroughly check the skin and scalp prior to commencing the colouring service
Incompatible products	Ask the client about any hair colouring products they may have used in between visits. Carry out an incompatibility test on the hair
Medical advice or instructions	Ask the client during consultation about any medical issues they may have that could prove problematic. If necessary, ask for notification from their GP
Evident hair damage	Carry out elasticity, porosity and colour tests prior to the service

In the salon

Allergy to colour

Margaret came into the salon for a colour service. She did not want a permanent colour, as the condition of her hair was quite poor due to several bleached highlight services. Her hair was very fine and below the shoulder in length, and her skin was quite pink in colour. She thought an overall colour might be more suitable until the condition of her hair had improved, and a quasi-colour was recommended. The stylist did not carry out a skin test, as she did not think it was necessary because she was not using a permanent colour.

The stylist applied the colour and, during the development, Margaret complained that her scalp felt quite sensitive and itchy. The stylist removed the colour immediately with cool water and noted the hairline and scalp were very red and looked quite 'angry'. However, she assured Margaret it would subside and not to worry. Margaret had in fact had an allergic reaction to the colourant.

- How could this have been avoided?

Influencing factors

Influencing factors should never be overlooked. Giving full consideration to these will help to produce perfect colouring results.

Temperature

As you have previously learned in your hairdressing training, the temperature of the salon will influence the processing time. A cold salon may slow down the processing time while warm temperatures will speed up the process. Use of heat to develop colours quickly is useful; however, the porosity and condition of the hair needs to be considered, as hair in poor condition will accept colour more readily. You should take extra care when developing lightening products using an additional heat source, as they may develop more quickly than you expected, resulting in over-processed hair.

Be professional ★★★

Always check the manufacturer's instructions to establish whether the colouring products should be developed using additional heat.

Body temperature plays an important role when carrying out a full head colour, as the colour on the roots of the hair will process more quickly than the colour on the end. This is because its development is speeded up by the addition of body heat. Therefore, when carrying out a full-head lightening or full-head red application, you should apply the colour to the mid-lengths and ends first, and the roots last. This will prevent the colour being too light at the roots (in the instance of a lightening application) and will prevent root glare when using 'reds'.

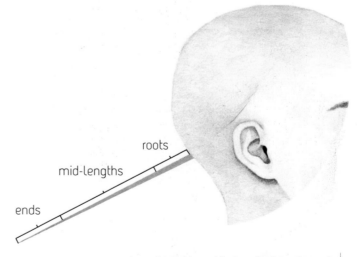

roots

mid-lengths

ends

Colour should be added to the lengths and ends of the hair first to prevent root glare

Existing colour of hair

The depth of hair colour needs to be considered, as permanent tint will only lift three to five shades. Therefore, if you have chosen a colour that needs to be lifted six or seven shades, this cannot be achieved by permanent colouring and a lightening service will have to be advised. You should always consider the capabilities of the products you are choosing from, for example, a quasi-permanent colour is not designed to lighten the hair, but is intended to add tone to the existing hair colour. Determining the hair's existing colour is important to ensure you choose the correct colour to apply and the correct hydrogen peroxide strength.

If the hair has previously been coloured, this must also be taken into consideration, as it will both affect and determine the choice of colouring products that you may use. Test cuttings are very useful in these instances.

Hair condition / hair porosity

It is essential that you determine the condition of the client's hair, as it will affect your colour choice and development times, and possibly your method of application. You must also consider whether the hair's condition is actually good enough to accept the service, as in some cases the addition of more chemicals will cause the condition to deteriorate. In this instance, you may need to use a pre-colouring treatment, or ask the client to wait until the condition of their hair has improved. Pre-colouring treatments even out the porosity of the hair and help to rebuild the internal fibres.

As previously stated, hair in poor condition accepts colour more readily; however, if the hair is in good condition, there is a greater chance of resistance. If you feel the hair may be resistant to the colour application, then you should consider pre-softening the hair to open the cuticle scales, allowing the colour molecules into the cortex. The hair's condition will also influence the advice you give regarding care of the hair. For example, the use of a good-quality shampoo and conditioner for colour-treated hair will help the colour to retain its vibrancy and tone.

In the salon

A funky colour?

John was very busy in the salon and had fallen behind due to several late clients. Suzanne arrived at the salon to have bleached highlights. As John was very busy, he did not carry out a thorough consultation. Suzanne's hair was 'mousy' brown and he felt bleached highlights would be fine. He applied the foils quickly and left the colour to develop whilst he finished his previous client.

He went back to Suzanne to check on the colour development and discovered her blonde highlights were in fact pale pink. He then asked Suzanne if she had coloured her hair recently, to which she replied, 'No.' After lots of searching questions, Suzanne finally admitted that she had in fact coloured her hair black and did not like it so she bleached it blonde. After a few weeks, she decided she did not want to be blonde any more, so she coloured it brown. Fortunately, John was able to correct the colour for Suzanne, who eventually left the salon quite a few hours later.

- What went wrong?
- How could this situation have been avoided?

Length of hair

You need to consider the length of the client's hair before colouring as it may affect the price and the time allocated for the colour treatment. For example, long hair will require more product and more of your time, whereas shorter hair will be quicker to complete and use less product; this should be reflected in the price. Another factor is the technique you use to apply the colour. If a client has very long hair and requires bleached highlights, you will need to bear in mind that bleach develops at varying times. Consideration would have to be given as to where on the head you started and which technique you used. Alternatively, if a client had very short hair, trying to wrap colour in foil packets could prove difficult and you may consider a polishing technique. Polishing is applying colour by placing it on a piece of foil and lightly brushing it over the hair, which deposits colour anywhere you choose.

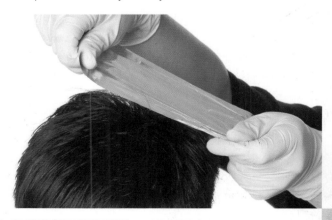

Polishing service taking place on short hair

Haircut

Colouring the hair should enhance and personalise a haircut. You should always balance the hairstyle with your colour choice. On completion, the colour should accentuate the features of the haircut and be working with the style. In addition, it should accentuate the client's best features, for example, the colour of their eyes.

Hair density

If a client has particularly thick, dense hair, then you will have to consider the cost of using more of the products and the time it may take. Again, the technique may be affected; if you need to apply the colour quickly, will you be able to on thick hair? Alternatively, if the hair is sparse and fine, then great care needs to be taken to prevent staining of the skin and scalp, which would be clearly visible through fine hair.

Be professional ★★★

When selecting colour, the hair density should be considered. Colour on thick, dense hair may appear darker than the same colour used on fine, sparse hair, as there is a greater concentration of colour present. When adding high or low lights, you should also consider the thickness of the weaves or slices, as very fine weaves in dense hair will disappear!

Percentage of white hair

The percentage of white hair will influence the type of colour and hydrogen peroxide choice. As the hair has no colour pigment, you are always darkening it; therefore, 20 volume, or 6 per cent hydrogen peroxide, should always be used when colouring the hair permanently. You will also need to be able to determine the percentage of white and decide the ratio of base shade to tonal shade. This is especially important when using strong fashion tones, as failure to add base with the fashion tone may lead to a more vibrant result, especially on the white hair. The table below shows the basic rules for mixing colour for use on white hair; however, always check with the product manufacturer's recommendations.

Percentage of white hair	Ratio of base shade to tonal
25–50%	25% base to 75% tonal
50–75%	50% base to 50% tonal
75–100%	75% base to 25% tonal

Be professional ★★★

- Remember that white hair can often be more resistant and the use of pre-softening can prove to be beneficial, especially on an area of concentrated white hair, such as around the front hairline.
- Some manufacturers have a permanent colour range specifically for resistant hair to ensure good coverage; this may affect your choice of product.

Skin tone

The colour you choose for the client should always enhance their skin tone, as this will give a more flattering effect. Skin tones fall into two categories: warm and cool. Warm skin tones tend to be peach coloured and suit warmer colours whereas cool skin tones are pink and look best with cooler colours.

Using the correct tone on a client's hair will enhance the colour of their eyes and give them a healthy glow. Some shade charts clearly indicate which colours are warm and cool.

Remember

It can sometimes be difficult to establish whether your client has warm or cool skin tones if they regularly use 'tanning products' or wear corrective make-up.

Lifestyle

You should consider your client's lifestyle when deciding on the type of colouring service to be carried out. Some professions require a more subtle look and this would have to be reflected in your choice of colour and technique. If your client is an active sports person, you need to consider the implications for the maintenance of the colour, for example, if the client is a regular swimmer, lightening products may not be suitable as the hair may discolour.

Tests and testing

The results from the tests that you carry out on the hair will play an important role in any colouring decisions you make. If the outcome of any test proves to be undesirable, this will have a restrictive effect on the services you can offer. For example, redness and itching of the skin following a skin test would prevent you from using permanent colouring products on a client. The results of any tests carried out, either prior to or during the colour service, should be noted on the client's record card. If you have any doubts regarding the suitability of the client's hair, carry out pre-service testing.

The tests required before colouring include:

- skin test
- test cutting or colour test
- incompatibility test
- porosity test
- elasticity test.

See pages 40–2 of Unit G21 for more information on these tests.

When carrying out a skin test, it is essential that you follow the manufacturer's instructions. If you fail to follow the instructions and your client has a reaction to the colour, you may find yourself liable in a court of law. Some clients may be upset if they react to a skin test, as this will indisputably mean they may not have their hair coloured. However, if your salon carries more than one product range, it may be possible to try a different manufacturer. In all other cases, you must advise your client against the chosen colouring service and suggest an alternative, for example, a semi-permanent colour (remember to check the manufacturer's instructions, as some semi-permanent colours require skin testing prior to application).

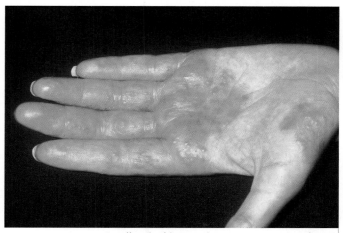

An allergic skin reaction to permanent colour

You should forewarn your client about the possibility of a positive reaction to a skin test and advise them accordingly. This may be to wash the area with warm soapy water and then apply a soothing lotion, such as calamine lotion. If this has no effect, they may need to seek medical advice. It is essential that you note on the client record card any positive reactions to tests, as the information must be communicated to any stylist who may intend to colour the client's hair in the future and also to comply with the requirements of the Data Protection Act 1998 (refer to page 62 of Unit G21 for more information).

Safe working practices

During colouring services in the salon there are several health and safety considerations that you must be aware of. Your own personal health and hygiene are important. If you are feeling unwell or rundown, then it will be difficult for you to keep up the pace in the salon and you run the risk of passing an infection on to others. You should keep yourself clean and fresh at all times to avoid causing offence to your clients or colleagues.

Your posture while working in the salon is another important consideration. You will soon become fatigued and stressed if you adopt an unhealthy posture whilst working. Bear this in mind and it will prevent any long-term stress or injury to your body. You should avoid standing in the same position for too long and move about as much as you can. If you are finding it difficult to access certain parts of the head during colour application, you must ask the client to assist you by moving their head. This will prevent you from working in an awkward position and help to maintain good posture.

The personal protective equipment that you need to use while colouring is essential to prevent the risk of harm or accidents to both yourself and the client. Permanent colourants are known to cause contact **dermatitis** and it is essential that you protect your hands when working. You can do this by wearing single-use gloves (vinyl or nitrile types) when working with colour and ensure they are not re-used. Make sure you dry your hands thoroughly and regularly apply hand cream to prevent the hands from drying out.

Dermatitis

an inflammatory condition of the skin (most commonly affecting the hands of hairdressers). It can result in dryness, itching, redness, flaking, swelling and blistering.

Check it out

As dermatitis is prevalent within the hairdressing industry, the HSE, HABIA and other organisations launched a campaign in November 2006 called 'Bad Hand Day'. The aim of this campaign is to raise the profile of dermatitis within the industry, thus reducing the number of hairdressers with work-related dermatitis.

Are you aware of the 'Bad Hand Day' campaign? If not, log on to www.habia.org for more information.

Colour hair using a variety of techniques **Unit GH17**

Personal protective equipment (PPE) will protect both the skin and clothes from staining. In addition, barrier cream should be available to protect the client's skin when applying colour, especially if the client has a history of sensitivity around the front hairline or if you are using a dark colour.

Check it out

Write a list of all the PPE that you use in the salon whilst colouring. Write down next to each one what its purpose is and what it serves to protect. Use the photo below as a prompt.

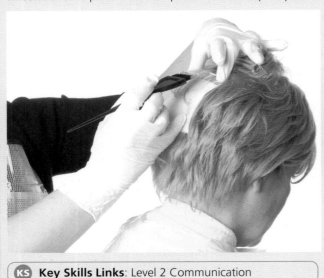

KS **Key Skills Links**: Level 2 Communication

Many clients are sensitive around the front hairline, but not on the scalp itself. This may be due to the fact that the hairline is cleaned along with the face several times a day, whereas the scalp should have a protective layer of dirt and grease to protect it from the colouring products. Care must be taken to avoid getting barrier cream onto the hair itself, as it will cause a barrier and the colour will not penetrate.

In addition to the above safe working practices, you have responsibilities under the COSHH Regulations and the Electricity at Work Regulations (see Unit G22, pages 6–7). In relation to the requirements of COSHH, there are specific safety considerations relating to the use of powder bleach. Powder bleach should be mixed in a well-ventilated area as inhalation of the powder may cause coughing, choking, and/or breathlessness. This could prove to be hazardous, especially in the case of someone suffering from asthma. Personal protective equipment should be worn at all times, as powder bleach is a known irritant and may cause skin sensitisation. A protective facemask may be worn when mixing the bleach to prevent inhalation of the powder. Most manufacturers now make 'dust free' powder bleaches to help alleviate the problem.

Check it out

Are you aware of your responsibilities under the current COSHH Regulations and Electricity at Work Regulations? If you are not sure, refer back Unit G22, pages 6–7.

Preparation of products, tools and equipment

The salon assistant will play a vital role in the preparation of products, tools and equipment used for colouring services. It is essential that you have trained him or her fully in how to prepare for all colouring services and this is best done, initially, by observing your working practices. As your assistant will have less technical knowledge than you, you must ensure any instructions given to your assistant are clear and accurate, as this will prevent any misunderstandings and potential problems.

Be professional:
- When giving instructions to your assistant, ask them to repeat back to you what you have instructed them to do to clarify their understanding.
- When preparing and using colouring products in the salon, it is essential that you follow the manufacturer's instructions, as this will ensure optimum results. Failure to follow the specified instructions could lead to an unwanted or undesirable outcome.

Mixing colours

When mixing colours, you must ensure you measure the correct quantities of colour and hydrogen peroxide; nothing should be left to chance. Most product manufacturers indicate quantities of colour down the side of the tint tubes; others provide applicators, which also act as a measure that may be used for both the colourant and the oxidant. When measuring liquids such as hydrogen peroxide, this should always be carried out with the measuring cylinder on a stable flat surface that is at eye level, as this will give an accurate reading. When using cream hydrogen peroxide, make sure all the hydrogen peroxide is poured into the mixing bowl. As the cream hydrogen peroxide is of a thicker consistency, it is very easy to leave 10 ml of hydrogen peroxide in the measure, meaning your working mixture has not been prepared to the manufacturer's specifications.

Remember

Some lightening products have different mixing ratios and therefore you have a choice of which to use. This may be down to personal preference or the type of work you are carrying out, for example, you may want to use a thicker consistency for panel work or a small re-growth (to ensure it doesn't run) and a looser consistency when covering a larger area.

Check it out

Check the manufacturer's instructions for the mixing ratios of lightening products used in your salon.

Be professional ★★★

When applying a full-head colour or bleached highlights on long hair, you will need to mix a second (or possibly third) batch of product to ensure the colourant you are using is fresh and working at full strength. Mix only the amount you need, as any leftover products will be washed down the drain along with your employer's money!

If you are not fully prepared when you begin the service, and have to keep leaving the client unattended to find what you need, this will present an unprofessional image and will waste your valuable time. You will need to be sure that the necessary products are available for you to use and that the tools and equipment used are clean and sterilised, as this will ensure you minimise the risk of cross-infection. (More detailed information regarding the sterilisation of tools and equipment may be found in Unit G22, pages 13–14.) All tools and equipment should be checked prior to use to ensure they are fit for purpose, which will minimise the risk of harm to yourself and others. They should be at hand to enable you to give a professional and efficient service and to avoid any unnecessary stretching or twisting of the body.

Check it out

Make a list of the products, materials, tools and equipment used in your salon for all the colouring services that you offer. State the purpose of each item on the list. This will ensure you are fully aware of everything available for use in your salon.

 Key Skills Links: Level 2 Communication

Colouring and lightening techniques

There are benefits for both the salon and the client when colouring and lightening hair. For the client, the benefits might be:

- to complement or accentuate a haircut
- to give individual or personalised results
- to create fashion effects
- to have an up-to-date service.

For the salon, the benefits might be:

- to create client loyalty
- profitability
- to enhance the salon's professional image
- to create variety in your working day
- to give job satisfaction
- to allow for inspiration in your work.

Check it out

Choose four different styles and decide how the hair should be coloured to accentuate the features of the haircut. Which colours would you use and why?

All of these benefits will help to motivate you in your colouring work and encourage you to be a successful colourist.

The effects of light and artificial lighting on the appearance of colour

In an ideal world, all colouring would take place in natural daylight, in the middle of the day, as this gives a truer indication of a colour result. However, as the day progresses towards dusk, the colour of the natural light alters to a warmer colour, altering the appearance of the hair colour.

In the salon, the lighting must be given special consideration to ensure the colours seen are as true as possible with no shadow. This is especially important when colour matching. Incandescent light, from an ordinary light bulb, can be quite yellow; and this would be undesirable within the salon, especially when colouring white or blonde hair. However, the higher the wattage, the whiter the light becomes. Fluorescent tubes are made in a variety of colours. Those marked as 'warm white' or 'warm white daylight' are most suitable for colouring work, as they give off a strong white light with some slightly warm tones.

The intensity of the lighting in the salon must be strong enough to judge colour without any glare. Many salons now use spotlights as a means of lighting the salon. Again, these are available in a variety of colours, including 'warm daylight'. However, spotlights can cast shadows and leave dark areas in the salon. This may be overcome by the use of specific types of reflectors.

The salon décor plays its own part in how you perceive colour. Afterimages and competing colours can influence and interfere with your colour vision. White is not considered ideal for walls, as it can be very bright and harsh. Softer colours such as beige, cream or pale peach are ideal for use in the colouring area.

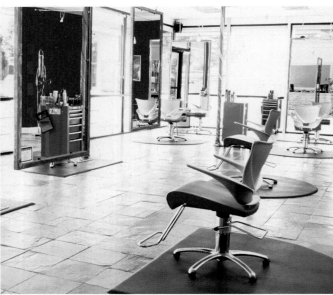

Correct lighting in a salon gives a truer indication of colour

Natural colour pigment

The hair's natural colour pigments are found in the cortex and are seen as such because the cuticles are colourless. The hair contains both melanin (black and brown pigment) and pheomelanin (red and yellow pigment) in varying degrees. Therefore, you could expect someone with dark hair to have more melanin than pheomelanin and someone with naturally fair hair to have predominantly pheomelanin.

However, when looking at the client's natural hair colour, remember that there may not be a uniform colour, but individual hairs that may be quite different, for example, a client with dark hair may have some individual hairs that are quite red. Hairs that have no melanin or pheomelanin are colourless but are seen by the naked eye as being white. This is usually due to age but may be attributed to illness or hereditary influences.

How natural pigmentation affects the colouring process

The hair's natural pigmentation must be considered to ensure the chosen colour is achievable. You must check the client's natural depth and tone. Darker hair may not lift as easily or as much as you would like and you will need to consider the products you are to use. If a client with naturally red/copper-coloured hair wants all vestige of warmth removed, you must consider your colour choice very carefully (reds are not always easy to tone down).

Principles of colour selection

Before applying any colouring products on a client's hair, there are a number of points that must be considered to ensure the best results for your client, such as:

- the hair's natural depth and tone
- the target shade (is it achievable given the hair's natural depth and tone?)
- the type of colouring service required (slices, woven highlights, etc.)
- the percentage of white hair
- strength of hydrogen peroxide needed
- the condition of the hair (elasticity)
- the porosity of the hair
- the hair texture
- the hair density
- previous chemical history
- the results of any tests carried out
- the length of the hair
- will the chosen colour complement the client's skin tones? (Warm skin tones suit warm colours, whereas pink skin tones suit cooler colours.)
- any contra-indications
- client image and lifestyle
- the haircut
- the temperature in the salon.

When you have answers to all of the above, you should have sufficient information to choose your colourant, oxidant and colouring technique.

The effects on the hair structure of different colouring and lightening products

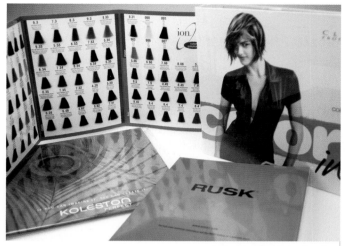

A range of colour charts

Semi-permanent colours

A true semi-permanent colour comes ready to use and is not mixed with any type of oxidant; always check the manufacturer's instructions first. Semi-permanent colourants work by depositing small colour molecules into the cuticle and outer part of the cortex. The colour will last between six to eight washes, unless the hair is porous, in which case it may last longer.

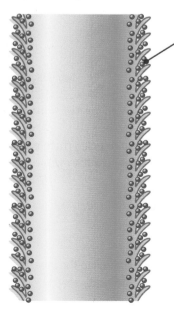

Small molecules are deposited into the cuticle and outer edge of the cortex

The effects of semi-permanent colour on the hair structure

Semi-permanent colours are not designed to lighten the natural hair colour, but to add tone and depth. Because they have a conditioning base, they add shine to the hair. They are not meant to cover large amounts of white hair, but many will cover up to 30 per cent. Remember, if the hair is unevenly porous, the result may be patchy and the colour molecules will remain in the hair for more than six to eight washes.

Quasi-permanent colours

Quasi-permanent colours are mixed with a low-volume oxidant, usually on a 1:2 ratio. They work in a similar way to permanent colour (see below), in as much as the colour molecules are oxidised. However, as the oxidant is very mild, the colour molecules do not become as large (as permanent colour molecules) and will wash out of the hair over a period of time. The colour is designed to fade gradually over 16–22 shampoos, without giving a pronounced re-growth.

Permanent colour

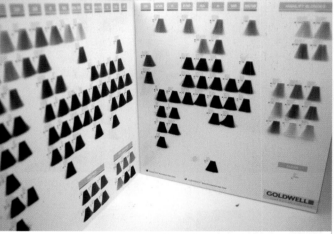

A permanent and quasi-permanent colour board

Permanent colours have a wide range of uses in the salon and are available in a variety of colours, from subtle, natural colours, through to striking and bold colours that add individuality and flair to your work.

Permanent colours can lighten or darken the hair and they can also be used to add tone. They may be used to achieve a number of different effects and are designed to cover white hair. Permanent colours may be mixed with 10, 20, 30 or 40 volume hydrogen peroxide, depending on the desired results. Remember to read the manufacturer's instructions to check which hydrogen peroxide strength will give the optimum results, given the base shade you are working on.

Permanent colours may also be referred to as para dyes

or oxidation tints. They work by depositing small (usually colourless) molecules into the hair cortex along with the hydrogen peroxide. The hydrogen peroxide (which is an oxidising agent) begins to break down, releasing nascent oxygen, which joins together with the small molecules to form larger, coloured molecules. As the molecules become larger, they are unable to pass back through the cuticle as they become trapped between the polypeptide chains within the cortex.

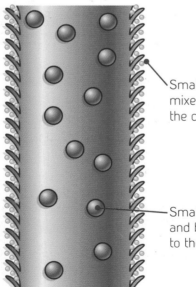

Using colour swatches during consultation

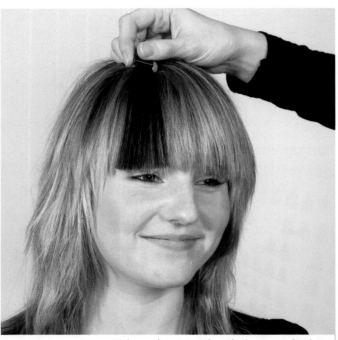

Small colourless molecules mixed with oxidant penetrate the cuticle, into the cortex

Small molecules swell and become larger due to the nascent oxygen

The effect of permanent colour on the hair structure

> **Remember**
>
> If the hair is too porous and the cuticles are damaged or have been destroyed, even the larger molecules may be washed out of the hair, resulting in colour fade.

Bleach / lighteners

Bleaching may occur through exposure to the sun and salt water, or artificially by using bleaching / lightening products in the salon. Bleach is usually used when other colouring products, for example, high-lift tints, cannot achieve the required amount of lift. It is also used when lightening hair that has already been coloured with tint and for pre-lightening.

Bleaching is the process of changing the natural colour pigments, melanin and pheomelanin, by a process of oxidation into colourless oxymelanin and oxypheomelanin.

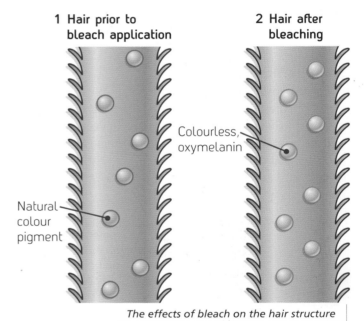

1 Hair prior to bleach application

2 Hair after bleaching

Colourless, oxymelanin

Natural colour pigment

The effects of bleach on the hair structure

Melanin (black and brown pigments) are oxidised more easily than pheomelanin (red and yellow), therefore the oxidisation process takes place in three stages:

1. The black and brown pigments are oxidised.
2. The red pigment is oxidised.
3. The yellow pigment is oxidised.

By watching the colour changes that occur during the bleaching process, the sequence of oxidation may be easily seen.

Hydrogen peroxide

Hydrogen peroxide is the **oxidising** agent used in permanent, quasi-permanent and lightening services. It comes in different strengths and each strength has a specific purpose.

Strength	Purpose
10 vol (3%)	Used for refreshing faded ends, giving maximum depth of colour (tinting darker than the natural colour)
20 vol (6%)	Used for permanent colouring when adding depth or tone, will give up to one shade of lift on a base 6 or lighter
30 vol (9%)	Used for permanent colouring, will give up to three shades of lift on a base 6 or lighter
40 vol (12%)	Used for permanent colouring when using high-lift tints, will give up to five shades of lift on a base 6

The above table is a guide to choosing the correct volume strength; however, you should always check the manufacturer's instructions.

Oxidation

the addition of oxygen to enable hair colouring preparations to work.

Hydrogen peroxide is made up from two parts of hydrogen and two parts of oxygen and is recognised as H_2O_2. It is classed as an unstable substance as it decomposes easily to form water and oxygen ($H_2O + O$). Stabilisers are added during its manufacture to avoid the loss of oxygen during storage. However, during colouring, lightening services and neutralising, the decomposition of the hydrogen peroxide is necessary as the newly formed oxygen (nascent oxygen) does all the work.

When mixing colouring products with hydrogen peroxide, you must follow the manufacturer's instructions regarding the mixing ratios. Some colourants are mixed on a 1:1 ratio, for example, 30 ml of oxidant to 30 ml of colourant, whereas others, such as high-lift tints and quasi-permanent colours, may be mixed on a 2:1 ratio, for example, 60 ml of oxidant to 30 ml of colourant.

There are occasions when the salon may not have the correct strength of oxidant in stock. Diluting the hydrogen peroxide with water may readily solve this problem. For example, if you only have 40 vol (or 12%) but need 30 vol (9%):

$$\frac{30}{40} = \frac{3}{4}$$

You would need to use three parts of 40 vol H_2O_2 to one part water to achieve 30 vol.

To dilute 40 vol (12%) to 20 vol (6%):

$$\frac{20}{40} = \frac{2}{4} = \frac{1}{2}$$ You would need to use one part H_2O_2 to one part water.

Lightening the hair

As part of this unit you need to be able to apply both a full head and re-growth service using **lighteners**. As the product will be in direct contact, it's essential that you chose a preparation that is designed to be used on the scalp.

Lighteners

Products that lighten the natural pigments of the hair changing melanin to oxy-melanin and pheomelanin to oxy-pheomelanin, without depositing artificial colour. Also known as bleach.

Salon life

A blistering performance!

Unit GH17 colour hair using a variety of techniques

Image by TONI&GUY

Gary's story

A new client came into the salon for a re-growth application. During my consultation I gauged that her natural base was a 3 so I wouldn't be able to achieve the lightness required unless I used a lightening product.

Earlier in the day we had run out of our usual lightening product and my colleague had gone to the wholesalers to buy more. She brought back a different brand, but they all do the same job.

I carefully applied the product to the root area and let the colour develop for the full time, but I kept checking all the way through to make sure the client was OK and her hair condition wasn't deteriorating. As the lightening product started to dry out, I knew it wasn't working as efficiently so decided to remove it, but the colour wasn't light enough, so I did a second application and used heat to make sure I achieved the right result this time.

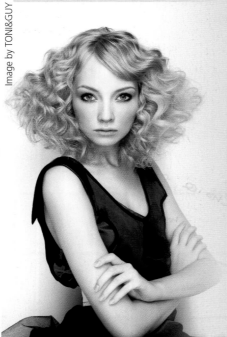

After a short time the client told me her scalp was burning, so I said the lightener needed to come off straight away. She refused as the colour wouldn't be light enough. We ended up having a huge argument – she said she'd sign a disclaimer, I said absolutely not; the product had to come off now. Eventually the client allowed me to remove the product. Her scalp was red and hot, so I used cool water and very gentle massage to remove the product.

Afterwards the client wasn't happy as the colour wasn't light enough and demanded I put on a toner. I had to say no, her scalp was just too angry for any more products. She left the salon very unhappy and vowed never to return.

Be professional ★★★

- When applying a re-growth lightening application, make sure you don't overlap onto previously lightened hair as this will cause it to become over-sensitised. You must make sure you place the product right up to the demarcation line, as failure to do this will result in small dark 'spots' on the hair.
- When applying lightening products, begin where the hair is darkest, as this hair should take longer to lighten.
- Make sure you carry out regular strand and elasticity tests during development to ensure the hair condition isn't deteriorating.
- After a lightening service, it's important to use an anti-oxidant conditioner before toning as this will prevent any deterioration of the cortex and stop the oxidising process. If the bleaching process is not 'stopped' the toner may not be satisfactory and the condition of the hair may be compromised. Although you can use permanent colours for toning, it's preferable to use semi-permanent or mildly oxidising products as they also have staining action, which may benefit porous, lightened hair.
- Although you can't test for bleach, a skin test should be always be carried out before the service as it is rare to leave bleached hair in its raw state – without some form of toner. Most insurance companies would be more inclined to support any litigation if a skin test is recorded.

ASK THE PROFESSIONALS

Q *What could I have done to prevent this from occurring?*

A Firstly, make sure your stock control system is effective, so you don't run out of products. Then, read the manufacturer's instructions before using any products you haven't used before and if they're lightening products, make sure they can be used on the scalp (as some are not designed for this). You should also check whether added heat is recommended.

Q *Should I have left the lightening product on and let her sign a disclaimer?*

A No!! I very much doubt this would stand up in a court of law, as you had been negligent in the first place!

Block colour and slicing techniques: a step-by-step guide

1 Before the service.

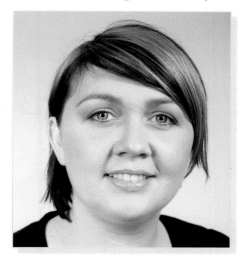

2 Section hair into triangular sections and secure.

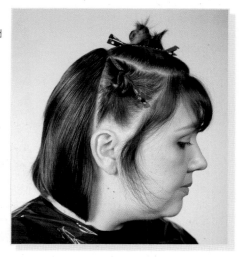

3 Leave the front hairline out of the sectioning pattern.

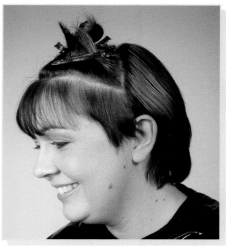

4 Apply colour to the back section and isolate using wraps.

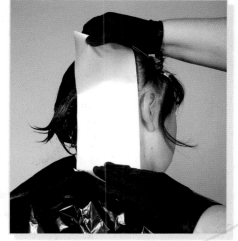

5 Apply back to back slices (permanent colour).

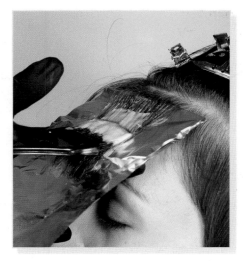

6 Apply back to back slices (lightening product).

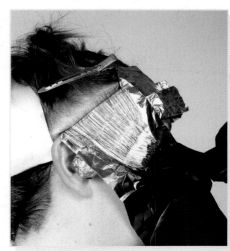

7 Complete the slices and mask off with wraps and foil.

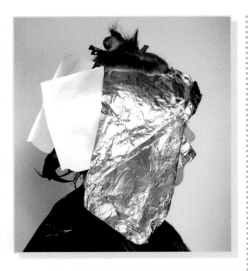

8 Development time can be reduced with the use of a climazone.

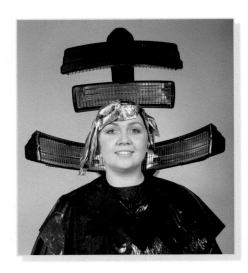

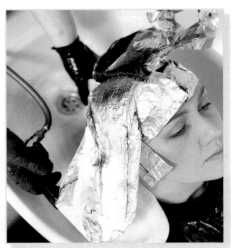

9 Remove dark areas first to prevent colour bleed.

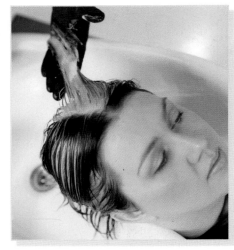

10 Apply toner at the backwash basin.

11 The finished look.

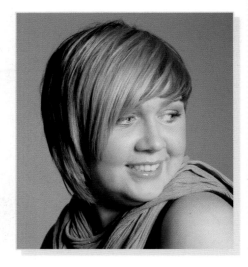

12 The finished look.

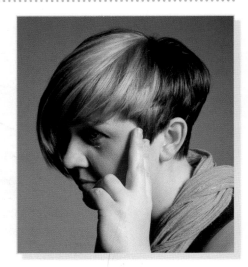

Weaving and slicing: a step-by-step guide

1 Before the service — the hair was pre-lightened.

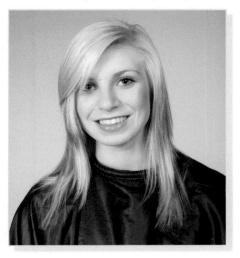

2 Section from above the left eye to the nape on the right-hand side of the head in a horseshoe pattern.

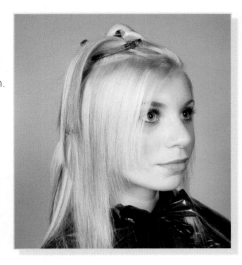

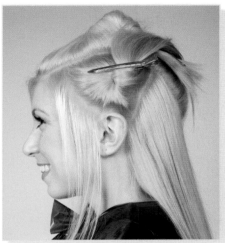

3 Section hair on the opposite side into a triangular section leaving the hairline out.

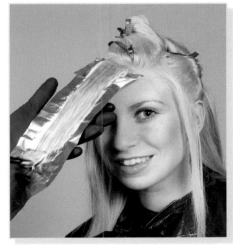

4 Place back to back slices in the foil following the curved section.

5 Complete the curved section.

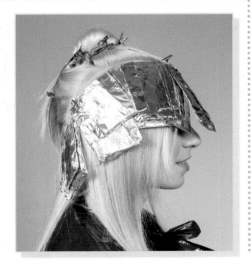

6 Begin to work through the triangular section using a woven and slicing technique in a diagonal pattern.

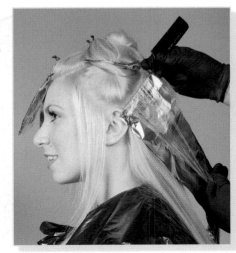

Colour hair using a variety of techniques **Unit GH17**

7 Apply the product.

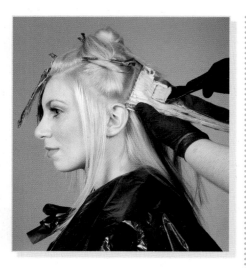

8 Complete the triangular section.

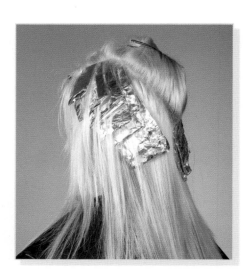

9 The effect of the pink, purple and blue weaves.

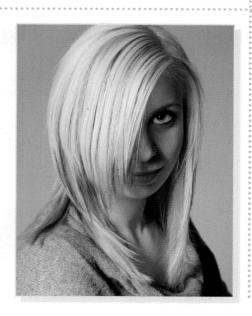

10 The finished look.

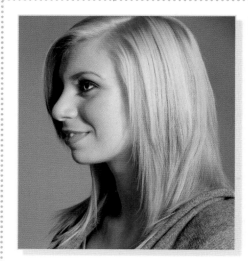

11 The finished look.

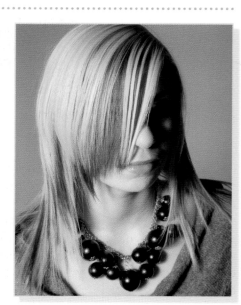

12 The finished look.

The table below shows some of the materials / tools used for colouring.

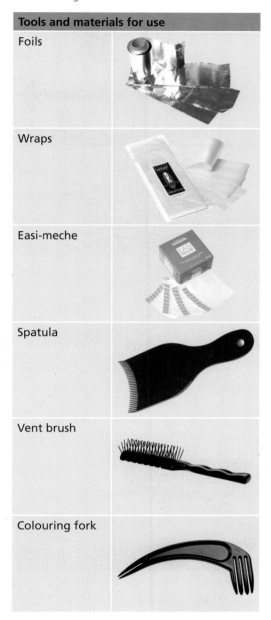

Tools and materials for use	
Foils	
Wraps	
Easi-meche	
Spatula	
Vent brush	
Colouring fork	

Monitoring development and removing colour

Careful monitoring of the colour development must be carried out, especially when using bleaching / lightening products, as they do not always have a set development time and may easily over-process if not checked frequently enough. If a client has very long hair and requires bleached highlights, you will need to bear in mind that bleach develops at varying times. Consideration would have to be given as to where on the head you started and which technique you used.

You must also consider that the bleach may be fully developed at your starting point before you have completed the whole application and would need to be removed with extreme care so as not to disturb the areas that are still developing. When using bleach and permanent colours, care must be taken so the permanent colour does not 'bleed' into the bleached hair. This may be achieved by removing the permanent colour first, taking care not to disturb the bleached areas.

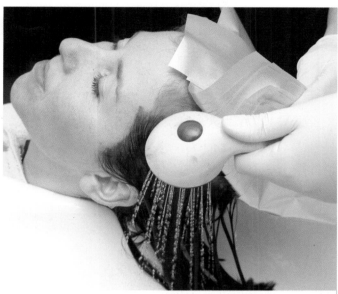

Take extra care when removing lightening products and permanent colours

When the colour has fully developed, it must be entirely removed from the hair and scalp. Failure to do so will cause scalp irritation. Always remove colour following the manufacturer's instructions.

In the salon

A colour run

Philippe, the stylist, had completed a full head of foil highlights using alternate slices of bleach and a vibrant red permanent colour. When the colours had developed, he asked Jenny the junior to remove the colour and shampoo the client's hair. Jenny was used to removing foils, but she had only ever removed permanent colour. Philippe was now busy with his next client and left Jenny to it. She removed all the foils and then began to rinse the colour from the hair. During the shampooing process she noticed the hair looked quite pink in places and called Philippe over to look at the client's hair. The red colour had bled into the bleach, leaving pink slices where the bleach should have been.

- What went wrong?
- How could this have been avoided?

pH values of colouring products

The pH value indicates the level of acidity or alkalinity within a product. The pH value of colouring products is an important factor to consider, as acidic products are kinder to the hair since they help to close the cuticles, whereas alkaline products will open the cuticles.

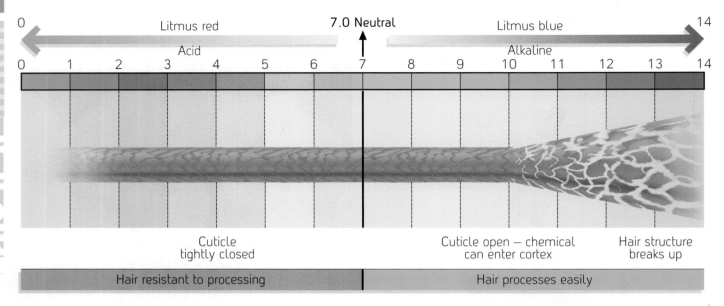

pH values and their effects on the cuticles

The more alkaline the product, the more damage it will cause to the hair; therefore, you should consider the products you are using and the potential damage they may cause.

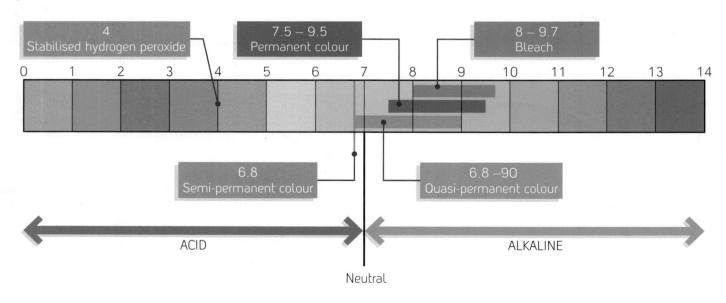

pH scale showing the approximate values of colouring products

As most colouring products are alkaline (they open the cuticles), it is essential that an anti-oxidant conditioner be used after the colour has been shampooed off the hair. An anti-oxidant conditioner will:

- return the hair back to its normal pH of 4.5–5.5 (slightly acid)
- add moisture to the hair
- stop any further oxidation taking place (continuing oxidation will cause unnecessary damage to the hair)
- close the cuticles.

Remember

Remember to keep the salon clean and tidy throughout the service, as this will maintain your professional image and help to prevent cross-infection. All remaining colouring products and used materials must be disposed of correctly.

Solving colouring problems

There may be times when colouring or bleaching problems occur in the salon and it is essential that you know why the problems have occurred and how they may be rectified. If you do not have a good understanding of why the problems have occurred, it may prove very difficult to remedy the situation to produce a satisfactory result.

There are several problems that you may encounter while colouring that are easily solved, such as restoring depth and tone or neutralising colour tone. However, if you feel the level of colour correction is above your ability, then you may need to refer the client to another stylist in the salon for specialist correction work. When dealing with a colour problem, you need to accurately identify the hair's condition and what has previously been used on the hair. You will need to use questioning and / or observation in addition to testing the hair to establish the exact nature of the problem and determine the best course of action.

Check it out

List the tests you might carry out on a client's hair prior to colour correction work. State the purpose of the test and what the expected outcomes might be (see Unit G21, pages 40–1).

Once you have determined the problem and assessed your client's needs, you can present to him or her the options available to resolve the predicament. Ensure you present all the options and thoroughly discuss the outcomes and consequences of each to enable yourself and your client to agree a course of action.

Remember

Accurate sectioning of the hair will ensure you work methodically and achieve an even coverage.

Restoring depth and tone

Depth and tone may be lost for several reasons, for example, a client may have been on holiday and exposed his or her hair to the sun. Another reason might be that the client has very porous hair that cannot hold on to colour. If the cuticles are badly damaged or non-existent, the hair may not be able to 'hold' the colour molecules in the cortex, resulting in colour fade. This may also occur if permanent colour is not left on the hair for the full development time, as the molecules do not have sufficient time to join together to form the larger molecules and may be 'washed away'.

If the client has lost depth and tone out of their hair colour, you have several options available to help with this problem. If the hair is sensitised, in order to prevent any further chemical damage, the use of temporary or semi-permanent colours may be necessary. These will stain the cuticle layer and will not affect the elasticity of the hair. Remember that if the hair is extremely porous, they may last longer than a few shampoos.

The most commonly used solution is to refresh the tired hair with the usual colour. Several product manufacturers now produce their own colour refreshers; however, other companies still use the method of diluting their permanent hair colours. There may be instances where the loss of depth and tone is so great that pre-pigmentation is necessary prior to the usual colouring service.

Be professional ★★★

Always follow the product manufacturer's instructions. If you are unsure, telephone the technical helpline.

Neutralising colour tone

From time to time you may come across a client who has developed unwanted tones in his or her hair. This can be due to a number of influencing factors, for example, smoking can leave a yellow tinge in the hair and swimming in water containing chlorine can place a green cast on the hair. In your initial colour training, you will have learnt about the colour star and the fact that opposite colours neutralise each other; however, you must remember to consider the intensity of the colours.

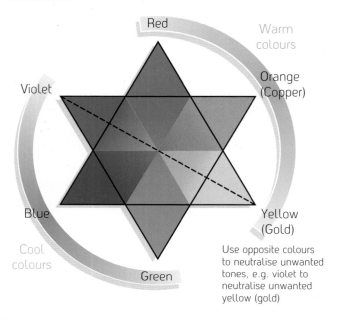

Use opposite colours to neutralise unwanted tones, e.g. violet to neutralise unwanted yellow (gold)

You will need to be aware of this when using a colour to neutralise unwanted tone. There are shampoos available to neutralise colour tone, the most common being a purple shampoo that neutralises yellow. If you do not already retail these, consider stocking them for sale, as it would provide a good selling opportunity. Due to the high levels of pollution in our towns and cities, most clients with blonde colours in their hair will benefit from infrequent use of 'brightening' shampoos.

Be professional ★★★

Take care not to use a darker or more vibrant colour tone than is necessary or the outcome could be undesirable. Assess the depth of the client's hair colour and use a slightly lighter depth, but make sure that the intensity of the tone is the same, for example, if you wanted to remove nicotine staining on white hair, you would use a silver colour rather than a colour with intense violet tones.

Colouring resistant hair

The resistance of a client's hair is due to the cuticle scales being flat and smooth; this is usually found in hair in good condition. Some hair, such as Oriental hair, falls into this category, as it has more layers of cuticle scales than either European or African type hair and does not allow the colour to penetrate into the cortex and develop. You can overcome this by pre-softening the hair, which lifts the cuticle scales, allowing colour molecules to enter the cortex.

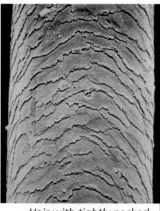
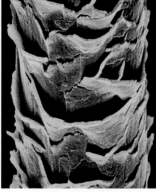

| *Hair with tightly packed cuticles* | *Hair with raised cuticles* |

Pre-softening the hair is a relatively quick and simple process. It involves applying neat 10 vol or 3% hydrogen peroxide to the resistant areas, drying the H_2O_2 into the hair, and then proceeding with the colouring service. You may find it easier to use cream hydrogen peroxide as it has a thicker consistency and is therefore easier to work with.

You will need to carefully assess the hair's porosity to determine its resistant tendencies. Consider also that naturally white hair is often more resistant and this can be overcome not only by pre-softening, but also by the use of permanent colour with extra depth added. Most product manufacturers now produce colours with intense depth for improved coverage on resistant white hair.

Using bleach to pre-lighten the hair

If you cannot achieve the required amount of lift using permanent colour or a high-lift tint, it may be necessary to pre-lighten the base using bleach. However, many hairdressers make the mistake of bleaching the hair to almost white before applying the target colour. This will cause unnecessary damage to the hair. The hair should be lightened only to the corresponding depth and used as an undercoat. The target shade should then be applied on top of the undercoat.

A client with a natural depth of 4 (medium brown), who wants highlights of 7/43, would need to be pre-lightened only to an orange/yellow base as this corresponds to the depth of 7. However if pre-lightening hair that is to be coloured blue, it is essential to bleach the hair to almost white first. If there is any yellow left in the hair, it will give a green result when it is mixed with the blue colour!

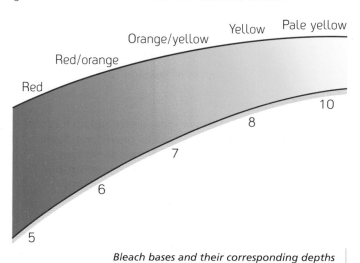

Bleach bases and their corresponding depths

Pre-pigmentation

Pre-pigmentation is the term used to describe restoring lost pigment to pale hair that needs to be made darker and/or warmer. An example of this is a client with bleached hair who wishes to go back to their natural colour. As bleaching / lightening hair removes the warm tones (red and yellow) from the hair, these tones must be replaced prior to applying the target shade or the finished result will have a green cast.

Pre-pigmenting may be done using temporary, semi-permanent, quasi-permanent or permanent colour; however, the porosity of the hair must be taken into consideration when choosing the correct product. The pre-colour may be either red,

copper or gold, depending on the depth of the target shade, for example, a light colour would usually require a gold pre-colour, whereas darker hair would require a red pre-colour. Look at the illustration below left of bleach bases and corresponding depths for an indication of the correct colour to use. Always remember to follow the manufacturer's instructions.

> **Be professional ★★★**
>
> When taking clients back to their natural colour, always use one shade lighter than the target shade, as you can add colour to the hair at any time, but it is more difficult to remove colour from previously treated hair.

> **Check it out**
>
> Which pre-service tests should be carried out prior to taking a client back to their natural colour?

Pre-pigmentation may be carried out in a number of ways and this should be checked using the manufacturer's instructions. Below is a simple and effective method of pre-pigmenting the hair.

1 Prepare yourself and the client.
2 Make all the necessary preparations as per any colour application.
3 Prepare the hair (by shampooing) if required.
4 Apply the correct pre-colour evenly to the hair, avoiding the re-growth area.
5 Allow the colour to develop fully.
6 Wipe off any excess colour using cotton wool.
7 Mix permanent colour (one shade lighter than target shade) following the manufacturer's instructions and apply directly over the pre-coloured hair and develop as normal.
8 Remove the colour and apply an anti-oxidant conditioner.

This method is tried and tested; however, with experience this process may be carried out in one stage, where the warm (pre-pigmenting) colour is added to the target shade. This may be as a 'mix tone' or a warm colour that corresponds to the type of warmth needed.

> **Be professional ★★★**
>
> This method yields better results if the undercoat is warm. If not, the results may not be stable and possibly uneven.

Colouring problems do occur from time to time and it is essential that you have a good understanding of the common faults that may arise.

Below is a table of common colouring problems and remedies.

Problem	Cause	Remedy
Over-processing	Usually caused by incorrect timing during the development of the colour/lightening product, e.g. the colour has been left on too long	Remove colour immediately; use a restructuring conditioner to help rebuild some of the internal fibres; cut off as much of the over-processed hair as possible; give the client effective and accurate after-care advice
Under-processing	Usually caused by incorrect timing, e.g. the colouring product has not been left on long enough	Check the condition of the hair and reapply if the condition allows
Skin staining	This may be due to several reasons: poor application; seepage of products; excessively dry skin that has not been protected (especially when using dark or red colours)	Use a skin stain remover
Deterioration of hair condition	This may be due to several reasons: the product used was too strong; the colour has been over-developed; the condition of the hair prior to colour application was poor	Remove colour immediately; use a restructuring conditioner to help rebuild some of the internal fibres; give the client effective and accurate after-care advice
Uneven results	This may be due to several reasons: the application was uneven; the sections taken were too large; when mixing two or more colours together, the colours weren't mixed sufficiently, giving an uneven result	Spot colour the darker or uncoloured areas
Product seepage	This may be caused by: using too much product which then seeps out of the foil / packet; incorrect mixing, e.g. the product is too runny	Spot colour the areas of seepage
Scalp sensitivity	This may be caused by: an allergy to the products used; high strength of hydrogen peroxide used on the scalp or the over-use of chemicals on the scalp, e.g. permanent colour used directly after a lightening service	Rinse immediately with cool water and no further chemical processing should be carried out. Some product manufacturers have scalp sensitivity products that may be used for this purpose, but ensure there is no evidence of broken skin

You should also be aware of other potential problems, such as those which may occur when using colouring products and lighteners on previously chemically treated hair, for example, deterioration of the hair condition, possibility of incompatible products on the hair, breakage, uneven result, etc.

After the service

When any colour service is complete, it is imperative to give the client the correct advice. This will serve to ensure long-lasting results and client satisfaction. It is also a good selling opportunity; following any colour treatment, the correct hair-care advice will give your client the optimum, long-lasting result.

Once the colour treatment is complete, you must discuss with your client how to care for the hair and the colour. During the initial and ongoing consultation, you will have determined your client's lifestyle and given advice about how often to shampoo and condition. You should make sure the client understands the importance of looking after their hair in order to maintain the colour. It's also worth discussing the use of heated styling equipment and instilling the importance of using a heat protection spray to prevent the hair from becoming dehydrated and to protect the cuticles.

Discuss the features and benefits of the shampoo and conditioning products that have been specifically designed for use after colour treatments. Ensure the client understands not only how these products help to maintain their hair in good condition, but how and when to use them.

Many clients believe all colour shampoos and conditioners will achieve the same results, therefore you need to educate them by explaining how the products work and also highlighting the products to avoid, such as any silicone-based shampoo or conditioner as this may prove to be problematic with subsequent colouring services.

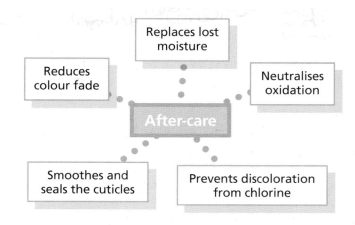

Reduces colour fade

Replaces lost moisture

Neutralises oxidation

After-care

Smoothes and seals the cuticles

Prevents discoloration from chlorine

Remember

Remember to advise your client against using shampooing products with tones, unless you feel it's the correct product for them to use. If so, make sure you give the client clear and accurate advise on its usage.

Check it out

What products does your salon retail that will help the client to maintain the colour intensity between visits?

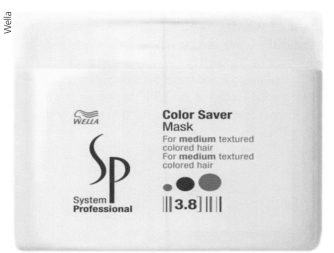

Wella

Color Saver Mask

For **medium** textured colored hair
For **medium** textured colored hair

||3.8|| ||

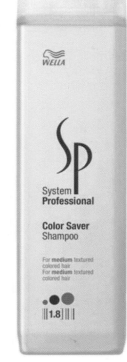

WELLA

SP System Professional

Color Saver Shampoo

For **medium** textured colored hair
For **medium** textured colored hair

||1.8|| ||

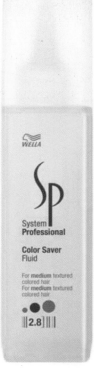

WELLA

SP System Professional

Color Saver Fluid

For **medium** textured colored hair
For **medium** textured colored hair

||2.8|| ||

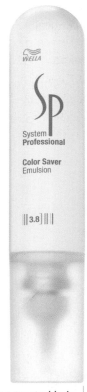

WELLA

SP System Professional

Color Saver Emulsion

||3.8|| ||

You should recommend that your client uses products for colour-treated hair

Intervals between colour appointments

The client's hair growth and the type of colour treatment will determine the length of time between the colour appointments. Most clients hate to see their re-growth visible and are usually counting the days until their next colour appointment. However, this is not always the case and if a client has a large re-growth when they return to the salon, then there are implications for this. For instance, the hair ends will have changed colour over time and an accurate colour match may be more difficult. Implications such as these should be explained when giving advice on the client's return visit.

Temporary colours usually last only one shampoo and the client will need this treatment each time their hair is blow-dried or set. Semi-permanent colours will last between six and eight shampoos; therefore, consideration will need to be given to how often a client shampoos their hair in determining the next colour appointment. A quasi-permanent colour can last on the hair between sixteen and twenty-two shampoos, giving the client the option of a colour treatment every few months. These colours are designed to fade and they should not leave a visible re-growth. If your client is having a quasi-permanent colour every four weeks, you should ask yourself whether your product choice is correct. Permanent colours and bleach both grow out of the hair and the next colour treatment will be determined by the client's hair growth. However, most clients will require a re-touch every four to six weeks.

Encourage your clients to make their next appointment before leaving the salon, as this will help to reinforce the professionalism of the salon and ensure a return visit.

Completion of the record card

Completion of a record card can prove to be useful if there are any repercussions following a colour treatment. It is your responsibility to ensure the card is completed both accurately and legibly. Not only is it vital to be able to read and understand the information on it for the next appointment, but it could also be needed as proof of your professionalism. The information contained on the client record card must be clear to other stylists who may colour the client's hair in the future and should include:

- the client's name, address, and contact number
- their hair's natural depth and tone
- the percentage of white hair and whether the white hair is scattered across the head or confined to one area
- the date of the client's skin test
- the results of any pre-service tests that have been carried out
- the colour(s) used
- the volume or percentage strength used with each colour
- how or where the colours were used (e.g. alternate slices of colour)
- the length of time the colour(s) was developed
- the final result
- any retail sales made.

> **Check it out**
>
> List your responsibilities under the Data Protection Act.
>
> **Key Skills Links**: Level 2 Communication

You should also consider your responsibilities under the Data Protection Act. Remember that you have to store and use this information in line with the requirements of the Act.

Disposal of waste

At the end of the colour service, any waste products and materials must be disposed of carefully and in a safe manner. You have legal and moral responsibilities under the Environmental Protection Act 1990 to dispose of waste in a safe manner that will not cause harm to others or the environment

Check your knowledge

The following questions will help you to check your understanding of this unit. The answers can be found on page 418. Take care, as there may be more than one correct answer for some questions.

1 Which of the following are true?
   a A warm room will speed up the development of lightening products
   b A cold room will speed up the development of lightening products
   c The temperature of the room is irrelevant to the speed of colour processing
   d The use of added heat will speed up the development of lightening products

2 Alkaline hairdressing preparations will:
   a close the cuticle
   b penetrate into the medulla
   c have no effect
   d open the cuticle

3 Under-processing of a colour is likely to be due to:
   a poor application
   b the colour not being left on long enough
   c the colour being left on too long
   d excessively dry skin

4 Why is it important to remove all colouring / lightening products from the hair and scalp when the development is complete?
   a To avoid damage to the hair and scalp
   b To prevent anaphylactic shock
   c To stop any further development taking place
   d To prevent atmospheric moisture from entering the hair shaft

5 Why would you need to pre-soften the hair?
   a To avoid any further damage
   b To fix the melanin into the cortex
   c To keep the hair in optimum condition
   d To raise the cuticles of resistant hair

6 Why would you need to pre-pigment hair?
   a To restore lost pigment to pale hair that needs to be made darker or warmer
   b To prevent further oxidation from taking pace
   c To keep warm tones on porous hair
   d To open the cuticles of resistant hair

7 What makes hair resistant to colour?
   a Tightly packed cuticles
   b Over-use of chemicals
   c Product build-up
   d Over-use of heated styling equipment

8 The international colour chart may be used to:
   a identify the depth and tone of colouring products
   b open the cuticles to aid colour penetration
   c identify the hair's natural depth and tone
   d help choose the colour

9 It's important to return the hair to its normal pH of 4.5–5.5 after the full development of a colouring
   or lightening service:
   a to help prevent colour fade
   b to close the cuticles
   c to add moisture to the hair
   d to restore the natural pH balance of the hair

10 When colouring hair, you should take accurate sections:
   a to ensure good coverage
   b because the client might notice
   c to enable you to work methodically
   d to ensure the correct colour is used

Assessment guidance

You must demonstrate in your everyday work that you have met the standards for colouring hair using a variety of techniques on either men or women.

You will be assessed on at least six different occasions and you will have to prove that you can competently carry out:

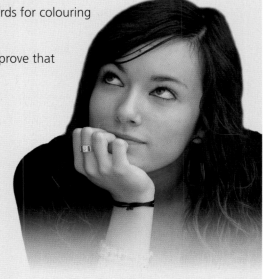

- a full-head application using a lightening product
- a re-growth application using a lightening product
- a basic colour correction
- three creative colouring looks, using two or more colours on each head.

One of the above colouring services must include the use of a toner.

Simulated activity is not allowed for any part of this unit.

Provide colour correction services

What you will learn:

- How to prepare the client
- How to prepare for the colour correction service
- How to correct a colour problem
- How to proceed after the service.

Royston Blythe

Introduction

Colour correction is carried out in order to:

- lighten the hair
- darken the hair
- change the tone of the hair.

Hair colour problems can occur no matter how experienced you are as a stylist. The majority of colour problems are the result of human error, which stresses the importance of following the correct procedures. Colour problems can be varied and there are no hard and fast solutions to correcting these problems, as the desired outcome and influencing factors will differ from client to client. This unit is about the advanced skills you will need to develop in order to determine and correct complex colouring problems.

You the stylist

This unit aims to give you possible solutions to colouring problems but you must make your own decisions regarding the most suitable course of action to take in a range of different circumstances. You must always ensure that your clients are aware of the length of time required to perform this kind of service and the cost.

Preparing the client

Thorough consultation to determine the problem

One of the most important factors to consider is a thorough and effective consultation in order to determine the problem. This will ensure that you have all the necessary facts to enable you to select the most appropriate products and techniques to perform the service to a satisfactory standard. You will need to draw on your communication skills to ensure you elicit the correct information from your client. If you fail to gain all the necessary information, you may not achieve a satisfactory result. You must establish:

- the nature of the colouring problem
- the extent of the problem
- the condition of the client's hair and scalp
- the extent of artificial and natural colour on the hair
- the results the client would like to see (using visual aids may help at this point)
- the most suitable products and techniques to achieve the desired result
- if the client's desired result is achievable — if not, you will need to discuss and negotiate with your client until you reach a satisfactory outcome.

This information may be obtained by asking the client a series of probing questions to find out the exact nature and the extent of the problem. You must also establish whether your client has any known contra-indications. Some contra-indications are easily identified by observation; however, others may not be so apparent. Therefore it is essential that you question your client beforehand and any responses must be logged on the client's record card. This is not only good practice but may also be required at a later date should the client decide to start legal proceedings against the salon. You should at this point establish the client's requirements regarding the expected outcome.

You should make reference to the client's existing record card, as this should hold the client's complete colouring history (providing the client is an existing client). This information may affect the colour correction service you are able to offer and the products you may use, for example, the client's natural base shade and products previously used on the hair.

> **Be professional ★★★**
>
> The information contained on a record card should be accurate and up to date to comply with the Data Protection Act 1998. This includes the responses from your clients when questioned about contra-indications, etc. See Unit G11 (page 98) for more information on the Data Protection Act 1998.

The extent of the problem may be identified by observation. In addition you should question your client to gain their perspective on the problem, using both factual and feeling questions. As an experienced hairdresser, you should be able to recognise a number of different colouring problems.

In this unit, the problems you must effectively correct are:

- removing artificial colour on a full head
- removing bands of colour
- re-colouring bleached / lightened hair using pre-pigmentation and permanent colour over at least 60% of the head
- re-colouring hair that has had artificial colour removed by reduction on a full head
- correcting highlights and lowlights.

Plan and agree a course of action to correct colour

Once you have all the necessary information, you must decide on the most suitable course of action to take. This should include the products and techniques you intend to use to achieve the optimum result for your client. There may be more than one possible course of action, in which case these should be presented to your client using non-technical language that they can readily understand. Explain to your client the reasons behind your recommendations, in other words, the results of your analysis. Be honest with them and explain the likelihood of achieving the colour result they want. There may be times when you know it is highly unlikely that you will be able to achieve the required colour and it is better that the client is aware of this from the onset than for it to be a shock at the end of the service. This also gives both of you the opportunity to explore other possibilities with a more acceptable outcome. You must also discuss maintaining the colour result; this should include plenty of home-care advice on product usage and general maintenance.

You must explain to your client the implications that the colour correction service may have on future hairdressing services, for example, following colour removal by reduction and subsequent re-colouring of the hair, a permanent wave would be unadvisable as the hair may not be able to withstand further chemical treatments.

Contra-indications and influencing factors

Contra-indications

A contra-indication is something that would prevent you from continuing with the service. Therefore you must question your client and record the responses.

Contra-indications should always be carefully considered. Below is table of contra-indications and the reasons how and why they can affect the delivery of colour correction services.

Be professional ★★★

> When the client is in possession of all the facts regarding the colour correction service (e.g. the products you intend to use, the cost and duration of the service and the expected outcome), and you have their consent to continue, this should be recorded on their record card. In the event of an unexpected problem occurring, you have documented evidence to prove you have followed the correct procedures.

Contra-indications	How and why they can affect the delivery of colour correction services
Skin sensitivities	Every client must have a skin test prior to a colouring service to test for an allergic reaction to the colourant. Any reaction to the colourant would result in the colouring service not being able to take place or possibly an alternative product needing to be used. You should ask your clients if they have ever had any sensitivity to hairdressing products and record their answers on the client record card
Previous history of allergic reaction to permanent colouring services	Once a client has developed sensitivity to permanent colouring products, this is unlikely to ever change. If placed in this situation, you will need to use non-permanent colouring products, but you must carry out a skin test using the products you intend to use
Known allergies	Some allergies may prevent services taking place. You should ask your clients: • if they have any known allergies • if they have ever been referred to see a dermatologist for patch testing and if so, the number of known allergies they may have. A client with a history of allergies or sensitivity is more likely to react to hairdressing products
Skin disorders	Any skin disorder must be identified prior to application. An infectious skin disease would obviously mean that you could not carry out the colour correction service. With others, such as psoriasis, the service may continue as long as the skin is not broken. If in doubt, ask for confirmation from the client's GP

Provide colour correction services **Unit GH18**

Contra-indications	How and why they can affect the delivery of colour correction services
Incompatible products	Any products used prior to the colour correction service that contain metallic salts will have an adverse reaction when mixed with hydrogen peroxide. Therefore, any products that contain or are mixed with hydrogen peroxide must not be used
Medical advice / instructions	Certain drugs / medication may affect the final outcome of the colour correction service. Therefore you should ask your client for confirmation from their GP that their medication will not affect the outcome before you colour the hair
Evident hair damage	Carry out elasticity, porosity and colour tests prior to the service

Influencing factors

An influencing factor may not necessarily prevent you from performing a colour correction service but must be considered in all the decisions you make both prior to and during the service. Some of the influencing factors are also contra-indications.

Temperature

The temperature of the salon will influence the processing time. A cold salon may slow down the processing time and warm temperatures will speed up the process. The use of heat to develop colours quickly is a good technique; however, the porosity and condition of the hair needs to be considered, especially during colour correction services, as careful monitoring of colour development may be necessary to prevent additional problems such as over-processing.

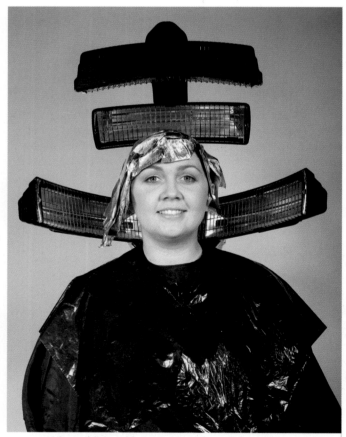

Using additional heat can speed up the colouring process

Existing colour of hair

The existing colour of the client's hair, both the natural colour and any artificial colour present, must be taken into consideration when carrying out a colour correction service. The outcome of the consultation will determine the most suitable products to use to enable you to achieve the required result. For example:

Hair's natural base	6
Colour on mid-lengths and ends	4.45 (medium warm brown)
Target shade	7.1

Permanent colour would not be an option here, as a tint will not lighten another tint. The options open to you in this instance would be to remove the artificial colour by either reduction or oxidation.

You must be aware of the potential problems that may arise when colouring hair that has previously been coloured, for example, deterioration of the hair condition or, on occasion, unexpected results due to the presence of incompatible products. However, if all pre-service testing has been carried out, these problems can be kept to a minimum. Test cuttings are very useful in these instances.

Hair condition / hair porosity

It is essential that you determine the condition of the client's hair before the colour correction service, as it will affect your colour choice and development time, and possibly your method of application. You must also consider whether the hair's condition is actually good enough to accept the service, as in some cases the addition of more chemicals will cause the condition to deteriorate. In this instance you may need to use a pre-colouring treatment. These treatments even out the porosity of the hair and help to rebuild the internal fibres. Hair in poor condition accepts colour more readily but if the hair is overly porous, there is a good chance the hair won't hold the colour and it will fade very quickly. This is because when the cuticles are open or non-existent, there is nothing to trap the colour into the cortex.

If the hair is in good condition, it may be resistant to colour; this would necessitate pre-softening the hair to open the cuticle scales allowing the colour molecules into the cortex.

This is an ideal opportunity to give your client advice on how to maintain their colour and condition, as it essential after a colour correction service.

Test results

The results of any pre-service testing must be considered, as this will enable you to take the most appropriate course of action. You will need to think about the choice of products you can use or even the possibility that the colour correction service cannot be carried out due to poor hair condition, or the presence of incompatible products. All test results must be recorded on the client's record card.

Length of hair

The length of the hair will dictate the time you need to allocate for the service and the price you should charge for the service. The mid-lengths and ends of longer hair will be more porous, therefore this may affect your method and sequence of application and determine the most appropriate products to use.

Hair density

The hair density will also determine the amount of product you need to use. A client with an abundance of hair will require more product than a client with sparse hair. The size of your sections must also be considered. When colouring the hair of a client with a great density of hair, the size of the sections should be finer to ensure a thorough application. It may also affect your application techniques.

Percentage of white hair

The percentage of white hair must be taken into consideration, especially the re-growth area, as although you may not need to colour correct the roots, they may be resistant to the subsequent colour being used. In this instance you may need to pre-soften the re-growth area or use a colorant specifically designed for use on resistant hair.

Sequence of application

When applying colouring products, you may need to consider the sequence of application. Body temperature plays an important role when carrying out a full-head colour. The colour on the roots of the hair will process more quickly than the colour on the ends because its development is speeded up by the addition of body heat. Therefore, when carrying out a full-head lightening or full-head red application, you should apply the colour to the mid-lengths and ends first, and the roots last. This will prevent the colour being too light at the roots (in the instance of a lightening application) and will prevent root glare when using 'reds'.

However, when carrying out a colour correction service, such as removing colour by reduction, you may need to start your application at the darkest point.

Scalp sensitivity

Scalp sensitivity may affect your choice of product or application technique. A client with sensitivity to permanent colouring products will obviously limit your choices.

> **Remember**
>
> Don't forget to ask your client about any scalp sensitivity during your consultation.

Strength of hydrogen peroxide

The purpose of the different strengths of hydrogen peroxide is discussed later on in this unit; however, you must also remember that you could be using different strengths of hydrogen peroxide on different areas of the head when correcting colour, for example, 12% through the mid-lengths and ends (to lift artificial colour) and 6 or 9% on the roots.

Ideally you shouldn't be using more than 6% on the scalp when using bleach. When removing depth, use the lowest oxidant possible, as if the artificial colour is removed too quickly it tends to leave a 'brassy' result.

> **Remember**
>
> - The more slowly the hair is lifted, the cleaner the colour will be and the condition of the hair won't be compromised.
> - When planning a colour correction service, you must consider your client's lifestyle, as this may affect the finished result. For example, if your client is a regular swimmer and has heavily coloured hair, especially if lightening products have been used, the hair may discolour and fade quickly.

Pre-service tests and examinations

It is essential that you establish the condition of the client's hair, skin and scalp prior to performing a colour correction service. You should carry out a thorough examination of the hair, skin and scalp, checking for cuts and abrasions and any other known contra-indications to ensure suitability.

You are also required to carry out pre-service tests. The results from the tests that you carry out on the hair will be an important factor in any decision you make. If the outcome of any test proves to be undesirable, this may limit the services you can offer. For example, if when testing the elasticity of the client's hair, it stretches, but does not return to its original length, this indicates damage in the cortex. Extreme caution should be observed, as use of the incorrect product may cause the hair condition to deteriorate still further. The results of any tests carried out should be noted on the client's record card. Refer to Unit G21 (pages 40–2) for more information on pre-service tests.

Maintain effective and safe methods of working when correcting hair colour

Personal protective equipment

When carrying out any colour correction, it is essential that personal protective equipment is worn by both you and your client. You must ensure your client's clothing is protected throughout the whole of the service to prevent any colouring products from staining their clothes. Barrier cream may also be applied around the hairline to prevent skin staining, especially when using dark colours or if the client has very dry skin. You should be wearing gloves to protect your hands from the colouring products; and to prevent skin irritation (**dermatitis**). You should also wear an apron to protect your own clothes from staining.

> **Dermatitis**
>
> an inflammatory condition of the skin (most commonly affecting the hands of hairdressers). It can result in dryness, itching, redness, flaking, swelling and blistering. See page 16 in Unit G22 for more information on dermatitis and how to avoid developing it.

> **Check it out**
>
> Are you aware of the 'Bad Hand Day' campaign? If not, log on to www.habia.org for more information.

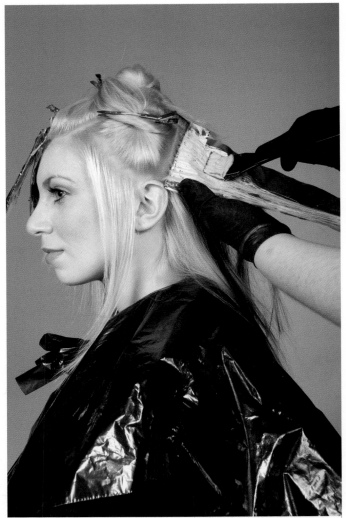

You must wear the correct personal protective equipment, and ensure the client also has protective equipment on

> **Check it out**
>
> What are your salon's requirements for client preparation?

Working safely in the salon

When working with any colouring products, you must ensure compliance with COSHH regulations. Your responsibilities in relation to this piece of legislation are to:

- maintain your protective equipment and report its loss or demise to your employer
- comply with your salon's policies for safe handling, usage, storage and disposal of hazardous substances
- report any hazards you cannot deal with yourself to the designated person within your salon
- follow the manufacturer's instructions relating to the colouring, lightening and bleaching products you are using.

There are specific safety considerations relating to the use of powder bleach under the COSHH regulations. Powder bleach should be mixed in a well-ventilated area as inhalation of the powder may cause coughing, choking and / or breathlessness. This could prove to be hazardous, especially in the case of someone suffering from asthma. Personal protective equipment should be worn at all times as powder bleach is a known irritant and may cause skin sensitisation. A protective facemask may be worn when mixing the bleach to prevent inhalation of the powder. Some manufacturers now make 'dust free' powder bleaches to help alleviate the problem.

All tools and equipment that you use during the service must be checked prior to use to make sure they are safe and fit for purpose. This includes items of electrical equipment used to aid the colouring process, for example, clymazone, rollerball, etc. Using tools and equipment for their intended purpose will reduce the risk of damage to such equipment and minimise the risk of harm or injury to yourself and others.

Here is a checklist for preparing your work area.

What to do	Why / how?
All the necessary tools and equipment for the service should be prepared beforehand	Saves time and conveys a professional image to the client
Any products needed for the service should be available and ready to use	Regular and effective stocktaking will ensure that all products are available
Work areas must be clean and tidy	Prevents accidents occurring, reduces risk of cross-infection and promotes a professional image
Instruct junior staff to prepare the work areas correctly	Saves time. Make sure that you clearly communicate what is required – a short list of instructions may be given to junior staff
Tools and equipment should be clean, sterilised and fit for the purpose	The appropriate method of sterilisation should be used (for further information see Unit G22, pages 13–14) and the equipment should be checked for defects
Electrical equipment should be used in compliance with health and safety legislation	Ensure all staff are complying with the safe use of electrical equipment (see Unit G22, page 6). This is your responsibility

Use this checklist for personal health and hygiene.

What to do	Why / how?
Make sure your body and clothes smell clean and fresh	The client will feel more comfortable in your presence. Daily washing and the use of a good deodorant are essential
Make sure your breath is fresh	Use a breath freshener. This will help to combat odours from strong smelling foods or smoking
Do not work if you are feeling unwell	Infections can be spread in the salon. Keep yourself fit and healthy to ensure that you produce the best work possible
Maintain a good posture while working. Think about whether your client is positioned correctly for your needs as well as their own comfort	This will minimise the risk of injury or fatigue. Make sure you keep your back straight and balance your weight evenly. Having your tools and equipment close to hand will prevent you from over-stretching

Maintaining stock levels

Stocktaking should be carried out on a regular basis. This may be weekly, fortnightly or monthly, depending on the amount of stock you carry / use and the amount of storage space available in the salon. When carrying out colour correction services, you may not necessarily know precisely which products and / or materials you will be using. Therefore it is essential that you maintain adequate stock levels at all times.

Remember

- Use all colouring products economically; prepare only the amount you actually need, as this will ensure you are working cost-effectively and minimising the wastage of the products.
- If necessary, adjust the position of your client to enable you to gain access to all areas of the head. This will not only make your job easier, but also prevent you from working in awkward positions that have the potential to cause you injury.

Preparing for the colour correction service

Your client's hair should be prepared for the colour correction service. You must consider the products you will be using, for example, are they applied to dry hair or hair that has been shampooed and towel dried? All products must be prepared (mixed and measured) and used following the manufacturers' instructions to ensure the best results. You should be able to estimate the amount of product you will need to enable you to carry out the service. It is important that you use products economically (but use a sufficient amount to achieve the desired results) as this will have a positive effect on the salon's finances. The hair should then be sectioned off in a way that is suitable for the colour correction service. Your sectioning should be clean to enable you to work efficiently and precisely throughout the colour correction service.

Colouring products

You must be aware of the full range of colouring products available for use in the salon and their effects on the hair structure. Your choice of product will depend on:

- the intended result
- the condition of the hair, both elasticity and porosity
- the existing hair colour
- the products previously used on the hair.

> **Check it out**
>
> List the products, tools and equipment that may be used when colouring hair and state the reasons why you would use them. Refer to Unit GH17, page 157 if you need a reminder.
>
> **Key Skills Links**: Level 2 Communication

Principles of colour correction

Before applying any colouring products on a client's hair, there are a number of points that you must consider to ensure the best results for your client.

- The hair's natural depth and tone.
- The target shade (is it achievable given the hair's natural depth and tone?).
- The type of colouring service required (slices, woven highlights, etc.).
- The percentage of white hair.

- Strength of hydrogen peroxide needed.
- The condition of the hair (elasticity).
- The porosity of the hair.
- The hair texture.
- The hair density.
- Previous chemical history.
- The results of any tests carried out.
- The length of the hair.
- Will the chosen colour complement the client's skin tones? (Warm skin tones suit warm colours, whereas pink skin tones suit cooler colours.)
- Are there any contra-indications?
- Client image and lifestyle.
- The haircut.
- The temperature in the salon.

When you have answers to all of the above, you should have sufficient information to choose your colourant, oxidant and colouring technique.

Reduction and oxidation

Oxidation is the term given to a chemical process that involves the addition of oxygen. In hairdressing, oxygen is used during permanent colouring processes, bleaching and when neutralising a perm. It is also used in some quasi-permanent colours. The oxygen used in these processes comes from hydrogen peroxide.

Hydrogen peroxide is made up from two parts of hydrogen and two parts of oxygen and is recognised as H_2O_2. It is classed as an unstable substance as it decomposes easily to form water and oxygen ($H_2O + O$). The additional part of oxygen (nascent oxygen) is necessary when colouring the hair. The stronger the volume or percentage of hydrogen peroxide, the greater amount of nascent oxygen can be found.

Reduction is the opposite of oxidation. A process of reduction sees the addition of hydrogen and the removal of oxygen. Artificial colour may be removed from the hair by using a colour reducer that works by a process of reduction. As permanent colour works by a process of oxidation, it may be removed by using the opposite kind of chemical reaction.

Melanin

The hair's natural colour pigments are found in the cortex and are seen as such because the cuticles are colourless. The hair contains both melanin (black and brown pigment) and pheomelanin (red and yellow pigment) in varying degrees. Therefore, you could expect someone with dark hair to have more melanin than pheomelanin and someone with naturally fair hair to have predominantly pheomelanin.

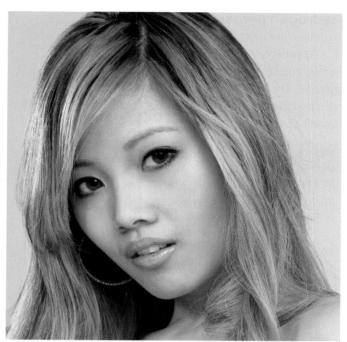

Sometimes it is not easy to tell what your client's natural colour is

However, when looking at the client's natural hair colour, remember that there may not be a uniform colour, but individual hairs that may be quite different, for example, a client with dark hair may have some individual hairs that are quite red. Hairs that have no melanin or pheomelanin are colourless but are seen by the naked eye as being white. This is usually due to age but may be attributed to illness or hereditary influences.

Light and lighting

In an ideal world, all colouring would take place in natural daylight, in the middle of the day, as this gives a truer indication of a colour result. However, as the day progresses towards dusk, the colour of the natural light alters to a warmer colour, altering the appearance of the hair colour.

In the salon, the lighting must be given special consideration to ensure the colours seen are as true as possible with no shadow. This is especially important when colour matching. Incandescent light, from an ordinary light bulb, can be quite yellow and this would be undesirable within the salon, especially when colouring white or blonde hair. However, the higher the wattage, the whiter the light becomes. Fluorescent tubes are made in a variety of colours. Those marked as 'warm white' or 'warm white daylight' are most suitable for colouring work, as they give off a strong white light with some slightly warm tones.

The intensity of the lighting in the salon must be strong enough to judge colour without any glare. Many salons now use spotlights as a means of lighting the salon. Again, these are available in a variety of colours, including 'warm daylight'. However, spotlights can cast shadows and leave dark areas in the salon. This may be overcome by the use of specific types of reflectors.

How natural pigmentation affects the colouring process

The hair's natural pigmentation must be considered to ensure the chosen colour is achievable. You must check its natural depth and tone. Darker hair may not lift as easily or as much as you would like and you would need to consider the products you are to use. If a client with naturally red / copper coloured hair wants all vestige of warmth removed, you must consider your colour choice very carefully (as reds are not always easy to tone down).

Effects on the hair structure of different colouring products

Semi-permanent colours

A true semi-permanent colour comes ready to use and is not mixed with any type of oxidant; always check the manufacturer's instructions first. Semi-permanent colourants work by depositing small colour molecules into the cuticle and outer part of the cortex. The colour will last between six and eight washes, unless the hair is porous, in which case it may last longer.

Semi-permanent colours are not designed to lighten the natural hair colour, but to add tone and depth. Because they have a conditioning base, they add shine to the hair. They are not meant to cover large amounts of white hair, but many will cover up to 30 per cent. Remember, if the hair is unevenly porous, the result may be patchy and the colour molecules will remain in the hair for more than six to eight washes.

Quasi-permanent colours

Quasi-permanent colours are mixed with a low-volume oxidant, usually on a 1:2 ratio. They work in a similar way to permanent colour (see overleaf), in as much as the colour molecules are oxidised. However, as the oxidant is very mild, the colour molecules do not become as large (as permanent colour molecules) and will wash out of the hair over a period of time. The colour is designed to fade gradually over 16–22 shampoos, not giving a pronounced re-growth.

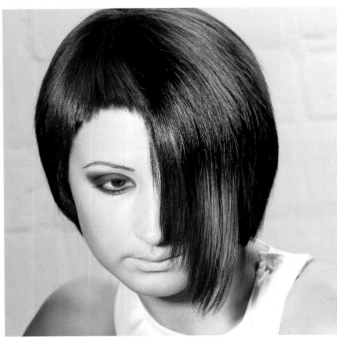

Bold colours can add flair to your work

Permanent colour

Permanent colours have a wide range of uses in the salon and are available in a variety of colours, from subtle, natural colours, through to striking and bold colours that add individuality and flair to your work.

Permanent colours can lighten or darken the hair and they can also be used to add tone. They may be used to achieve a number of different effects and are designed to cover white hair. Permanent colours may be mixed with 10, 20, 30 or 40 volume hydrogen peroxide, depending on the desired results. Remember to read the manufacturer's instructions to check which hydrogen peroxide strength will give the optimum results, given the base shade you are working on.

Permanent colours may also be referred to as para dyes or oxidation tints. They work by depositing small (usually colourless) molecules into the hair cortex along with the hydrogen peroxide. The hydrogen peroxide (which is an oxidising agent) begins to break down, releasing nascent oxygen, which joins together with the small molecules, to form larger, coloured molecules. As the molecules become larger, they are unable to pass back through the cuticle as they become trapped between the polypeptide chains within the cortex.

Remember

If the hair is too porous and the cuticles are damaged or have been destroyed, even the larger molecules may be washed out of the hair, resulting in colour fade.

Hydrogen peroxide

Hydrogen peroxide is the oxidising agent used in permanent, quasi-permanent, lightening and bleaching services. It comes in different strengths and each strength has a specific purpose. The table below is a guide to choosing the correct volume strength; however, you should always check with the manufacturer's instructions.

Hydrogen peroxide strength	Purpose
10 vol (3%)	Used for refreshing faded ends; giving maximum depth of colour (tinting darker than the natural colour)
20 vol (6%)	Used for permanent colouring when adding depth and / or tone; will give up to one shade of lift on a natural base 6 or above
30 vol (9%)	Used for permanent colouring; will give up to three shades of lift on a natural base 6 or lighter
40 vol (12%)	Used for permanent colouring when using high-lift tints; will give up to five shades of lift on a natural base 6

Be professional ★★★

When measuring hydrogen peroxide, if you accidentally pour out too much, you must pour it down the sink. Putting it back into its original container may cause the hydrogen peroxide to start to deteriorate.

As previously mentioned, hydrogen peroxide is made up from two parts of hydrogen and two parts of oxygen and is recognised as H_2O_2. It is classed as an unstable substance as it decomposes easily to form water and oxygen ($H_2O + O$). Stabilisers are added during its manufacture to avoid the loss of oxygen during storage.

However, during colouring, bleaching and neutralising, the decomposition of the hydrogen peroxide is necessary as the newly formed oxygen (nascent oxygen) does all the work.

When mixing colouring products with hydrogen peroxide, you must follow the manufacturer's instructions regarding the mixing ratios. Some colourants are mixed on a 1:1 ratio, for example, 30 ml of oxidant to 30 ml of colourant, whereas others, such as high-lift tints and quasi-permanent colours, may be mixed on a 2:1 ratio, for example, 60 ml of oxidant to 30 ml of colourant.

There are occasions when the salon may not have the correct strength of oxidant in stock. Diluting the hydrogen peroxide with water may readily solve this problem. For example, if you only have 40 vol (or 12%) but need 30 vol (9%):

$$\frac{30}{40} = \frac{3}{4}$$

You would need to use three parts 12% / 40 vol H_2O_2 to one part water to achieve 30 vol.

To dilute 40 vol (12%) to 20 vol (6%):

$$\frac{20}{40} = \frac{2}{4} = \frac{1}{2}$$ You would need to use one part 12% / 40 vol H_2O_2 to one part water.

pH

The pH value indicates the levels of acidity or alkalinity within a product. The pH value of colouring products is an important factor to consider; acidic products are kinder to the hair as they help to close the cuticles, whereas alkali products will open the cuticles. The more alkaline the product, the more damage it will cause to the hair, therefore you should consider the products you are using and the potential damage they may cause.

As most colouring products are alkali (they open the cuticles), it is essential that an anti-oxidant conditioner be used after the colour has been shampooed off the hair. An anti-oxidant conditioner will:

- return the hair back to its normal pH of 4.5–5.5 (slightly acid)
- add moisture to the hair
- stop any further oxidation taking place (continuing oxidation will cause unnecessary damage to the hair)
- close the cuticles.

Remember

Remember to keep the salon clean and tidy throughout the service, as this will maintain your professional image and help to prevent cross-infection. All remaining colouring products and used materials must be disposed of correctly.

Correcting the colour problem

Removing the colour

There will be times during colouring services when some of the hair has achieved the desired result and therefore the colour needs to be removed to prevent over-processing. This is particularly true when carrying out a full head of bleached foil / packet highlights. Great care must be taken when removing the foils that have reached the desired degree of lift, to ensure that the hair that is still processing is not disturbed. If care isn't taken, the colour may bleed (causing an unnecessary colour correction service to take place).

It is important when removing colouring and lightening products from the hair that the hair and scalp are thoroughly clean and devoid of any residual products. Failure to ensure the hair and scalp are clean can lead to scalp irritation and chemical damage.

If you have a junior member of staff working with you, it is essential that this and other relevant information be given clearly and accurately to them, as this will ensure a good final result. Failure to give clear and accurate information to less experienced members of staff will ultimately lead to mistakes and client dissatisfaction.

Using different products to remove artificial colour

Removing artificial colour
Artificial colour is usually removed from the hair because the colour is too dark. It is much easier to add depth to hair that is too light, but removing artificial colour requires knowledge and skill. As tint will not generally lighten hair that already has tint on it, the tint must be removed first. Artificial colour may be removed from the hair either by reduction or bleaching.

Removing colour by reduction
This involves removing artificial colour (tint) from the hair. As you already know, permanent colour works by depositing small colourless molecules into the cortex along with the hydrogen peroxide. The hydrogen peroxide (which is an oxidising agent) begins to break down, releasing nascent oxygen, which joins together with the small molecules to form larger, coloured molecules. As the molecules become larger, they are unable to pass back through the cuticle as they become trapped between the polypeptide chains within the cortex.

Unit GH18 Provide colour correction services

The process of removing the permanent colour requires the colour reducer to penetrate the cortex and break down the large molecules into smaller molecules that can then be passed through the cuticles and rinsed away.

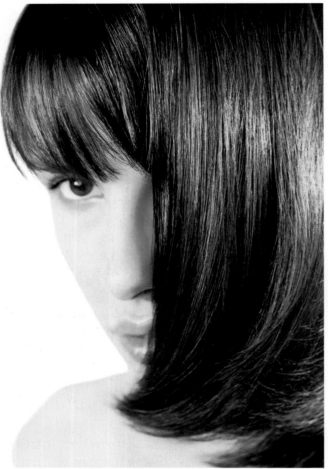

Use reduction or bleaching to remove colour that is too dark

This service is usually carried out if the hair has a build-up of colouring products or it is too dark. The client's hair may be too dark due to applying an incorrect colour or because the client has decided to change the colour of the hair to a lighter shade. Before carrying out a colour reduction service, all tests should be performed and results assessed, especially porosity and elasticity tests, to ensure the hair is strong enough to endure the harsh treatment that will follow. This should be continued throughout the service, so that you are aware of any sudden deterioration in the hair's condition.

Be professional ★★★

Test cuttings (or a colour test) carried out prior to the application will give a good indication of the outcome of the service.

As a general rule, colour reducers may be mixed with either water or hydrogen peroxide, depending on the amount of lift required. You must assess the condition of the hair, as the more damaged the hair, the weaker the mixture would normally be.

To 'clean out' a build-up of colour, the colour reducer would usually be mixed with either water or 3 per cent hydrogen peroxide. However, if you need to remove the colour to lighten the hair, 6 per cent or 9 per cent hydrogen peroxide may be used. When using colour reducers, the manufacturer's instructions must always be followed.

The application of the colour reducer should always be started where the colour is darkest and / or the hair most resistant. This is to allow more time for the colour reducer to work in these areas. Your application should be carried out as quickly as possible, but taking care to apply the colour reducer methodically to ensure all intended areas are covered. Care must be taken to avoid the re-growth area.

Be professional ★★★

Use strips of cotton wool between the sections to ensure the re-growth area doesn't come into contact with the colour reducer.

It is highly unlikely that you will achieve an even base to work on. As the hair's porosity will have been uneven before application, the colour will be removed more quickly from the areas that are most porous, thus giving an uneven result.

While the colour reducer is developing, you should remain with your client and monitor the development as the colour may lighten unexpectedly. When development is complete, remove the colour reducer by rinsing the hair with cool water and shampoo the hair thoroughly. The hair should now be dried and the results assessed to ensure a satisfactory result. The colour is likely to be very warm and this may be quite alarming to your client. Therefore you may need to reassure your client that this is not the end of the service and not to worry. At this point the colour result may not be satisfactory and remedial action will be necessary before applying the target colour.

1 If the result is patchy, it may be necessary to re-apply the colour reducer to the darker areas to even out the colour.
2 If the result is excessively warm you may either:
   ● use a mild bleach mixture to remove the warm tones in the hair
   ● choose a matt / ash tone to neutralise the warmth.

Re-colouring the hair

Removing colour by oxidation

All pre-service tests must be carried out prior to the application to ensure the hair is suitable for the service. Test cuttings taken before the service will give a clear indication of the final colour result and the condition of the hair afterwards.

Removing colour by oxidation is carried out in much the same way as removing colour by reduction, in that the darkest or most resistant areas are treated first. The main difference is the products that are used work by oxidation. These products are bleach preparations and they will not only lighten the artificial colour, but also the natural hair colour as well. For this reason, the re-growth area should be avoided. An even base may not be achieved on the first application and it may be necessary to re-bleach any darker areas with a second application to ensure an even base.

If your client requests a warm target shade, you may bleach the hair to its corresponding depth, and then apply the target colour.

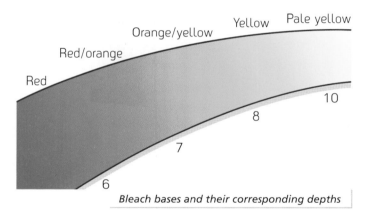

Bleach bases and their corresponding depths

However, if the client chooses an ashen or matt tone, the hair should be bleached lighter to remove excess warmth from the hair. In both instances, you may wish to add a little base to the target colour to ensure the colour adequately covers the hair and does not result in a translucent effect.

This method of removing artificial colour from the hair is most commonly used to 'break up' a full-head colour; for example, highlights. Throughout the service you must check the elasticity of the hair at regular intervals to ensure the hair condition is not deteriorating. After the service, the client's hair will be extremely porous and the internal fibres may have experienced some distress; therefore it is essential you give the client extensive after-care advice on how to maintain the colour and condition.

Removing bands of colour

Bands of colour usually appear as a direct result of incorrect application or choice of colour when selecting or matching the existing hair colour. The banding may be either darker or lighter than the rest of the hair and needs to be corrected. When carrying out any colour correction service, pre-service testing and research into the client's chemical history should be carried out. This includes even the most experienced hairdressers. If the bands of colour were lighter than the rest of the hair, spot colouring the hair using a tint to match would correct this; however, you must consider whether it is necessary to add warm tones into the hair (this may be necessary if the banded hair is lacking warmth, possibly as a result of a bleach application).

If the colour is too dark, it will need to be lightened sufficiently to match the existing hair. This may be carried out in several ways, depending on the degree of lift required. Many manufacturers recommend using their lightest tint, usually a 10/0 mixed with either 6, 9 or 12 per cent hydrogen peroxide and applied to the darker bands. Development must be closely monitored and when the colour reaches the desired shade, blot off any excess product and apply your target shade.

Darker banding may also be removed from the hair by mixing powder bleach with water and a little shampoo to give a good consistency to work with. This is then applied to the darker bands and must be monitored carefully until the desired amount of lift has been reached. The key to correcting banding has to be precision in your product application, in other words no overlapping.

Re-colouring hair after the reduction process

Before re-colouring the hair, you must consider the condition of the hair. The hair will be very porous and therefore you should choose the colouring products you use very carefully. Immediately after the colour reduction service, the cuticles of the hair will be open and receptive to colour. On occasion this may result in the final colour result being darker than expected. Therefore it may be wise to opt for a slightly lighter shade to ensure client satisfaction.

The condition of the client's hair will have suffered during the process and effective after-care advice must be given.

Remember

All product manufacturers have help lines for hairdressers who are experiencing difficulties with certain products or who need assistance. These help lines are manned by experienced technicians, who are usually able to answer any queries you may have regarding the correct usage of their products.

Re-colouring bleached hair using pre-pigmentation and permanent colour

Pre-pigmentation is the term used to describe restoring lost pigment to pale hair that needs to be made darker and / or warmer. An example of this is a client with bleached hair who wishes to go back to her natural colour. As bleaching removes the warm tones (red and yellow) from the hair, these tones must be replaced prior to applying the target shade or the finished result will have a green cast.

Pre-pigmenting may be carried out using semi-permanent, quasi-permanent or permanent colour; however, the porosity of the hair must be taken into consideration when choosing the correct product. The pre-colour may be either red, copper or gold, depending on the depth of the target shade, for example, a light colour would usually require a gold pre-colour, whereas darker hair would require a red pre-colour. The diagram on page 181 indicates the correct colour to use. Always follow the manufacturer's instructions.

Be professional ★★★

When taking clients back to their natural colour, always use one shade lighter than the target shade. You can add colour to the hair at any time but it is more difficult to remove colour from processed hair.

Colour correction: a step-by-step guide

1 Before the service.

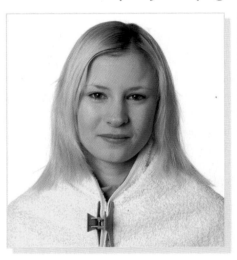

2 Apply a copper semi-permanent colour to the hair, avoiding the re-growth area.

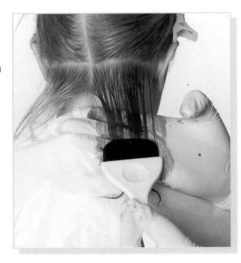

3 Place cotton wool between each section to prevent the colour from touching the re-growth area.

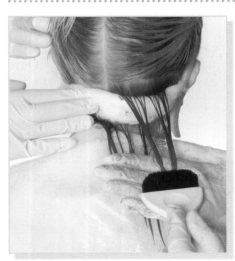

4 Leave the colour to develop.

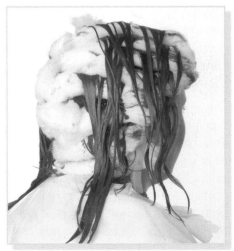

5 Wipe off excess colour to check development.

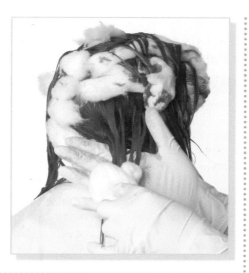

6 The hair after pre-pigmentation.

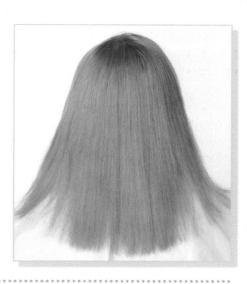

7 Apply a dark golden blonde permanent colour to the re-growth.

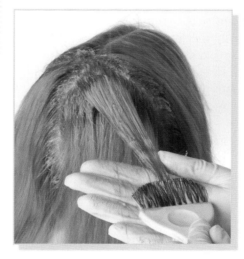

8 Apply the permanent colour to the mid-lengths and ends.

9 The finished result.

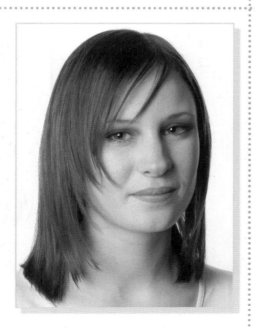

This method is tried and tested; however, with experience this process may be carried out in one stage, where the warm (pre-pigmenting) colour is added to the target shade. This may be as a 'mix tone' or a warm colour that corresponds to the type of warmth needed for the target depth. For example, if your client requires a warm light brown result, a light brown colour with red tones may be added with the target shade.

Correcting highlights and lowlights

There are several reasons why highlights or lowlights may need to be corrected. The most common reasons are stated below.

In the salon

Not as easy as it looks!

Cheryl was a very quiet, traditional client who attended the salon every three months for fine bleached highlights to brighten her hair, but she didn't want anything too noticeable. She cancelled her next appointment at the salon without giving a reason, but said she would phone again soon for a cut and blow dry. A few days later she telephoned the salon, asking for an immediate colour appointment. When she entered the salon, it appeared that she had a full-head bleach. She was very upset and proceeded to tell the stylist that she had bought a home highlighting kit and persuaded her friend to have a go, as it didn't look too difficult. The result was not at all as she expected! After carrying out all the pre-service tests and examinations, the stylist then proceeded to weave out sections of hair, to break up the colour and colour them to match her natural base, but with some added warmth to counteract the effects of the bleach (and prevent the colour from having a green cast). The result was good and Cheryl was very pleased with the result and decided she would leave colouring to the experts from now on.

Problem	Caused by	Remedy
High / lowlights give the effect of a full-head colour	Too many high / lowlights have been placed in the hair; more likely to occur on fine hair	Weave out sections of hair and apply a colour to match the client's natural base, giving the illusion of a highlighted effect
High / lowlights do not show	The wrong choice of colour. High / lowlights woven too finely. This is most common on clients with thick, dense hair. Not enough hair was coloured	The whole highlighting procedure should be carried out. If using bleach / lightening products, take care not to bleach / lighten the hair that has already been treated
Patches of colour at the roots	Product seepage from the foils or packets	Weave out sections of the affected hair and apply a colour to match the client's natural base. If the product that bled was bleach, you will need to add a little warmth into the base colour to prevent a green cast appearing

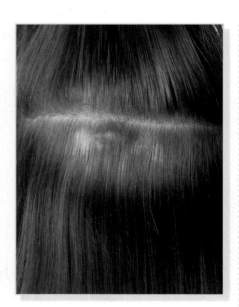

1 Seepage of product has caused a patchy result.

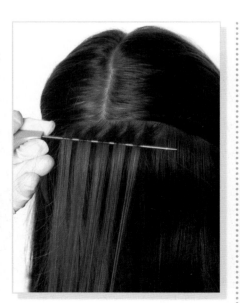

2 Weave out the affected areas and spot colour.

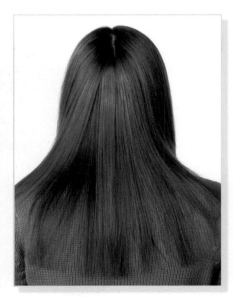

3 The finished result showing even highlights.

> **Be professional ★★★**
>
> When working with lightening / bleach products:
> - Don't overlap when applying a re-growth application as this will cause the previously lightened hair to become sensitised.
> - When applying a re-growth application you must make sure you colour right up to the demarcation line as failure to do this will result in small dark areas on the hair.
> - As a general rule, begin your application where the hair is darkest as this will take longer to lighten.
> - Make sure you take regular strand and elasticity tests during the development.
> - When removing the product (especially if it has been an 'on-scalp' application) make sure the water isn't too hot and don't massage too vigorously as this could irritate the scalp.

Pre-softening the hair

Hair will usually require pre-softening due to its resistant tendencies. The resistance of a client's hair is due to the cuticle scales being flat and smooth, usually found in hair in good condition. Some hair, such as Oriental hair, falls into this category as it has more layers of cuticle scales than either European or African type hair and therefore doesn't allow the colour to penetrate into the cortex and develop.

You may discover a client's hair is resistant to colour when you assess the final result of a colouring service. The indicators would be:

- the colouring product has not covered the natural hair colour
- the white hair has a translucent appearance; in other words it has been coloured but has not been covered.

White hair that is resistant to colour may be recognised by its 'glassy' appearance. You can overcome this by pre-softening the hair, which lifts the cuticle scales, allowing colour molecules to enter the cortex.

Pre-softening the hair is a relatively quick and simple process. It involves applying neat 10 vol or 3 per cent hydrogen peroxide to the resistant areas, drying the H_2O_2 into the hair and then proceeding with the colouring service. You may find it easier to use cream hydrogen peroxide as it has a thicker consistency and is therefore easier to work with. For common colouring problems and solutions, see pages 159–62.

Whatever colour correction service you have carried out, it is essential that you confirm your client's satisfaction at the end of the service. If you have given your client the correct information, both prior to and during the service, the outcome should be as expected.

After the service

When any colour service is complete, it is imperative to give the client the correct advice. This will serve to ensure long-lasting results and client satisfaction. It is also a good retail opportunity.

After-care advice

Once the colour correction service has been completed to the satisfaction of your client, you must advise the client on how to care for their hair and maintain the colour. You may also need to advise the client to visit the salon for further services in order to keep their hair in the best condition possible. This is essential if the client's hair shows more than minimal damage in the cortex. If you feel their hair cannot withstand any further chemical processing, you must inform the client of this and outline the possible consequences, for example, hair breakage.

During the initial and ongoing consultation you will have determined the condition of your client's hair and given advice on the most suitable products for home use, for example, shampoo and conditioner. You should ensure your client understands the importance of looking after their hair in order to maintain the colour and keep it in optimum condition. You should discuss the features and benefits of the shampoo and conditioning products that you have recommended and explain that they have been specifically designed for use after colour or colour correction treatments. This may include the use of a restructuring treatment that will help to rebuild the internal fibres in the cortex and improve the elasticity of the hair. You must ensure the client understands not only how these products help to maintain their hair in good condition but how and when to use them.

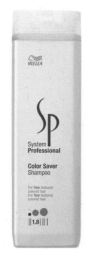
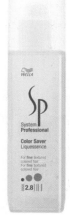
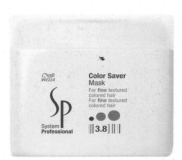

Wella

You need to advise your client on the most suitable products for home use

Check it out

List the retail products available for colour correction clients to purchase after the service.

KS **Key Skills Links**: Level 2 Communication

Many clients believe all colour shampoos and conditioners will achieve the same results, therefore you need to educate them by explaining how the products work and also highlighting the products to avoid, such as silicone-based products as these may prove to be problematic with future colouring services.

You must also explain to your clients that continued use of heated styling equipment may damage their hair further; however, the use of a good heat protection spray will reduce the damage and help to prevent further dehydration.

Remember

It is essential you discuss with the your client when they should return to the salon for further treatment, and if possible have them make the appointment before they leave the salon. This is not only professional but the client is more likely to return if their next appointment is pre-booked.

Completion of the record card

On completion of the service it is essential that you complete the client's record card. The information contained on the client record card must be clear to other stylists who may colour the client's hair in the future and include explicit details of the colour correction service.

Disposal of waste

At the end of the colour service, any waste products and materials must be disposed of carefully and in a safe manner. All unused colouring products should be disposed of, following the manufacturer's instructions. If you are in any doubt as to how the products should be disposed of, you should contact the product manufacturer and ask for their advice.

Check your knowledge

The following questions will help you to check your understanding of this unit. The answers can be found on page 418. Take care, as there may be more than one correct answer for some questions.

1 A colour correction service should be carried out if the client requires:
  a the hair to be lightened because it's too dark
  b highlights and lowlights
  c the hair to be darkened because it's too light
  d a change of tone

2 The term 'oxidation' refers to a chemical process that adds:
  a oxygen
  b hydrogen
  c nitrogen
  d sulphur

3 An example of a product that works by oxidation is:
  a colour stripper
  b semi-permanent colour
  c permanent colour
  d bleach / lightening products

4 When pre-softening hair, you should:
  a use a good quality conditioner
  b use stain remover
  c apply hydrogen peroxide to the resistant areas, then apply heat to open the cuticles
  d add warm tones to the hair

5 Why is it important to carry out a skin test before a colouring service?
  a To ensure the correct colour can be achieved
  b To find out whether the client is allergic to the products to be used
  c To ensure the tensile strength of the hair is good enough to take the service
  d To test the amount of damage to the cuticles

6 All electrical equipment should be checked before use in order to:
  a ensure that no electrons are emitted
  b prevent accidents or electrocution
  c make sure it's working properly
  d ensure it's the correct voltage

7 How should waste products from a colouring service be disposed of?
  a In the bin
  b Burned in a fire
  c Anyway you choose
  d Diluted with plenty of cold water, and then flushed down the drain

8 It's important to complete client record cards as this:
    a ensures you are complying with the Data Protection Act
    b will help the next stylist when the client returns
    c may be used in a case of litigation
    d ensures you are complying with all aspects of COSHH

9 If you needed to dilute 12% hydrogen peroxide to give you 6% you would:
    a mix 1 part hydrogen peroxide to 3 parts water
    b mix 2 parts hydrogen peroxide to 1 part water
    c mix 1 part hydrogen peroxide to 2 parts water
    d mix 1 part hydrogen peroxide to 1 part water

10 It's essential you give your clients effective after-care advice, as this will:
    a ensure your clients' hair remains in optimum condition between visits
    b ensure more commission for you
    c make the clients think you care
    d help to prevent colour fade

Assessment guidance

You must demonstrate in your everyday work that you have met the standards for providing colour correction services. These may be carried out on either men or women.

You will be assessed on at least four different occasions and you will have to prove that you can competently carry out:

- all the types of colour correction
- questioning your clients on all the areas of contra-indication
- all the tests in the range
- thorough and effective after-care advice to all clients.

Simulated activity is not allowed for any part of this unit.

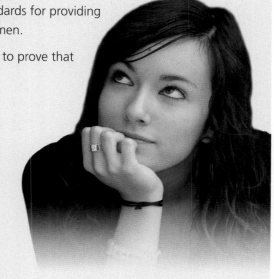

Provide colour correction services **Unit GH18**

Style and dress hair to achieve a variety of creative looks

What you will learn:

- How to prepare the client
- The different styling techniques and the effects that may be produced
- How to dress the hair
- How to proceed after the service.

Darren Ambrose

Introduction

There are many different ways that hair can be styled and dressed in a creative way; this includes setting, blow-drying, pin curling, finger waving and using heated styling equipment. You may also need to use added hair to create volume in the style, increase the length of the client's hair or to give a variety of colour. By combining some of the above techniques, your styling and dressing will become more exciting and innovative, making you a much-sought-after stylist.

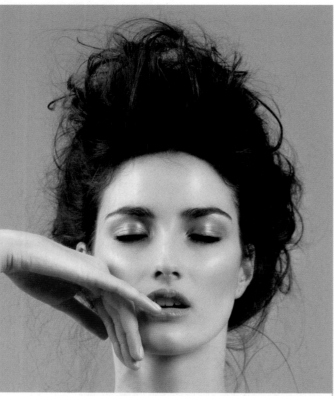

Different styling and dressing techniques are used to create innovative looks

You the stylist

Styling and dressing hair gives you a great opportunity to use your creative and artistic flair. Sadly, some hairdressers see this service only as a 'finish' to other services, for example, cutting, colouring or perming. Styling and dressing hair should be looked upon as an exciting opportunity for you to gain valuable insight into ways in which you can personalise your work to suit the individual and the occasion.

Preparing the client

Preparation for any service is essential; it reflects both your salon's image and also your professional approach towards your work. You will need to consider the tools and equipment you will need to carry out the service. To ensure compliance with health and safety legislation, your tools and equipment should be clean and sterile before use on every client to prevent cross-infection and infestation. Methods of sterilising tools and equipment can be found in Unit G22. Any electrical equipment should be checked prior to use to make sure it is safe and fit for purpose. This will safeguard against accidents and minimise the risk of damage to the equipment. Remember, your responsibilities under the Health and Safety at Work Act 1974 apply throughout your work in the salon, regardless of the service you are carrying out.

Check it out

What can you remember about the Electricity at Work Regulations and the COSHH Regulations? What are your responsibilities within these health and safety laws? If you are unsure, look back at Unit G22.

You should also be aware of your responsibilities under the COSHH Regulations in relation to using styling and finishing products, as well as your responsibilities under the Electricity at Work Regulations 1989 when you are using electrical equipment.

Personal health and hygiene

Your own standards of health and hygiene are important. If you attend work knowing that you have an infectious or contagious condition, you must consider the consequences of cross-infection to other people at work. Working while you are unwell will have a negative impact on the salon, regardless of whether or not you have infected a client or colleague.

In most hairdressing environments, you are working in close proximity to your clients, so your personal hygiene is important. It can be particularly unpleasant for clients to experience your second-hand garlic or onions from lunch. Equally, the smell of stale nicotine on your breath or clothes should be avoided. Basic good personal hygiene rules should be followed at all times to ensure you do not cause offence to your clients or colleagues.

Preparing the client for the service

When your client enters the salon, take a good look at her prior to gowning. You should be looking at the type of clothes she is wearing to give you an indication of her image and whether she is more likely to require conventional styling or something more adventurous. Before you begin the service, you must ensure your client is gowned appropriately and the towel is positioned correctly. Keep checking throughout the service to ensure the gown and towel are still positioned correctly and her clothes are protected from spillages.

Check it out

If you are applying coloured mousse or setting lotion, what should you be wearing to protect your hands and clothes from staining? How should you protect your client from accidental spillages?

Thorough consultation

You must make sure your consultations are thorough so that you can carry out your client's wishes accurately. Use a stylebook where necessary to make sure both you and your client fully understand each other and the outcome of the service. There are several influencing factors that need to be considered prior to styling and dressing:

- the desired look
- the hair texture, length and density
- the haircut, client's facial features and head and face shape
- any hair growth patterns and elasticity.

The desired look

You must take into consideration the desired look; the client may be going somewhere special and have preconceived ideas of how she wishes to look. Alternatively, she may have no ideas but is open to suggestions. You need to understand the potential of your client's hair to ensure the final look is appropriate to her age, personality, and the occasion.

The hair texture, length and density

There are many questions you need to ask yourself with regard to your client's hair to ensure optimum results, for example, will the client's hair length, texture and density allow me to create the style required? If the client's hair is too long, thick and heavy, there is the possibility the style will drop quickly; however, with the correct styling products, this may be avoided. If you feel the hair is unlikely to achieve the desired outcome, use your skill and expertise to suggest styles that are achievable.

The haircut and client's facial features

The client's haircut must be suitable for the style you wish to create and the head and face shape should suit the intended style. Any unusual facial features may be disguised by clever styling and dressing; ignoring these could lead to an unsuitable style and unhappy client.

Hair growth patterns and elasticity

If the client has any irregular hair growth patterns, such as a widow's peak or cowlick, this may affect the way the hair lies and should be taken into consideration during the consultation. Again, with clever styling and dressing, these may be disguised. Ideally, the hair should be styled and dressed to follow the natural fall of the hair, as this will prolong the life of the style and help reduce the possibility of the hair lying awkwardly the next day. The hair's elasticity must be considered because, if it is poor, you cannot guarantee a good result.

It is your responsibility to take all the influencing factors into consideration and, should there be any potential problems, discuss them with the client and agree a course of action prior to the service rather than 'hoping for the best'. This will ensure that your client receives a professional style and dress service and leaves the salon as a satisfied client.

Your salon is trying to portray a professional image, which should be reflected in the high standard of work it carries out. Only your absolute best is good enough. Once you are both happy with the outcome of the consultation, you need to decide on the most appropriate styling and finishing products for your client's hair. By this stage, the client should have been made aware of the cost and duration of the service.

Check it out

Find out the times your salon allows for you to complete your styling, dressing and finishing services. These timings should be commercially viable for your salon.

The client should now be prepared for shampooing. While your assistant is shampooing (using a good-quality shampoo to ensure thorough cleansing), you should utilise this time to ensure you have all the tools and equipment you will need close to hand and everything is clean and sterile. This will enable you to provide an efficient and professional service, as you will not have to keep your client waiting while you find whatever is missing.

Unit GH19 Style and dress hair to achieve a variety of creative looks

Salon life

A long stretch

Zaid's story

I was asked to carry out a blow-dry on a client with fine, one-length, over-bleached hair. As the client wanted her hair as straight as possible, I was blow-drying the hair with a fair degree of tension. With each section that I blow-dried, the hair was visibly stretching. The finished result was very uneven. I was extremely disappointed with the result, although the client wasn't too bothered as she said it always happened!

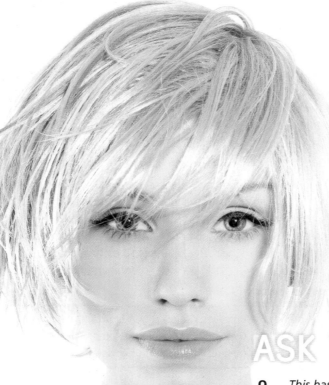

Be professional ★★★

- If in doubt, carry out an elasticity test! The hair should stretch and return to its original length when the pulling force is removed.
- A client with hair in such poor condition is obviously not taking very good care of their hair; therefore this is a great opportunity for you to recommend additional services and products.

ASK THE PROFESSIONALS

Q *This has never happened before, so what did I do wrong?*

A The client had highly bleached hair which had very poor elasticity (most probably due to the over use of bleach on the hair). The internal structure of the hair was damaged and the tensile strength of the hair was poor. If you think about it, the hair stretches more when it's wet but hair in good condition will always spring back to its original length.

Q *What could I have done differently?*

A Applied less tension to the hair but still made sure you kept the hair smooth, to ensure the result was good.

Q *What could have happened if I'd applied even more tension?*

A The hair could have reached its elastic limit (the point of no return) and the hair would have broken off.

Unit GH19 Style and dress hair to achieve a variety of creative looks

Different styling techniques and the effects that may be produced

To create variety and originality in your styling, use a combination of the styling techniques below, and remember that the techniques can be mixed and matched. You should not disregard any ideas at this stage; sometimes the results will amaze you!

In this section you will learn about the different styling techniques, how they work, and the results that can be achieved.

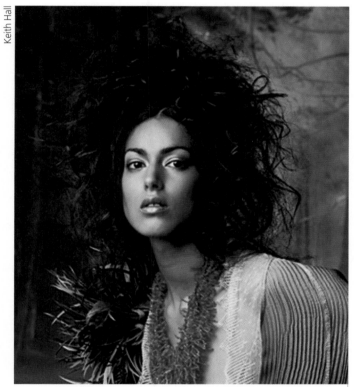

Keith Hall

A combination of styling techniques can create amazing results

The results of these styling techniques will cause a physical change within the hair. The change is temporary and will last only until the hair is wet or absorbs moisture from the atmosphere. The temporary changes that take place in the hair are usually classed as either:

- cohesive setting (wet – stretch – dry)
- temporary setting (heat – mould – cool).

Check it out

Which of the styling techniques covered in this unit are classed as cohesive and which are temporary?

Setting

The setting process enables straight hair to be made curly and curly hair made straighter. This is due to the way the hair is structured. As you already know, within the cortex lie a number of polypeptide chains, which run along the length of the hair. The chains are spiral-shaped (called an alpha (α) helix) and have cross-linkages that join them to their neighbouring polypeptide chains. Some of these linkages are permanent and others are temporary.

The hydrogen bonds, which are one of the temporary linkages, are the ones that enable us to set the hair. The hydrogen bonds are not only joined to their neighbouring polypeptide chain, but are also linked within the same polypeptide chain between the coils of the alpha helix. It is these hydrogen bonds that enable the hair to be stretched during setting, giving the hair its elasticity.

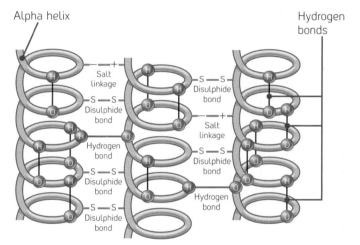

Before the hair is shampooed, the hydrogen bonds hold the coils of the polypeptide chains close together. The hair in this state is known as alpha (α) keratin. Once the hair has been shampooed, many of the hydrogen bonds are broken, allowing the hair to be stretched around the roller or brush (if blow-drying).

Once the hair has been stretched, fully dried and allowed to cool into the new shape, the hair is said to be in beta (β) keratin state. It is essential that the hair is fully dried and allowed to cool before brushing and styling. If the hair is still warm, some of the new shape may be lost.

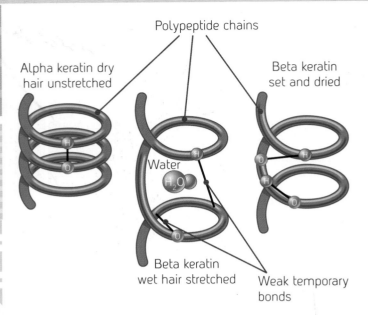

Polypeptide chains

Alpha keratin dry hair unstretched

Beta keratin set and dried

Water

Beta keratin wet hair stretched

Weak temporary bonds

The hair will stay in this new position until the hair is made wet or it absorbs atmospheric moisture. This is due to the hair being hygroscopic – it has the ability to absorb moisture from the atmosphere. Humidity levels (the degree of moisture in the atmosphere) will affect the length of time a set or blow-dry will last. The level of humidity in some salons may be quite high due to the evaporation of water from the hair, towels, and so on. This is also true during damp weather, therefore it is essential that good styling products be used, as this will help to prevent the atmospheric moisture entering the hair as quickly, prolonging the life of your styling.

Some styling products contain plastic resins, which are left as a film on the hair once the hair is dry. This plastic film helps to prevent the atmospheric moisture from being absorbed by the hair.

Temporary setting (heat – mould – cool)

As with cohesive setting, the hydrogen bonds need to be broken. When using heated styling equipment on dry hair, the hair's internal moisture breaks some of the hydrogen bonds; however, it is essential that the equipment be heated sufficiently to turn the internal moisture into steam. As the temporary setting utilises the natural moisture that is present in hair, overuse of heated styling equipment will cause the hair to dehydrate.

Check it out

Look at a client who uses straightening irons on a regular basis and test how brittle the hair feels. This is a good indicator of dehydrated hair, not to mention the damage to the cuticle!

Tools and equipment for setting

There is a variety of equipment that may be used when setting the hair, including rollers, Velcro rollers and Molton Browners (bendy rollers).

For this part of the unit you need to experiment with items that are not normally associated with setting but will alter the shape of the hair. This may include items such as pipe-cleaners, straws, foils, chopsticks, rik-raks, matchboxes and Toblerone boxes. The shape of the 'former' is the shape you will achieve, for example, if you use a Toblerone box, you will achieve angular curls.

Remember

Setting may be carried out on hair that is wet, that is, just shampooed, or hair that is dry. When setting dry hair, heat is required to mould the hair into its new shape.

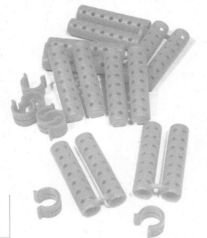

Double rollers may be used to produce spiral curls

When using items that are made from cardboard, the dry setting method should be used. If the hair is wet, the cardboard will become soggy! You must also ensure the shape of the item will not distort during use, as this would result in an incorrect form.

Many non-conventional items can be found at trade exhibitions, but that does not exclude you from designing your own. You need to consider the potential health and safety risks when choosing non-conventional items. For example:

- Are there any sharp edges that may cause discomfort to the client?
- Will it conduct heat under the dryer and burn the client?
- Is it flammable?
- Will it melt under the dryer?
- Can it be cleaned and sterilised?
- Is it safe to use and fit for purpose?

Using unconventional setting techniques: a step-by-step guide

1 A fine section of hair and double length of foil is taken. The foil is then pinned at the roots using pin curl clips.

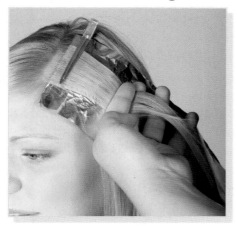

2 The foil is folded up to the roots and pinned in place. Then the foil is folded from the bottom, backwards and forwards to give a concertina effect.

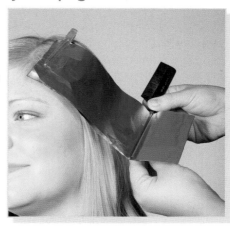

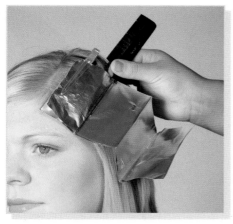

3 The concertina effect.

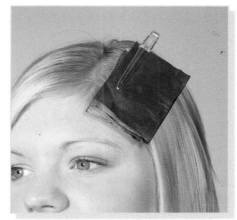

4 The first section is complete. Continue as in steps 1–3 throughout the head.

5 Straightening irons are placed over each foiled section, then the section is allowed to cool.

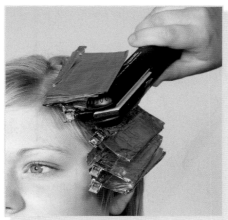

6 The finished look

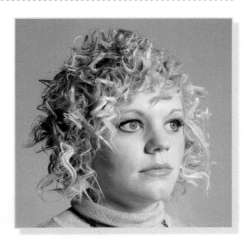

Check it out

Using a block, try setting the hair using everyday items not usually used for setting. Remember, you must consider the health and safety risks that may be associated with using non-conventional items. For example, a can of hairspray may give a good even round shape, but what are the potential risks when the aerosol goes under the dryer?

Winding techniques

Root to point

Root to point winding is usually carried out on hair that is shoulder-length or longer. The hair is wound on a long thin 'rod', for example, a straw, twig or chopstick, in a spiral manner, working down the 'rod' and taking care not to twist or buckle the hair.

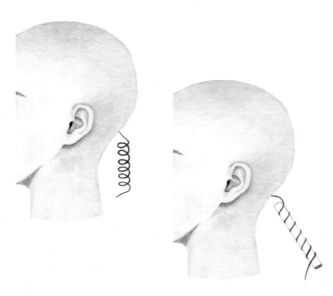

If the hair is wrapped around the rod in this manner, the diameter of the curl stays consistent throughout the length of the hair and produces an even spiral curl formation.

Point to root (croquignole) wind

Most conventional setting is carried out using this method of setting. Depending on the length of the hair, this method of winding will give a looser curl at the root than at the ends, as the hair is wound over the previous hair with each revolution.

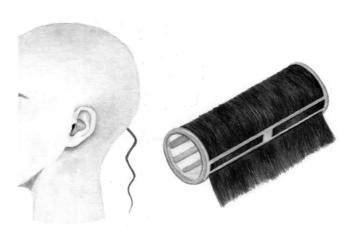

The roller size used is determined by the hair texture, density, and the amount of curl required. A general rule would be: the finer the hair, the smaller the roller. A client with fine hair in texture but abundant in mass may find the hair too curly if it is set on rollers that are too small.

Once you have decided on your style, you need to plan how you can achieve this. The direction in which you wind the hair will depend on the intended result (directional setting). You also need to consider the amount of lift required and whether you need to wind on or off base.

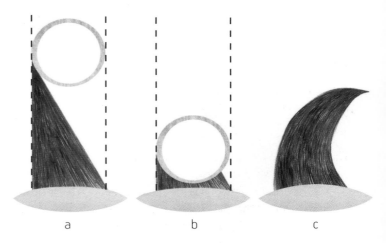

a   b   c

Hair wound to sit on its own base

To achieve normal root lift, the roller must be sitting on its own base. If the hair is dragged forward at an obtuse angle (greater than 90° angle) to the scalp, this will give increased lift.

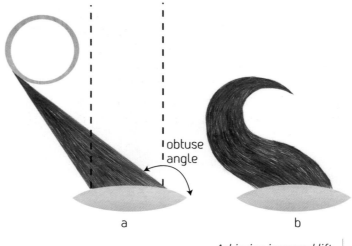

obtuse angle

a   b

Achieving increased lift

If the obtuse angle is increased (over-directed), the roller will sit off base. The result will give straight roots and curled ends, therefore gaining direction from the root area with some fullness at the ends. This type of setting may be used to create 'flicks' on the ends of the hair or to disguise a high forehead or hair that is receding at the temples.

If the hair is dragged back at an acute angle (less than 90°), the roller will sit off base. Hair with 'dragged' roots would usually be used at the sides and back of the head where the hairstyle requires less volume.

Once your set is complete, your client needs to be placed under the dryer. You must check the position of the setting pins (if used) to ensure they will not cause any client discomfort.

Be professional ★★★

If using metal setting pins, make sure they are not in contact with the client's scalp as they conduct heat and could burn the client's skin and scalp.

The length of time the client is under the dryer will vary depending on the length and density of the hair. If the rollers are removed before the hair is completely dry, the set will drop. However, if the client's hair is over-dried, this can cause the hair to become flyaway, making it difficult to dress. In addition, the unnecessary heat will cause the hair to become dry and dehydrated.

When the hair is completely dry, allow the hair to cool before removing rollers and pins, as the hair is still warm and soft at this point and the set may drop. When removing rollers, care should be taken to avoid causing the client any discomfort, especially if you have used a strong styling product that leaves the hair with a 'crispy' feel.

Roller marks should be removed by thorough brushing, which also stimulates the blood flow and sebaceous activity in the scalp. However, some styles do not require brushing. The rollers are removed from the hair and it is teased into shape with the addition of dressing products. Other sets are not brushed but merely combed through with a wide-tooth comb to maintain the curl.

By combining setting on and off base, you can create more personalised and innovative looks.

Blow-drying

Tools and equipment used for blow-drying

You will need:

- hairdryer
- nozzle or diffuser
- fingers
- radial brushes (various sizes available)
- paddle brush
- flat brushes, for example, Denman brushes
- vent brush (for more textured looks).

By now you should have used a variety of different brushes and other equipment and no doubt you will have decided which of these you find most comfortable to use and give the results you require. However, the industry is always making advances and producing new tools, so do not be afraid to experiment and try out other alternatives.

Drying techniques

By now you should have extensive experience of blow-drying a variety of different styles and determining which method of blow-drying, tools and equipment are most suitable for your client's hair texture. The techniques you learned and mastered during your initial training should now be adapted or modified to meet your clients' ever-increasing demands. Some examples of drying techniques are described overleaf.

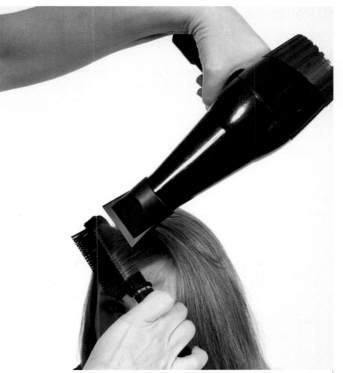

Drying hair from root to point

Root to point

This type of drying would be used where the main emphasis is shiny hair. To create smooth shiny hair, the hair should always be dried in a root to point direction, with the airflow following the lie of the cuticle.

Point to root

There are many reasons for drying hair in this way, but maximum shine will not be your priority.

When drying hair using a diffuser, the heat is travelling in a point to root direction. The results can vary from a tousled look to very curly.

When blow-drying fine hair that requires volume, you may need to direct the airflow against the lie of the cuticle so the cuticle becomes roughened and 'mattes' the hair together, giving the illusion of body. When 'blasting' hair to create volume, the same principle would be used.

When finger drying short hair, it is sometimes necessary to direct the airflow into the hair to ruffle the cuticle; this will add volume and give a less structured finish to your styling.

Creative blow-drying can produce a variety of different effects from smooth, straight looks to curly, unkempt looks. Your client's requirements should have been discussed at length prior to carrying out the service.

You must consider any influencing factors when preparing for a blow-dry service. Is it possible to create the style the client wishes?

Check it out

> Practise using your creative and artistic skills; experiment on a friend by blow-drying root to point and point to root and find out the different effects that may be achieved on differing hair types. Use products in the salon that you possibly have not used before and see the results that may be achieved. Above all, do not be afraid to try out new techniques and products – after all, this is one of the best ways to learn!

Pin curling

Pin curls may be used creatively to produce a variety of effects, including flat waves, curl and body. The effects are stunning, especially when used in conjunction with the other styling techniques mentioned in this unit.

Pin curls are not always suitable for frizzy or very long hair; you will achieve the best results using pin curling on medium, textured hair with a little natural movement. Take extra care when pin curling on hair that has been permed, tinted or bleached, as it marks easily and tends to buckle.

Types of pin curl

Barrel curl or stand-up pin curl

Gives the style lift and body. If using barrel curls in conjunction with rollers, you must ensure the diameter of the pin curl is the same as that of the roller.

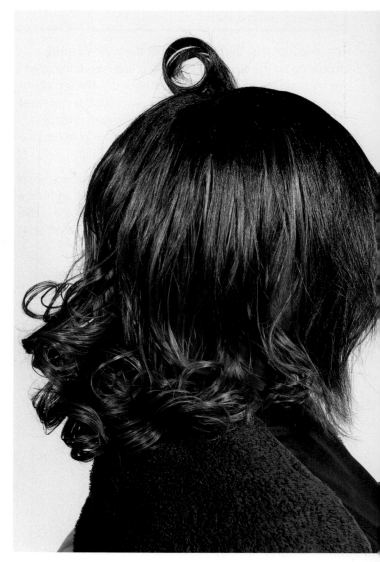

Half stand barrel curl

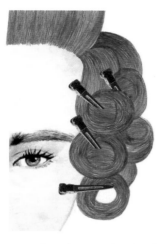

Creates springy, loose curls; ideal for use at the sides of the head as the curls move away from the head

Flat barrel curl

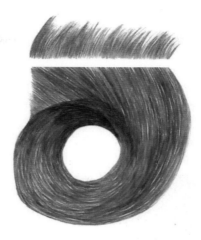

Used to create flat movements that lie close to the head. The flat barrel curl is used when carrying out reverse curling to produce waves

Flat barrel with the ends on the outside

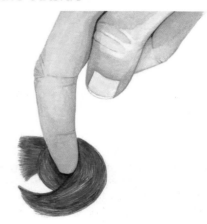

Used to create styles that require loose uncurled hair ends

Long stem pin curls

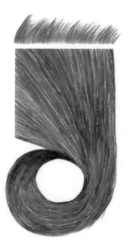

These pin curls are designed to sit 'off base'. They give a flat effect with curl at the ends and may be used to define the style in the nape, at the sides, or the front hairline

Sculptured curls

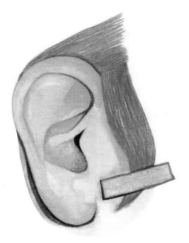

Again, these pin curls are designed to sit 'off base'. The hair is combed and moulded into position then either pinned or taped into place. These curls give very soft movement on short hair

Clockspring curls

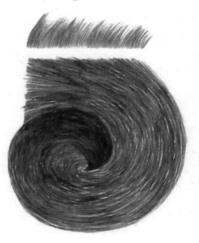

A clockspring curl has a closed centre and produces a tight curl on the ends with looser movement at the roots. It is generally used to create a curly effect in the nape of the neck

You must make sure the heads of the metal pins are not touching the skin, as this may result in burning the client's skin and scalp. If necessary, place a fine mesh of cotton wool underneath the offending pin; this will protect the client from burning.

Be professional ★★★

As with any hairdressing technique, the more you practise, the better you will get. For example, mastering pin curling might open up new avenues to creative styling!

Finger waving

Finger waving produces flat waves in the hair; no root lift is achieved when using this technique. The hair is moulded into 's'-shaped movements using the fingers and a straight comb. The use of strong styling products is essential when finger waving and the hair must remain wet (but not dripping) throughout the service. When finger waving, you should follow the natural fall of the hair and utilise any natural movement that may be present; this will help to prolong the life of the style.

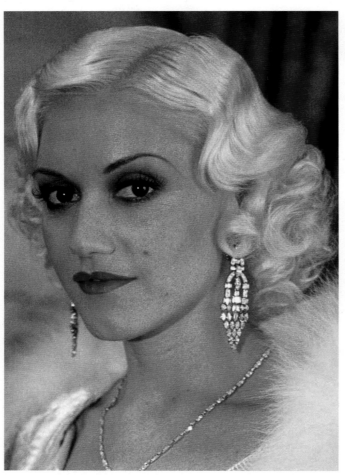

This type of styling is best carried out on hair that is medium to fine in texture and a reasonable length, especially on the crown. However, if using finger waving in conjunction with another styling technique, good results may be achieved by waving the sides or back, allowing the top area of the style to retain some fullness. Finger waves should be dried under a hood dryer, as the hair should be disturbed as little as possible.

When dressing waved hair, it is not usual to brush through the hair but to comb it using a wide-tooth comb to encourage the wave formation.

Use of heated styling equipment

Heated styling equipment comes in many different forms, which include:

- tongs
- straightening irons
- crimping irons
- Marcel waving irons
- heated rollers
- hot brush
- flexi curlers (heated bendy rollers).

Before using any type of heated electrical equipment, you should ensure it is fit for purpose and safe to use. You should also know how to use the equipment properly and in a safe manner to prevent accidents from occurring.

Be professional ★★★

Ask a senior stylist to show you how to use equipment that is new to you. Under the Electricity at Work Regulations, you should not be using equipment that you have not been trained to use.

Care must be taken when using heated electrical equipment. It is very easy to overheat the hair when using this type of equipment and this could lead to damage to the cuticle and dehydration of the hair. The equipment should be in contact with the hair for the minimum time necessary to achieve the desired result. You must ensure that you position your client in a way that enables you to access all areas of the hair without causing unnecessary discomfort or burning of the client.

In the salon

Blood, sweat and tears

Kath was tonging a client's hair in the salon. It was mid-August and the salon was very warm. The client removed her gown as she was becoming uncomfortably hot. The client was wearing a vest top with narrow shoulder straps. Kath was also becoming very warm and starting to perspire. Suddenly the tongs slipped out of her hands and dropped onto her client's shoulders causing a third-degree burn.

- Was Kath negligible in her duty to her client?
- How could this situation have been avoided?

Remember

Many styling products are flammable, so you must make sure no one is smoking in the near vicinity when you are using such products.

Heated styling equipment should be used on clean, dry hair that does not have excess products on it. Excess products may cause the hair to stick to the heated appliance causing discomfort to the client. It may also coat the appliance, which will then require thorough cleaning, or, at the very least, reduce the effectiveness of the equipment due to heat loss.

When using electrical styling equipment, you must make sure there are no **fish hooks**. Place the tongs close to the roots and slide the tongs down the length of the hair. This softens the hair prior to styling and also smoothes down the cuticle. The hair is usually easier to manage and it enables you to take the tongs right down to the points of the hair and secure them firmly within the barrel of the tongs.

Be professional ★★★

Electrically heated styling equipment shouldn't be cleaned using water due to the risk of electrocution, but wiped over with spirit.

Fish hooks

when the ends of the hair become bent over, which doesn't give a smooth finish

Types of heating styling equipment and their uses

Equipment	Types	Effects
Tongs	Small barrel	Gives small, tight curls if used on short hair; spiral curls if wound in a spiral manner on long hair.
	Large barrel	Gives curl and/or movement; may be used for spiral curling on long hair but will give a soft result
Spiral tongs		Gives spiral curls
Straightening irons	Metal plates	Temporarily straightens the hair
	Ceramic plates	Temporarily straightens the hair; less damaging to the hair than metal plates and also help to retain moisture
Crimping irons		Gives a crimped effect on the hair
Heated rollers	Various sizes	Gives curl. Adds lift and volume
Hot brush	Various sizes	Gives curl. Adds lift and volume
Flexi curlers	Various sizes	Gives a variety of effects, from large bouncy curls to spiral ones

Unit GH19 Style and dress hair to achieve a variety of creative looks

203

Positioning of self and client

Client comfort is essential throughout the service. You may need to adjust your client's position to enable you to reach certain areas of the head, for example, when tonging your client's hair in the nape, they should have their head down. This will enable you to get right into the nape area. You should always place a comb underneath the tongs to prevent them touching the skin.

Think about your own posture while you are working. Stooping or stretching will cause unnecessary stress on your body, causing aches and pains. Ideally, you should be standing with your feet at shoulders' width apart and your weight evenly distributed on both feet. Make use of hydraulic chairs, as these may be adjusted to suit the height of both yourself and your client, enabling you to maintain correct posture. Keep your tools and equipment close to hand and positioned in a way that does not require you to over-stretch to reach them.

Throughout the service your work area should be kept clean and tidy. This will help to promote a professional image and should also reduce the risk of cross-infection.

Added hair

Added hair has been around for many years. Its popularity has risen and fallen as fashions have changed. Added hair has been increasing in popularity over the last few years and has seen many younger clients and fashion icons favouring its use. This has had an impact on most age groups and added hair is now instrumental within the styling and dressing service, regardless of the age of the client. Currently there are many different forms of 'added hair' available. They range from clip-on hair swatches through to the more traditional postiche.

Added hair may be used for the following reasons:
- to add volume to fine hair
- to add length to the hair
- to add colour to the hair
- for special occasions, for example, weddings, graduation ceremonies, parties, etc.
- to cover scarring.

You should give considerable thought to the positioning of the added hair and how it may be incorporated most effectively in your styling. You also need to ensure that it blends effectively with the natural hair. The base or fixing of the added hair must be well hidden. More than one colour may be used for added interest or to create a contrast with the natural hair colour.

When using added hair, it is essential that it be secured properly. Your client must feel confident that the added hair will stay in place for the duration it is to be worn. For extra security, when adding a piece that is on a comb attachment, make a cross using two interlocking Kirby grips, then insert the comb underneath the grips.

Many hairdressers shy away from using added hair, especially if it is long. However, once the fear has been conquered, it opens up an exciting area of hairdressing that will enable you to stand out from the crowd. Most of the hairpieces available are made from synthetic fibres and the quality of these pieces is improving all the time. They come in a variety of colours and may be used to match your client's natural hair colour or add contrast.

Acrylic pieces come in a variety of colours and styles but there are limitations to their use. Heated styling equipment must not be used on acrylic pieces, as they will melt. They must only be cleaned in cold water using specialist products specific to acrylic hair. Conventional hairspray should not be used as they cause the fibres to stick together. If cutting is required, a razor should be used as this tapers the ends of the piece giving it a more natural appearance. Do not use your hairdressing scissors — acrylic pieces will blunt your scissors.

Pieces made from real hair have advantages and disadvantages. They may be styled using heated styling equipment. They are usually handmade to the client's specific requirements. They must not be washed, but should either be sent away or left with a reputable hairdresser who specialises in postiche for specialist 'dry cleaning'.

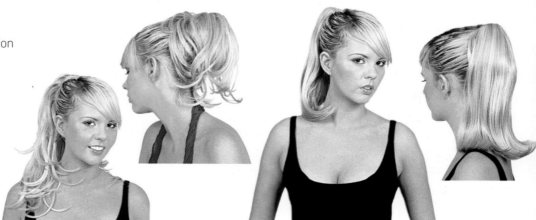

Using added hair to create a variety of effects

Dressing the hair

During the dressing process, you must continually check the direction, shape, volume and balance of the style. Re-confirm the desired look with your client before dressing, to ensure the correct result.

The direction you dress the hair should be the direction in which it is to be styled. If you try to dress the hair any other way, you will find it very difficult and unyielding. Continually check the shape, balance and volume as you work through. Check the dressing from every angle — it is important that the final result is superb.

> **Remember**
>
> The free advertising your clients convey to others may also be negative advertising if the quality of your work is not up to standard.

If the finished hair is not quite right, now is the time to address the issue. Do not wait until you have finished. Assess the dressing and make any amendments as soon as possible. Use your knowledge of finishing products and choose the most suitable product for your client's hair and the finished look that is required. The correct product will depend on the desired outcome. Check your finished result to ensure it complements your client's features, for example, does it suit her face shape and facial features? Is it in keeping with her total image?

When you are completely satisfied with the result and you feel it reflects your salon's standard of service, check your client is satisfied with the finished result. When you have their agreement, apply finishing spray to the hair to hold the style in place. If you apply the spray before confirmation and the client is unhappy, it is not always easy to rectify, as the spray will have already 'set'.

> **Remember**
>
> When applying finishing spray, provide a face shield for your client wherever possible, as this will protect their eyes.

Styling and finishing products

Each product manufacturer has its own vast range of styling and finishing products, each with a specific purpose. It is essential that you have a thorough understanding of the whole product range that is available to you so that you can ensure you are using the correct products to maximise the potential of your client's hair. Make sure you follow the manufacturer's instructions regarding the correct use of products and follow their recommendations concerning the most suitable products for specific hair types. Many styling and finishing products contain conditioning agents and UV filters to protect and condition your client's hair.

Mousse

Mousse comes in different strengths depending on the holding power required. It will help to prolong the life of the style by protecting it from humidity. Many also contain UV filters. Care should be taken when using mousse on very fine 'baby hair' as it may be too heavy for the hair and cause the style to drop.

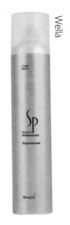
Wella

Setting/styling lotions

These are available in different strengths depending on the holding power required. They protect the hair from humidity, prolonging the life of the style. Very lightweight styling lotions are good for very fine hair, as they do not 'drag out' the styling.

Thermo-active sprays

These are used when dry-setting the hair with Velcro rollers. These sprays require the addition of heat to enable them to work efficiently. When setting short hair, they may be applied when the set has been completed. On long hair, they are better applied prior to setting to ensure an even distribution along the hair shaft.

Gels

Gels are usually stronger than mousse or styling lotion and are used for sculpting and moulding. Gel may be used on wet or dry hair, but read the manufacturer's instructions to ensure you are using it correctly.

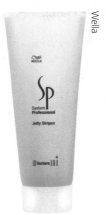
Wella

Moisturisers

These are used to help restore lost moisture and improve the strength and elasticity of the hair. It is a good idea to use these after blow-drying if you are to use heated styling equipment, for example, straightening irons, as they help to replace some of the moisture that is lost during the styling process.

Sprays

Sprays may be used during and after dressing to hold the style in place and protect the hair from atmospheric moisture. They come in different strengths depending on the amount of hold needed.

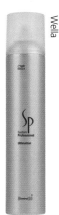

Wella

Shine sprays / glosses

These are used after dressing to give the hair maximum shine and UV protection. Care must be taken not to use excess amounts of these products, as this may cause the hair to look lank and greasy. If the client has a problem with static, the use of shine spray will help to reduce this.

Wax / dressing creams

These are used to define the finished style and are particularly good for texturising.

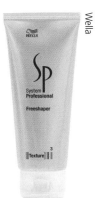

Wella

Straightening creams

These are used to defy the effects of humidity on the hair. Straightening creams are not designed to straighten the hair alone. It is the combination of the product and the blow-drying that produces straight results.

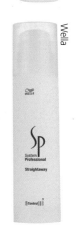

Wella

When using styling and finishing products, it is essential that you are aware of your responsibilities under the COSHH Regulations and have read the manufacturer's instructions on the products' safe usage. When using products, you should be economical with them to ensure you minimise waste and prevent the hair from becoming overloaded.

After the service

Before the client leaves the salon, you must make sure you have given them sound advice on the maintenance of the finished style. You should ensure your client is aware of the effects of humidity (they may go home and have a hot bath before going out), as this will cause the style to drop. Your client should be advised on the correct products to use at home to maintain the condition of the hair and the style that has been achieved. This will ensure the client's hair remains in optimum condition, the styling should last longer, and it shows an accurate reflection of the professional service your salon offers. It also gives you a great opportunity to retail, which will boost the amount of commission that you earn.

Encourage your client to book their next appointment before they leave the salon. The next appointment may not necessarily be a style and dress appointment, but may be a cut or colour service. Once the client has left the salon without an appointment, you cannot guarantee their return. However, a client is more likely to return if another appointment is pending. Even a satisfied client may opt to try another salon; this could result in the loss of a client. Once the client has left the salon, you should prepare your work area to ensure it is clean and tidy, ready for your next client.

You should now be ready to create some wonderful style and dress looks using some of the techniques you have learned throughout this unit. Photograph the work you do and track your progress as your skills develop. The photographs may be used as evidence within your portfolio.

> **Remember**
>
> Do not be afraid to try out new ideas or adapt previously learned concepts. Most of all, enjoy using your new-found knowledge and take pleasure in the results you will achieve.

Check your knowledge

The following questions will help you to check your understanding of this unit. The answers can be found on page 419. Take care, as there may be more than one correct answer for some questions.

1 It's a good idea to use styling and finishing products on the hair as this will:
   a make the hair sticky
   b protect the hair from the effects of humidity
   c increase the salon's profit margin
   d keep the style in longer

2 The hair should be allowed to cool down before dressing as this will:
   a prevent you from burning your fingers
   b give the hair more volume
   c allow the curl to set in its new shape
   d give a longer-lasting curl

3 Finger waving should be carried out:
   a on base
   b root to point
   c point to root
   d whichever way you like

4 Finger waving on wet hair is used to:
   a produce curls
   b make the style last longer
   c produce waves with specific direction
   d produce volume

5 Setting the hair from wet will produce:
   a a softer curl
   b increased volume
   c a firmer curl
   d less volume

6 When setting the hair to get minimum volume and drag, the hair should be wound:
   a on base
   b off base
   c from the top
   d from underneath

7 When styling hair it is important to consider the hair's elasticity as this will determine:
   a the finished style
   b the temperature of the tools used
   c the amount of tension to be applied
   d the styling products to use

8 Hazards relating to the use of heated styling equipment include:
   a trailing flexes
   b scalp burns
   c hood dryer left on for too long
   d switching off the appliance after use

9 The term 'hygroscopic' means:
   a a product to make the hair shine
   b has the ability to repel water
   c has the ability to absorb water
   d has the ability to absorb atmospheric moisture

10 The term 'beta keratin' refers to:
   a the hair's natural pigmentation
   b the hair's protein
   c hair in its natural unstretched state
   d hair that has been stretched and dried into a new shape

Assessment guidance

You must demonstrate in your everyday work that you have met the standards for creatively styling and dressing hair.

You will be assessed on at least five different occasions and you will have to ensure that:

- you create a different look on each of your clients
- you produce one look using accessories and / or added hair
- two of your observations include the use of different non-conventional items.

Simulated activity may not be used for any part of this unit.

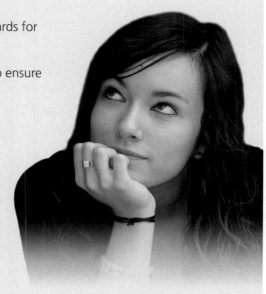

Unit GH20

Creatively dress long hair

What you will learn:

- How to prepare the client
- How to prepare the hair for the service
- How to creatively dress long hair
- How to proceed after the service.

Darren Ambrose

211

Introduction

Many hairdressers shy away from styling long hair, and tend to leave it for one particular member of staff to deal with. However, there is a large market for hairdressers who have the skills and imagination to create a variety of looks on long hair. There are many different ways long hair may be styled and dressed; this includes rolls, pleats, knots, twists, plaits, curls and woven effects. By combining some of these techniques, you will be able to personalise your styling and dressing service, thus promoting your specialist skills.

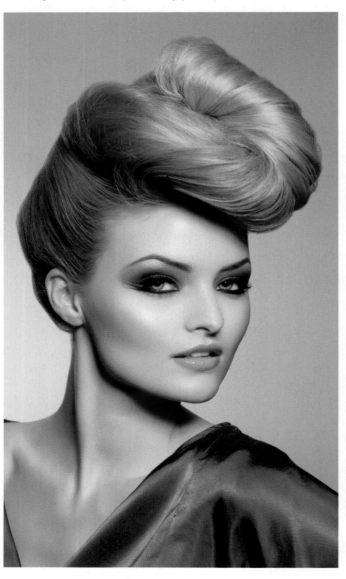

You the stylist

You need to be able to work safely whilst performing these services, ensuring compliance with all the applicable health and safety legislation.

Preparing the client

When carrying out any service, preparation is essential. You will need to prepare your work area, tools and equipment, and your client. You must ensure your client's clothing is adequately protected throughout the service. As a minimum your client should be wearing a gown and a towel. If your client's hair is to be dried under a hood dryer, the ears should be protected with disposable ear shields, which are designed to protect the ears from the heat. The use of a net may be necessary if the hood dryers in your salon have a fan, as any stray hairs, or those that may come loose during the drying process, may become caught in the fan, causing unnecessary harm to your client.

Preparing your work area

The table below provides a quick checklist for what to do and why when preparing your work area.

What to do	Why / how?
All the necessary tools and equipment for the service should be ready	Saves time and conveys a professional image to the client
Any products needed for the service should be available and ready to use	Regular and effective stock taking will ensure that all products are available
Work area must be clean and tidy	Prevents accidents occurring, reduces the risk of cross-infection and promotes a professional image
Instruct the junior staff to prepare the work area correctly	Saves time. Make sure that you clearly communicate what is required – a short list of instructions may be given to junior staff
Tools and equipment for dressing long hair should be clean, sterile and fit for purpose	The appropriate method of sterilisation should be used and equipment should be checked for defects
Electrical equipment should be used in compliance with health and safety legislation	Ensure that junior staff are complying with the safe use of electrical equipment (see Unit G22, page 16). This is your responsibility

Remember

When using heated styling equipment, it should be kept clean and free from product build-up, as this will prolong the life of the equipment and ensure it works efficiently. You also need to consider the risk of products transferring from one client to another, for example, oil-based products being transferred and making the hair greasy.

Personal health and hygiene

The table below provides a quick checklist on what to do and why in personal health and hygiene.

What to do	Why / how?
Make sure your body and clothes smell clean and fresh	The client will feel more comfortable in your presence. Daily washing and the use of a good deodorant are essential
Make sure your breath smells nice	Use a breath freshener. This will help to combat odours from strong-smelling food or smoking
Do not work if you are feeling unwell	Infections can be spread in the salon. Keep yourself fit and healthy to ensure that you produce the best work possible
Maintain a good posture when working. Think about whether your client is positioned properly for your needs as well as their own comfort	This will minimise the risk of injury and fatigue. Make sure you keep your back straight and weight evenly distributed. Having your tools and equipment close to hand will prevent you from over-stretching

Consultation

A thorough and effective consultation must be carried out with the client before commencing the service. The range of looks that are possible with long hair should be discussed so that the client is fully aware of the possibilities. The use of visual aids, such as stylebooks / hair magazines and journals may help to establish your client's exact requirements. This must be confirmed during the consultation procedure and you should check this throughout the service to ensure you are working towards the correct finished look. This will ensure client satisfaction.

Once you have established your client's exact styling requirements, you must consider which products, tools and equipment you should use to achieve the required look. You should also inform the client of the cost of the service and likely duration. All work carried out within this unit should be completed in a commercially viable time.

Check it out

You have responsibilities towards your clients and others in the salon under the Electricity at Work Act. Can you remember what your responsibilities are? List the kind of electrical equipment that is used when styling and dressing long hair.

Remember

When dressing long hair, any pins or grips used must not be placed in the mouth or opened with the teeth, as this may lead to permanent damage to your teeth, and portrays an unprofessional image to your client.

Check it out

Find out the time your salon allows for you to complete the styling and dressing of long hair. These timings should be commercially viable for your salon.

Preparing the hair for the service

Products

There are vast ranges of products available for styling and dressing long hair. The products you choose to use should be suitable for the hair type and texture you are working with, so you are able to achieve the optimum result. For more information on products that may be used when styling and dressing long hair, refer to Unit GH19, pages 205–6.

Influencing factors

The desired look

This must have been agreed during the consultation. You must ensure you re-confirm the look with the client during the dressing of the hair to ensure client satisfaction. The desired look may be for a specific occasion.

The occasion for which the style is required

There are many occasions when a client may require long hair to be styled and dressed. This may include weddings, balls, parties, etc. It is important that the styling is in keeping with the overall look the client is trying to achieve. If the occasion were a formal ball, then a current or classic look would be more appropriate than an avant-garde style. The clothing the client will be wearing for the occasion must be considered, for example, the style of the clothing (formal, alluring, etc.). Also, the neckline of the clothing may limit the types of dressing that will be suitable. The age of the client must be considered, as a young client would generally require a trendy hair-up style rather than a more formal one. All of the above will ensure the end result is not only suitable for the client, but exhibits your expert consultation skills.

The client may also require ornamentation or accessories in the hair to complement the outfit being worn and the make-up that is used. Ornamentation covers almost anything that may be placed in the hair to give added interest or another dimension to the styling. This may include feathers, chopsticks, flowers, ribbons or items of jewellery. However, you must remember that ornamentation should enhance the overall appearance of the finished look, rather than become the finished look. When using ornamentation, you must consider the health and safety aspects of the item, for example, is it flammable, excessively heavy, heat conducting, etc.

> **Check it out**
>
> Discuss with friends and / or colleagues items, including non-conventional items, which may be used to enhance long hair styling. Discuss the health and safety issues related to each one. What are the potential hazards?

Ornamentation or accessories may be secured into the hair in a number of different ways. They may be attached to pins, grips, combs, hair bands, etc. To ensure ornaments are firmly fixed, you may need to stitch or glue them onto the hair attachment.

It is important when planning possible styles for brides and bridesmaids to consider any headdresses or other hair accessories that may be worn. You must ensure that the finished style will sit correctly around the headdress and the elaborate part of the hairstyle will be on show.

Hair growth patterns

Hair growth patterns must be taken into consideration to ensure the best possible result is achieved. You should always try to work with the natural fall of the hair, as it will lie better and the styling will be more durable, and therefore easier for the client to maintain. The hair growth patterns in the nape area must be checked, as irregular growth patterns may not complement the finished look and you should therefore consider other techniques to mask any such imperfection. A widow's peak may be disguised by covering it with hair from the front hairline, creating a sweeping effect across the front of the dressing.

Hair elasticity

The hair's elasticity must be taken into consideration. Ideally, hair that is to be styled and dressed should be healthy and in optimum condition. Hair with very poor elasticity may be overstretched during the styling process, therefore rendering it likely to break. Hair with poor elasticity is often difficult to sculpt into specific shapes, for example, barrel curls, as the hair is often quite inflexible.

Head, face shape and features

Your client's head and face shape must be considered prior to starting to style and dress long hair. Clients with round faces will not look their best with all their hair off the face, especially if there is no added height to give the illusion of the 'perfect oval'. (For more information on head and face shapes, refer to Unit G21, pages 52–4.)

Facial features, such as a high forehead, large nose and heavy jaw line must also be considered. Failure to consider the above may result in a fantastic style that is marred by the client's features.

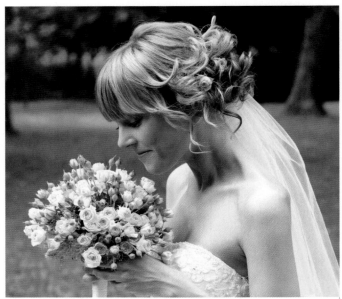

Hairpieces and accessories can enhance the overall appearance of the style

Hair texture

The texture of the client's hair should be considered when deciding on the style to be created. Coarse hair may need to be set first to smooth the hair, leaving it more manageable to work with. Products such as waxes and serums will be required to smooth the ends of the hair that would otherwise look dry and brittle. Fine hair has its own set of considerations. The style must be chosen carefully to gain maximum impact, for example, barrel curls may not appear full enough to create the intended look. Therefore a hairpiece may be needed to give the illusion that the client has more hair than she really has. It may be difficult to hide all the pins and grips used during the dressing, thus not showing your work to its best advantage. Your choice of securing materials must therefore be thought through carefully. Fine pins may be easier to disguise in fine hair, whereas grips may be required in thick, coarse hair to support the weight of the hair.

Salon life

A change of plan

Jason's story

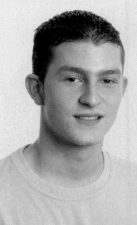

I was really excited to be doing my first wedding. I had been round to see the bride and bridesmaids for a trial – the bride and one of the bridesmaids were having their hair up with flowers intertwined and the other two bridesmaids were wearing their hair down. I made sure I had everything I was going to need; this wedding was planned like a military operation.

I arrived on Saturday morning, and did the bride's hair; she looked fantastic. I'd decided to use a bun ring to create a good shape that would remain secure throughout the day and evening. The first bridesmaid's hair was next and again it looked amazing. The other two bridesmaids then decided they wanted their hair up too. I knew I didn't have time to buy some more bun rings but I didn't panic as I thought back-combing and lots of strong styling and finishing products would do the trick. The first went up really well with lots of back-combing and looked great. The last bridesmaid had very dense hair, but I decided I would just use extra products, grips and pins and loads of back-combing. It looked ok.

I had been invited to the evening reception and was looking forward to the accolades about my fantastic creations. When I arrived at the reception I was horrified, the last bridesmaid's hair looked like she'd been dragged through a hedge backwards!! The style had fallen down and it looked dreadful. The bride was very upset and angry with me and told me I had ruined her photographs and her day. I was so sure I did everything right, I just feel really disappointed and guilty.

Be professional ★★★

- Make sure you have everything you need. It's better still to slightly over-stock to ensure total client satisfaction.
- Make sure you carry out a thorough consultation, which should include all influencing factors.

ASK THE PROFESSIONALS

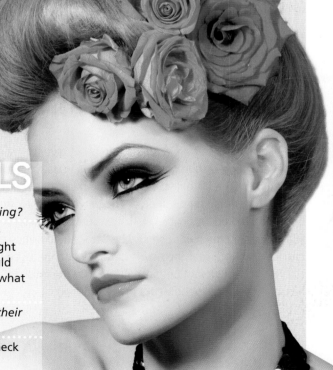

Q *Is there anything I could have done to prevent this from happening?*

A It's very difficult to tell an excited bridesmaid that she can't have what she wants, but in this instance, you were aware of the weight of her hair and should have taken this into consideration. It would have been better to explain to the client why she couldn't have what she wanted than to do her hair and hope!!

Q *I'm not telepathic, so how do you deal with clients that change their minds?*

A It's a good idea to call round the day before the wedding and check that everything is as you have agreed.

Hair length

Very long hair may be difficult to manage if you are dressing the hair in an 'up style'. Equally, hair that has been curled may drop very quickly due to the weight of the hair. Plaiting and twisting works well on very long hair and prevents these potential problems. When working with very long hair, try to dress small sections at a time wherever possible, as this will make life easier for you.

With shorter hair, you may need to create the dressing lower down the head, if the hair is too short to reach the crown. Twists work nicely on hair that is shorter, as the ends of the hair are held together in the twist.

Hair density

The amount of hair that you will be working with must be taken into consideration when planning a style. As with long hair, very heavy hair can be difficult to work with, especially if it is to be dressed up. Strong products must be used to give the hair support and manageability. If dressing the hair into a roll, plenty of overlapping grips should be used to ensure the dressing remains secure. You must check the dressing to ensure the amount of hair you are working with hasn't created more volume than you required!

If the hair is sparse, your choice of styling will be limited, as an incorrect choice of technique may leave pins and grips exposed and the client looking as if they do not have much hair. Additional pieces may be necessary to give the illusion of plenty of hair.

Styling and dressing techniques

Depending on the finished style requirements, the way the hair is prepared may differ. This may be decided by the style requirements of the client or preference of the stylist. Look at the table opposite to see how to prepare for different dressing techniques.

The hair may be wet-set and dried; this will give the hair a firmer and long-lasting curl. However, it is usual practice to dry the hair off a little first as this will reduce the length of time the client is under the dryer and prevent the hair from becoming too bouncy, which will then make it difficult to work with. If setting the hair, it should be set in the direction of the intended styling, so if the hair is to be styled into a vertical roll, the rollers should be placed following the finished result. This will prevent breaks in the dressing.

> **Remember**
>
> Remember to allow the hair to cool down properly after the drying process before you start to dress the hair, as this will ensure the hydrogen bonds are firmly fixed in their new position, thus making sure the styling will last as long as possible.

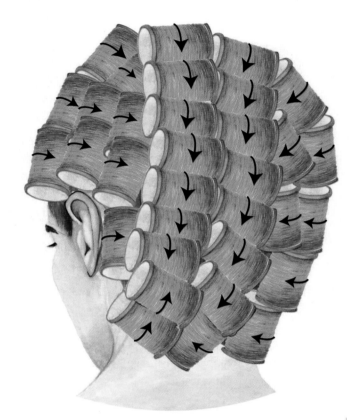

Rollers positioned for a vertical roll

The hair may be washed and blow-dried, then styled using heated electrical appliances, such as tongs, heated rollers, straightening irons, etc. Using different heated appliances will produce a variety of results.

The hair can be washed and blow-dried straight and then dressed, but the hair is usually very soft and difficult to manage. This may be helped by the addition of hairspray before styling, as this will make the hair less soft and therefore easier to work with. Many stylists prefer to work with hair that was shampooed the previous day, as this makes it easier to work with. If this is the case, you must ensure you inform the client prior to the service taking place.

The following table gives you a guide as to how the hair should be prepared for each of the dressing techniques and effects in the range.

Dressing techniques and effects	Preparing the hair
Rolls	The hair may be blow-dried, set or dry-set using Velcro rollers or heated rollers, depending on the amount of curl required
Pleats	The hair may be blow-dried, set or dry-set using Velcro rollers or heated rollers, depending on the amount of curl required
Knots	The hair should be dried straight
Twists	The hair should be dried straight
Plaits	The hair may be dried straight or plaited into wet hair. However, care must be taken if plaiting wet hair as the hair will shrink when dry and this may cause discomfort for the client and the possibility of traction alopecia
Curls	The hair may be wet-set, dry-set or tonged, depending on the amount of curl required
Woven effects	The hair should be dried straight

Creatively dress long hair

If you are looking for inspiration and ideas for creatively styling long hair, taking a look back through the history of hair styling and fashion can prove to be useful. As fashion is cyclical, you will notice many of the 'current' looks are just a variation of a look from the past. The ideas have been tried and tested, but you should be looking to interpret them in an up-to-date way. You may also look at cultural influences.

Check it out

Using the Internet, libraries, books and magazines, produce your own 'style file' of dressed looks. This may also be used in the salon to give your clients ideas of different looks.

When styling and dressing long hair, it may be useful to have a junior member of staff available to assist you to pass pins and grips, etc. Many stylists like to work with the same junior member of staff when carrying out this type of work as they become accustomed to the needs of the stylist. This type of relationship usually develops over a period of time. The advantage of working with the same member of staff is that it should reduce the time you take to complete the task and also give the junior stylist a good insight into styling and dressing long hair.

Check it out

List the tools and equipment that may be used for styling and dressing hair. Find out how to use them. If you are unsure, ask your tutor or trainer to demonstrate for you.

Be professional ★★★

When dressing up long hair it is essential that you maintain even tension throughout to ensure optimum results. If the tension is not maintained, the result will be uneven. Working with small amounts of hair may help you to maintain even tension.

Unit GH20 Creatively dress long hair

Pleats

The French Pleat is a quick and easy way to dress hair up. It has remained popular over the years, especially for formal occasions.

1 The hair being sectioned.

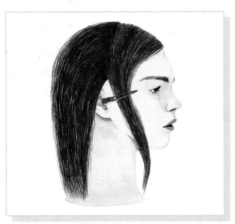

2 The hair being combed across and interlocking grips up the middle of the head.

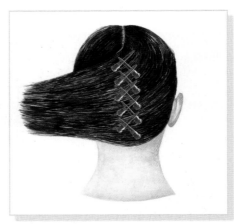

3 Brush the left side to the middle and twist the hair upwards.

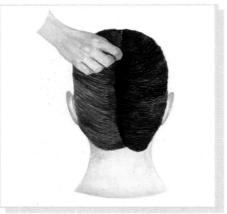

4 The pleat being made.

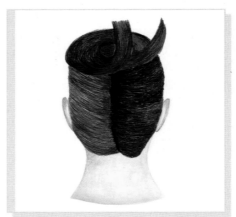

5 Pinning the hair into place.

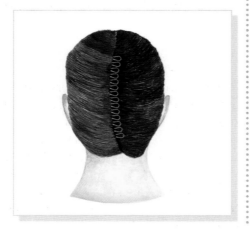

6 Back-comb the ends of the hair (either tucked in for a more formal look or fanned out and possibly tonged to create a barrel curls look).

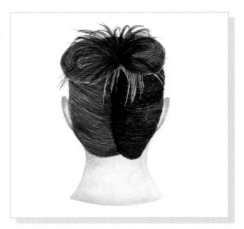

The front area may then be swept, twisted, plaited, etc., as requested by the client. If your client requests a woven effect (see pages 220–1), this should be done before the pleat.

Be professional ★★★

Make sure you have a range of different coloured grips and pins, as this will enable you to match them to the client's hair, thus enabling you to hide them more easily.

Rolls

Rolls maybe used anywhere on the head depending on the effect to be achieved. A chignon is a good example of a roll / rolls in the nape of the neck.

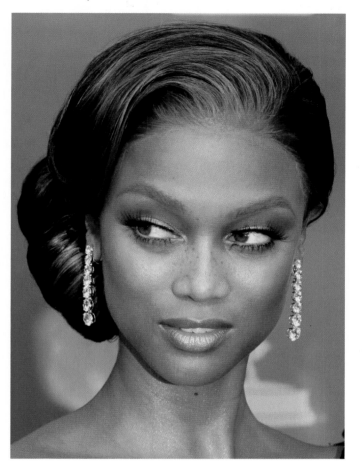

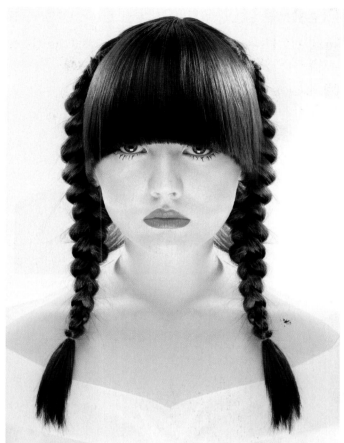

Plaiting can be carried out in a variety of different ways, each giving a different effect

The ends of the plaits may be secured in several different ways, for example, using suitable bands, threads, ribbons, hair, etc. Ornamentation, such as beads, may then be added. Coloured ribbon, thread or hair may be woven into the plait to create a greater impact.

Plaits

Plaits can be used in a variety of ways to produce a number of different effects. As there are numerous different plaits to choose from, the scope is almost endless. They may be used in conjunction with other techniques or on their own.

Scalp plaiting creates a very visual effect and adds texture to the styling. However, to gain maximum effect, your sections should be accurate and of the required width, whether the plaits are intended to be straight or curved. Plaiting off the scalp may be used to create a wide range of effects and, again, will add texture to your styling.

Whichever plaiting technique you choose, it is essential that your tension remains even throughout, thus maintaining the uniformity of the plait.

Twists and knots

When creating twists, your sectioning should be accurate and the required width, whether the twists are intended to be straight or curved. The tightness of the twist will depend on the effect you are creating and your client's wishes. When securing the twist, the hairgrip should be hidden (unless the client specifies otherwise). This may be done by holding the grip in the same direction as the twist, hooking a few hairs at the end of the twist, and then turning the grip until it slides through the twist.

Knots may be used to finish a twist or they may be used independently to create a number of different effects.

Goldwell

Unit GH20 creatively dress long hair

Creative styling: a step-by-step guide

1 Before the service.

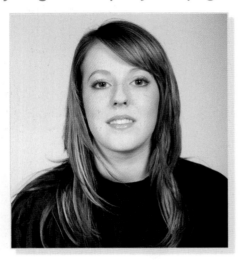

2 The crown area is sectioned off and placed in a ponytail. The front and back left are sectioned.

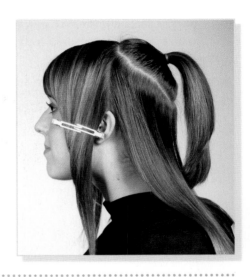

3 Take a one inch thick horizontal section from the front hairline.

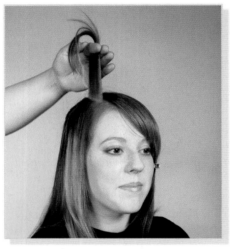

4 Weave the section. Hold the woven out hair securely and allow the remaining hair to fall.

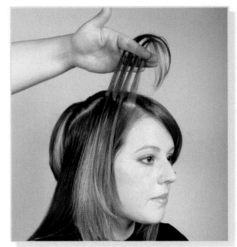

5 Take back a square-shaped section from the front hairline and draw back towards the ponytail, then grip to secure.

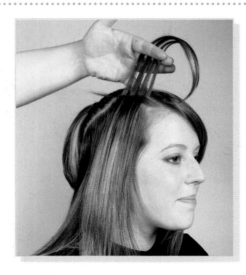

6 Continue with steps 3–5 until the side is complete. The hair will have a chequered appearance.

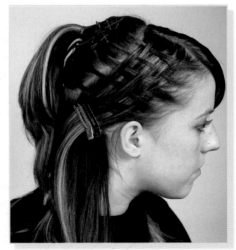

7 Back brush the front section of the hair to create height and volume.

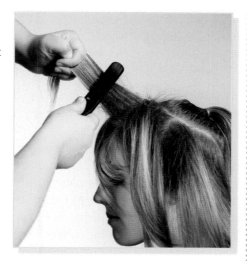

8 Barrel curl the ponytail and grip into place to hide the grips from the woven area.

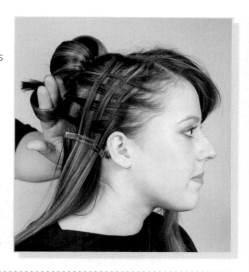

9 Sweep the 'tails' of the weave around and grip them under the barrel curls. Then, twist the bottom section over to the opposite side.

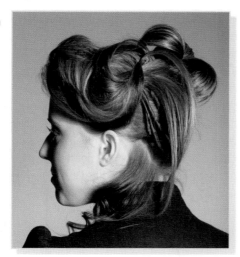

10 Dress the front and sides to sweep back.

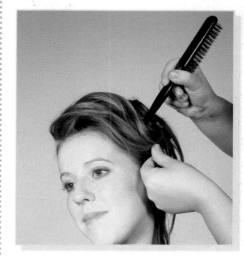

11 Tong the bottom and left-hand section to fall over the shoulder.

12 The finished look.

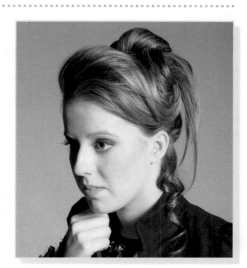

Curls

In addition to dressing the hair up into curls, the curls may be left loose and gently teased out into tendrils. You must remember to use products to separate the curls, for example, wax, serum, dressing creams, etc.

> **Check it out**
>
> If you are unsure how to carry out any of the techniques that have been mentioned, ask your tutor or trainer to demonstrate them to you.

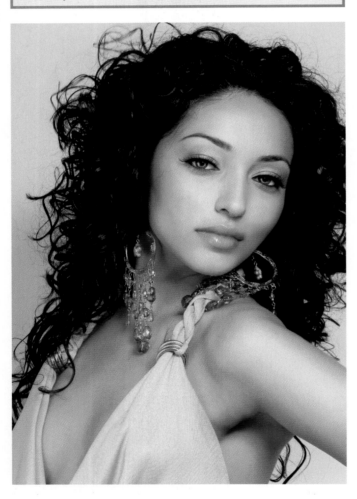

Added hair

Added hair has increased in popularity over the last few years and has seen many younger clients and fashion icons favouring its use. This has had an impact on most age groups and added hair is now instrumental within the styling and dressing service, regardless of the age of the client. Currently there are many different forms of 'added hair' available. They range from clip-on hair swatches through to more traditional postiche.

The reasons for using added hair are:

- to add volume to fine hair
- to add length to the hair
- to add colour to the hair
- for special occasions, for example, weddings, graduation ceremonies, parties, etc.

You should give considerable thought to the positioning of the added hair and how it may be incorporated most effectively in your styling. You must consider the shape you want to create and work around this shape to decide the most appropriate position for the added hair. You also need to make sure that it blends effectively with the natural hair. The base or fixing of the added hair must be well hidden. More than one colour may be used for added interest, to complement the outfit or to create a contrast with the natural hair colour.

When using added hair it is essential that it be secured properly. Your client must feel confident that the added hair will stay in place for the duration it is to be worn. For extra security, when adding a piece that is on a comb attachment, make a cross using two interlocking kirby grips, and then insert the comb underneath the grips. For more information on added hair, refer to Unit GH21, pages 237–8.

When dressing long hair, any pins, grips or bands used should be hidden, unless it is a style requirement for them to be on show. When using fine hair-pins, to ensure they remain firmly in the hair, bend the ends of the pins back on themselves to form a fishhook. This will prevent them from working loose and falling out.

Using back-combing and back brushing

Back-combing may be used for several reasons during the dressing of hair. The method you use will depend on the result you wish to achieve. Back-combing may be carried out as a means of supporting the root area of the hair when creating lift and volume. Comb a mesh of hair up from the scalp, holding the ends firmly in one hand, and comb down the hair from points to roots. Some of the hairs within the mesh will be pushed downwards towards the root area, producing a supporting pad of hair at the roots. This type of back-combing should be done close to the roots, on the underneath of the section using the fine teeth of the comb, as it is not intended to be seen.

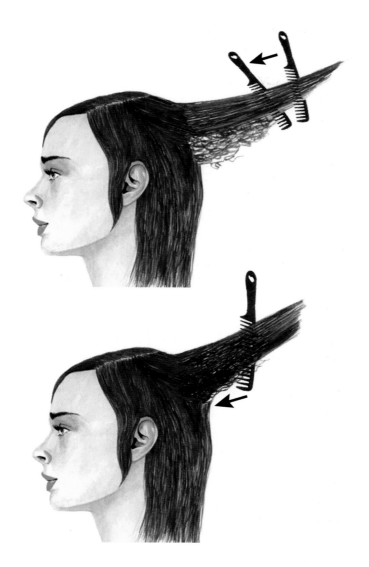

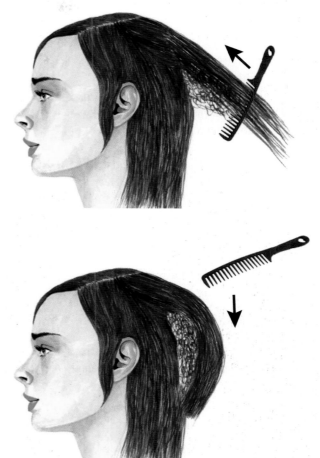

Back-combing along the whole length of the hair is sometimes carried out if plenty of volume is required, for example, with fine hair. It may also be used if the hair is too soft to work with, as it raises the cuticles so the surface of the hair is roughened. 'Teasing' the hair is the name given to gentle back-combing done on the top of the section to blend the hair during dressing.

Back-brushing is carried out in much the same way, except using a brush, rather than a comb. It is more suitable for long hair as it doesn't create too much lift. This may be done on the top or underneath the section, depending on the desired results.

Many stylists prefer to add volume to the hair during dressing by the use of hair pads. These may be bought or made to match the client's hair colour, thus making them easy to disguise.

Avoiding damage to the hair

Care must be taken as physical damage to the cuticles or tearing of the hair may occur through excessive back-combing / brushing, using poor-quality tools or by using an incorrect technique. It is essential that you use techniques that will minimise the amount of damage caused to long hair. Pins, grips and bands must be placed with care to avoid tearing the hair. If using bands to create a ponytail as a base for further dressing, the bands must be of the covered variety. To further ensure no damage occurs, place a grip at either side of the band, hold the ponytail firmly in your hand, insert one of the grips into the ponytail and then wrap the band around the hair until it feels firm, then insert the other grip through the ponytail. Failure to use the correct securing equipment may result in trichorrhexis nodosa (see page 50).

The effects of heat and humidity on the hair

As hair is hygroscopic (it will absorb moisture from the atmosphere), it is essential to use hair products that will help to prolong the style. Most styling and finishing products contain plastic polymers that coat the hair and help to prevent the absorption of atmospheric moisture. They also contain UV filters to protect the hair from the harmful effects of the sun. You must advise your client of the effects of having a hot bath or entering a damp environment after styling and dressing the hair, as this will ultimately cause the dressing to drop. For more information regarding the effects of humidity on the hair, see Unit GH19 page 196.

Excessive use of heat may cause the hair to become dehydrated, as it will cause some of the natural moisture to be lost. It may cause damage to the cuticles if electrically heated appliances are left in contact with the hair for too long. In addition, it may cause scalp burns if used too close to the skin or without due care.

Throughout the dressing service you should be continually checking the progress of the dressing with the client. This gives the client the opportunity to express her opinions and any necessary alterations may be made on an ongoing basis.

On completing the look, you must ensure the shape and balance of the finished style is correct; using the mirrors in the salon will help you to do this. There may be areas of the dressing that require modification, for example, if the style doesn't balance. You must also check the volume of the finished style is as the client intended. Check this in relation to the client's features, for example, does it accentuate the client's large nose or make the head look too big in proportion to the size of the body?

You must ensure that the total dressed look is a true reflection of the client's wishes and your professionalism. Only when you are completely happy with the result should you confirm the client's satisfaction with the finished look. Any finishing products should now be applied to the hair to ensure it remains in the intended style for the maximum length of time.

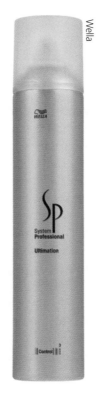

After the service

Before the client leaves the salon, you must make sure you have given them sound advice on the maintenance of the finished style. You should ensure your client is aware of the effects of humidity (for example, they may go home and have a hot bath before going out), as this will cause the style to drop. Your client should be advised on the correct products to use at home to maintain the condition of the hair and the style that has been achieved. This will ensure the client's hair remains in optimum condition; the styling should last longer and give an accurate reflection of the professional service your salon offers. It also gives you a great opportunity to retail, which will boost the amount of commission that you earn.

You must advise your client on how to remove pins, ornamentation, added hair and back-combing. Failure to do this may result in the client dragging pins, etc. from the hair thus causing unnecessary damage. Added hair should be removed carefully to prevent damage to the client's hair and also to minimise unnecessary wear and tear on the hairpiece (especially if it belongs to the salon and the client has it on loan!). Back-combing should be removed from the hair by gently combing the hair using a wide-tooth comb, starting at the ends of the hair and working gradually up the length of the hair to the roots. This way, any knotting in the hair will not become intensified, thus causing additional problems later.

If you have clients who regularly wear their hair in tight braids, twists or ponytails, you must be vigilant for signs of traction alopecia; this will be more evident at the point of tension (see page 47).

Clients with braids and / or twists are likely to show signs of traction alopecia around the hairline, whereas clients who regularly wear their hair in a ponytail may show signs around the base of the ponytail. You must inform your client immediately it becomes evident and advise them to remove all tension from the hair until it grows back. Even then, extreme care must be taken to prevent a recurrence.

You must ensure your clients are aware of the potential effects on the hair, skin and scalp of wearing their hair up over a long period of time. The potential effects are:

- traction alopecia (caused by excess tension on the hair in the follicle)
- hair breakage (especially if uncovered bands are used)
- hair becoming knotted, matted and tangled
- headaches or scalp sensitivity caused by muscle trauma
- infestations (in severe cases this may include cockroaches!).

Encourage your client to book their next appointment before they leave the salon. The next appointment may not necessarily be a style and dress appointment, but may be a cut or colour service. Once the client has left the salon without an appointment, you cannot guarantee their return. However, a client is more likely to return if another appointment is pending. Even a satisfied client may opt to try another salon; this could result in the loss of a client.

Once the client has left the salon, you should prepare your work area to ensure it is clean and tidy, ready for your next client.

Check your knowledge

The following questions will help you to check your understanding of this unit. The answers can be found on page 419. Take care, as there may be more than one correct answer for some questions.

1 When using ornamentation, you should consider health and safety factors such as:
  a whether it conducts heat
  b whether it adds colour
  c whether it adds length
  d whether it has sharp edges

2 When producing 'woven effects', the hair should be prepared by:
  a setting
  b tonging
  c straightening
  d blow-drying

3 Hair should always be correctly prepared before styling and / or dressing because:
  a it's easier
  b it looks professional
  c it's quicker
  d your boss says you should

4 When dressing long hair you must ensure that the hair has been:
  a cut
  b coloured
  c brushed and thoroughly de-tangled
  d set

5 When dressing long hair it is important to keep the correct tension because this will:
  a make it easier
  b prevent sagging
  c make it quicker
  d ensure the style is well balanced

6 Back-combing the hair results in:
  a a mess
  b the cuticle scales being roughened
  c added volume
  d weight gain

7 When discussing with your client how to remove back-combing from the hair, you should advise them to:

   a tug hard

   b brush the hair starting at the points and work gradually up towards the roots

   c brush the hair starting at the roots and gradually work down to the points

   d shampoo the hair first

8 Great care should be taken when using grips, pins and combs etc., because misuse may cause:

   a pediculosis capitis

   b fragilitis crinium

   c trichorrhexis nodosa

   d diffuse alopecia

9 If too much heat is applied to the hair, this may result in the hair becoming:

   a scorched

   b wet

   c discoloured

   d over porous

10 Traction alopecia may be recognised by:

   a a receding hairline

   b total baldness

   c lack of hair around a scar

   d raised follicles

Assessment guidance

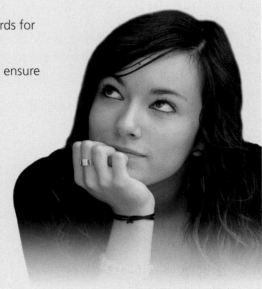

You must demonstrate in your everyday work that you have met the standards for creatively styling and dressing hair.

You will be assessed on at least five different occasions and you will have to ensure that you:

- create a different look on each of your clients
- produce one look using accessories
- create one look using added hair
- produce one look with at least 40 per cent of the hair dressed up and the remainder dressed down.

Simulated activity may not be used for any part of this unit.

Unit GH21

Develop and enhance your creative hairdressing skills

What you will learn:

- How to plan and design a range of images
- How to produce a range of creative images
- How to evaluate your results against the design plan.

Darren Ambrose

Unit GH21 Develop and enhance your creative hairdressing skills

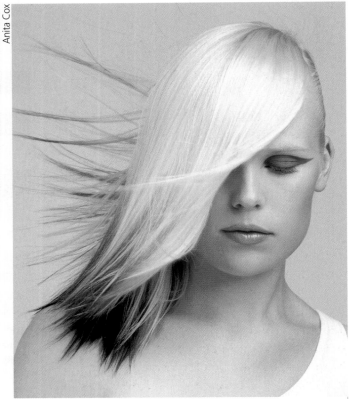

Anita Cox

To create exciting new styles you will need creative hairdressing skills

Introduction

This unit is about developing your creative hairdressing skills in a way that enhances your own professional profile. You will need to carry out research and planning, while exploring a variety of different hairdressing techniques, in order to create a range of images that demonstrate the diversity of your skills. You will also need to be able to work as part of a team as you will be working in conjunction with others. Once you have created the images, you must carry out an evaluation of your results. Finally, you will be expected to look at ways that your images may be adapted or modified for commercial use.

You the stylist

To succeed in developing and enhancing your creative skills, you need to have belief in your own ability as well as confidence in exploring new techniques. Think about the opportunities that you may have for this in the salon. For example, many salons carry out activities on a regular basis, which enable the staff to develop and enhance their creative skills. This may be an annual hair show, which seeks to raise the profile of the salon and increase salon

business. The salon may also choose to use this type of activity to launch the season's new look or introduce the salon's new collection. This may be carried out in conjunction with photographic work, for example, the collection is then photographed and displayed in trade magazines such as the *International Hairdressing Journal*.

Other salons use competition work to encourage the staff to show off their creative talents. There are competitions to suit all levels of hairdressers, from trainees through to very experienced stylists.

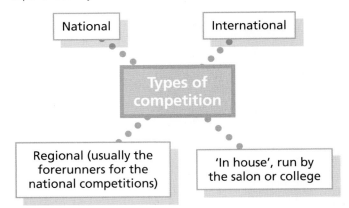

Plan and design a range of images

You must first decide which of the activities you intend to carry out. This will be dependent on your level of ability, the support networks within the salon, the resources available to you and the financial assistance that you will be given. The activities you may choose from are:

- photographic work
- hair shows
- competition work.

Whichever activity you choose to undertake, planning has to be the key factor. Detailed and accurate planning will ensure everything runs smoothly. Without meticulous planning and attention to detail, the activity may prove to be disappointing. You should leave nothing to chance and work on the principle of good time management, which means that nothing is left until the last minute.

Be professional ★★★

Think carefully about your level of ability and that of others involved. Planning to the best of everyone's ability will help to guarantee success.

Design principles and presentation

When creating your image, you should be aware of the basic principles of design as this will enable you to produce images that are aesthetically pleasing, well balanced and express your visual ideas. You need to think about a number of basic elements including colour, shape and texture.

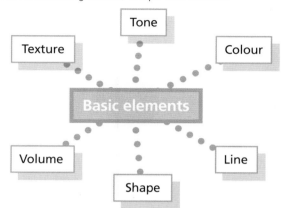

All of the above elements relate not only to the hair you are working with, but also the fabrics, make-up, etc.

You should now consider the design principles and how you can achieve the best effects possible. The following principles should be considered: emphasis, harmony, unity, opposition and balance.

Emphasis may also be described as the centre of interest. It relates to dominance and influence. Do you want to have one major focal point of interest, or do you hope that all parts of the work will be equally exciting? One major focal point could be used for competition or photographic work; however, for a hair show, all the work should be equally exciting to hold the audience's attention.

Harmony describes complex but pleasing visual combinations. This should apply to any work you perform.

Unity could best describe a whole image with no distractions. Again, in relation to competition or photographic work, unity is ideal, as it does not detract from the main point. However, unity without any variation can be uninteresting, especially within the realms of a hair show.

Opposition is based on contrasting visual concepts, for example, rough and smooth, dark and light, curved and straight, etc. – and may be applied to any of the activities in this unit.

Balance refers to the consideration of visual weight and importance on both sides of the image. Asymmetrical balance is usually more interesting and dynamic. All images should have good balance (but not necessarily symmetry) to be aesthetically pleasing.

Once you have been given information regarding the theme for the activity, you may need to carry out some research, especially if your creative styling is based on historical or cultural influences, to ensure accuracy in your design. This information may be sought from the library, trade journals, magazines, television or the Internet.

When you have several ideas, discuss them with friends and colleagues in order to gauge the opinion of others. Remember to use open questions if you require a full answer to any questions you may ask. You may be required to use a varied vocabulary when discussing ideas with friends, especially those who do not have a hairdressing background, as you must ensure your ideas are fully understood by all involved. Your friends may be able to give you additional ideas or information that you may not have thought of, and this may include your interpretation of the theme.

When receiving information you should actively listen to the speaker and ask relevant questions to show that you value his or her thoughts and ideas. When you feel you are in possession of all the necessary facts, you should summarise the key points to clarify your understanding, with a view to developing these areas more fully, but always making sure you remain focused on the purpose of the conversation. This will enable you to develop your ideas further. (See Unit G21, pages 29–32 for further information on communication.)

Be professional ★★★

Keep notes and sketches of all your ideas, as it is easy to go off at a tangent and forget what you should actually be doing! This evidence may be used as a record of your planning. If you are good at graphic design, a computer-generated image is an excellent medium for you to work from. You may modify and adapt your original ideas, while keeping an overview of your intended image.

You will be required to create a design plan that should contain sufficient information and be explicit in its content. Your design plan must include:

- your intended activity
- your objectives (what you want to achieve)
- images that are suitable for the activity
- the roles and responsibilities of the people involved
- the budget you have to work with
- a comprehensive list of the resources you will require
- ways in which health and safety risks may be reduced
- any foreseeable problems and a contingency plan where possible
- the venue requirements, if applicable.

Develop and enhance your creative hairdressing skills **Unit GH21**

Unit GH21 develop and enhance your creative hairdressing skills

The objective of the activity

The objective of any activity is what you hope to achieve as a result of undertaking the task. There may be many reasons for carrying out this type of activity, including:

- positive advertising for the salon, thus increasing revenue
- to increase your personal profile
- to improve your employability
- self-fulfilment.

Whatever your desired outcome, it must be quantifiable in some way. Therefore, when planning your objectives, consideration must be given to the way it can be measured after the event.

Suitable images for the activity

There are two types of image that must be covered:

- thematic, that is based on a theme
- avant-garde.

You should have explicit guidelines that indicate which of the above you are expected to cover. An avant-garde image is a look that is a forerunner of fashion or a style beyond what would be commercially expected.

However, you may create an avant-garde style that is based on a theme, thus covering both of the images together. The theme you may be working towards can be virtually anything, for example, bridal work, historical figures, moods and / or emotions. Some are more prescriptive than others, so you may need to use your own interpretation of the theme.

There are many options for you to explore, depending on the objectives you are planning to achieve.

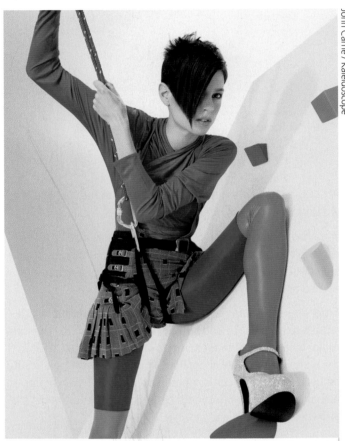

John Carne / Kaleidoscope

A look based on the theme of 'kaleidoscope' from John Carne's collection

Darren Ambrose

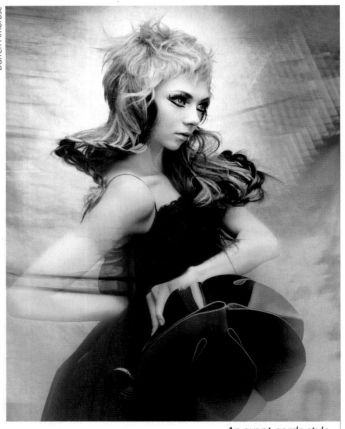

An avant-garde style

Be professional ★★★

If you opt for competition work, it is essential that you thoroughly understand the rules of the competition. Many competitors are taken aback on reaching the competition floor, only to find their design doesn't abide by the rules. This is very disappointing when you have spent many hours practising and preparing for the event.

The roles and responsibilities of others

You will need to enlist the help of others to enable you to carry out your work effectively. Each member of the team should know their own roles and responsibilities and those of the others involved. Whilst working with others it is essential that you communicate effectively to ensure the complete understanding of all of the people involved. Effective communication should ensure mistakes are avoided and nothing is overlooked as being somebody else's responsibility.

When giving instructions to other members of the team, you should ensure their understanding by asking them to confirm what you have said to them. Remember this if you are asked to carry out a task; you should confirm your own understanding of the task in hand. You will need to have regular meetings with the people involved in the activity to discuss the progress each person is making and to ensure there are no problems. The meetings may be informal or formal (with an agenda of items to be discussed). Remember, if a member of your team is having difficulties regarding their specific duties, you should offer support and advise them how to resolve their difficulties. This may be indicated to you by their manner and tone of voice, for example, they may appear quite forlorn and speak quietly. You, in turn, should think carefully before you speak to ensure you don't turn the situation into a huge problem! For each problem encountered, there should be a number of solutions. Your role may be to find the most appropriate and workable solution to the problem.

> **Check it out**
>
> Write a list of all the people involved with your activity and note their roles and responsibilities. Distribute a copy to everyone involved and include a copy on the wall in the staff room. This will help to ensure that nothing is forgotten.
>
> **Key Skills Links**: Level 2 Communication

The importance of working to a budget

Once the budget has been set it is important that you keep your outgoings within the budget. Any activity must be cost effective for the salon, that is, it will not cost more to carry out than the expected long-term revenue the salon can expect to receive. The amount of money you have to spend will vary depending on the budgetary constraints of the salon. Within your plan, you should be able to get a good idea of the amount of money you will need to cover your expenditure. You must be realistic and able to keep your expenditure to a minimum (unless of course the salon has an unlimited budget for this kind of activity). Failure to produce a plan containing sufficient details of possible expenditure will undoubtedly lead to you exceeding your budget. All those little things that spring to mind at the last minute will undoubtedly end up sending your expenditure soaring.

Resource requirements

In your design plan you must state all the resources that you will require. The budget that you are set will impact on the resources that you are able to purchase. Therefore you may need to look at other ways to obtain the necessary resources that you require. Make-up artists should provide their own make-up, although you may wish to obtain specific items the make-up artist does not carry. This must be checked and confirmed prior to the activity, to ensure that you have all the necessary items on the day.

You must remember to include any hair products that you may need to use, both prior to and during the activity. Your salon will most probably provide these; however, it may be useful to contact a product manufacturer or other large business to enquire about sponsorship. Additional media, such as clothing and accessories, may be acquired from other people or hired for the purpose. Your local theatre company may lend you costumes and accessories, although there may be a nominal charge. Check with designer retailers to see if they would be willing to supply you with clothing and accessories for the activity (with a little publicity for them of course!).

If you require props for the activity, these must be included in your plan, but consideration must be given to the health and safety implications of any such items being used.

Health and safety requirements

When carrying out any type of creative activity, health and safety must not be forgotten just because you are not in the normal salon environment. You must still abide by:

- the Health and Safety at Work Act
- COSHH (when dealing with products covered by this legislation)
- the Electricity at Work Act (when using electrical equipment)
- the Manual Handling Operations Regulations (when moving equipment and props around, etc.)
- the Personal Protective Equipment Regulations.

> **Check it out**
>
> Are you aware of your responsibilities under the legislation listed here? If not, see Unit G22, pages 5–7.

You must remain alert to the presence of hazards while working in other venues, in order to avoid accidents. This may necessitate you carrying out a risk assessment. It is likely that the venue will have a designated person responsible for health and safety. However, this does not mean that you can afford to be unaware of any potential hazards, just because the responsibility lies with someone else. You should clarify with the venue manager the areas they are responsible for and those for which you are responsible.

> **Be professional ★★★**
>
> Even if the venue assumes responsibility for health and safety, the salon should carry out its own risk assessment and implement steps to reduce any identified. This shows a professional attitude towards health and safety. You must not overlook your duty of care towards others for whom you have responsibility.

Some possible hazards may include unstable equipment, trailing wires, or stairs the models and stylists need to use to gain access to the stage area, all of which should be considered prior to the event and control measures put into place to reduce the risk (as far as is practicable).

> **Check it out**
>
> List the potential hazards you would need to consider when carrying out:
> - a competition
> - a photoshoot
> - a hair show.
>
> **Key Skills Links**: Level 2 Communication

> **Check it out**
>
> Are there any local by-laws, or other legislation, that may limit your use of tools and equipment that you should be aware of when working in venues other than your salon?

When using any additional media such as props, you should identify any potential hazards that may occur, for example, if using props, are they likely to fall and injure someone, or are they highly flammable? Wherever possible you should try to use alternative media that are less hazardous or ensure that any props used are sturdy in design. This will necessitate you carrying out a risk assessment of each additional piece of media used.

As stated above, most venues have their own health and safety procedures, which cover fire and first aid. You must ensure that you are familiar with these procedures when working in any venue, so that you are able to act safely in the event of an accident or emergency.

Insurance must also be given consideration. In the event of an accident occurring, you must be confident that your insurance will cover any eventuality. You must have public liability insurance and possibly an entertainment licence, but check with the venue and your insurance company to ensure no other insurance is required.

Problems and ways to resolve them

Problems may occur in even the best-planned events; however, being aware of some of the more common faults and ways in which they may be resolved should help to prevent problems from occurring during your activity.

Photographic shoots	
Common problem	**How to resolve them**
Model doesn't turn up for the shoot	Have a stand-in model(s)
Model is pretty but not suitable for the look	See photographs of all models beforehand. Have stand-in models
Weather	Arrange suitable alternatives if the photoshoot is to be held outdoors
Equipment breakdown	Always carry spares
Running out of film	Always carry spares
Time overruns	Stick to the agreed plan
Clothes do not fit the model	Ask the models to bring their own clothes, but make sure they are in keeping with the finished look. Have fittings beforehand to make sure the clothes fit properly. Ask the models to send you details of their measurements.

Hair shows	
Model doesn't turn up for the show	Make sure you have sufficient 'back up' models
Model is late	Within your preparation time, you must allow much more time than you anticipate you will need. You should still have time to prepare your model
Models not ready on time, e.g. hair still wet, run out of hair grips etc.	Ensure plenty of time for preparing models
Equipment breakdowns	Always carry spare hairdryers, etc.
Show overruns	The show should be rehearsed until it is 'time perfect'
Pauses in the show	Rehearse everything until the show is 'time perfect'
Electrical problems, e.g. lighting too low, microphone distortion	Ensure everything is thoroughly checked before the show
Poor seating, audience not able to see the show	Make sure you check there are no blind areas prior to the show
One of the make-up artists doesn't turn up	Re-allocate the work amongst the other make-up artists
Poor choreography	Make sure there have been sufficient rehearsals
Hair and make-up don't look as good under the stage lighting as they did when done in the make-up room	Check hair and make-up under show lighting
Model(s) are allergic to the false eyelash glue	Carry out sensitivity testing (glue) 24–48 hours before the show

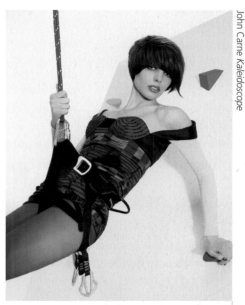

John Carne Kaleidoscope

Clothes are an important part of the finished look

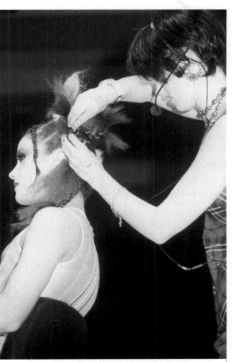

Thoroughly check everything, including accessories and hairpieces, before the show

Competitions	
Model doesn't turn up for the competition	Ensure there are suitable stand-in models
Not adhered to the competition rules	Ensure you have read the rules thoroughly. If there are any areas you do not understand, ask for clarification from either an experienced colleague or contact the competition organisers
Left some equipment or products behind	Ask other competitors for help
Run out of time	Practise until you are 'time perfect'
Equipment breakdowns	Always carry spares / ask other competitors for help

Competition work

Venue requirements

During your planning, you should check the venue to ensure there will be no foreseeable complications on the day. This may include the use of basins for shampooing models, sufficient plug sockets in the correct place and whether the venue's electricity supply can accommodate the possible surge of electricity. If you require refreshments for your audience, does the venue have a licence or the facility to provide food? You must also consider public liability insurance when presenting a show. Are you responsible for this, or is it the responsibility of the venue?

You may need to set up the venue prior to the activity; check whether you can have access to the venue beforehand. If planning a hair show, do you require staging for the models to use as a catwalk? If so, can the venue provide suitable staging for your requirements? Will the staging be large enough to fulfil your requirements?

> **Remember**
>
> You must always remember the 5 Ps:
> Poor Planning Produces Poor Performance.

> **Be professional ★★★**
>
> You should test and evaluate your ideas now and ask yourself three basic questions:
> - Does it work?
> - Does it meet the design brief?
> - Does it need to be modified in any way?

When you are happy with the outcome, all your planning has been carried out, and you are sure you have covered every eventuality, you should take your design plan to your line manager for approval. Any modifications or alterations must be carried out and shown as amended on your design plan. Only when you have your line manager's consent should you go ahead and produce your range of creative images.

Produce a range of creative images

When carrying out this type of work it is essential that you communicate effectively with all the people you are working with. This will ensure that there are no misunderstandings which could lead to problems later on. It is essential that all the people involved maintain confidentiality regarding the activity. This will help to prevent plagiarism by competing salons. If staging a show, it will heighten the impact of the show by adding an air of mystery.

> **Be professional ★★★**
>
> Lighting and music play an important part in any show. The lighting must be bright enough to clearly show your creative work, but must not dazzle the audience. The music used to accompany your work should be in keeping with the image you are trying to portray.

Additional media

Your use of appropriate additional media can add dynamic emphasis to the work you create. The clothing you use must complement the image you wish to portray.

The make-up used should be in keeping with the overall image and should be used to enhance and complement the total look. When choosing a make-up artist, ask to see their portfolio of work, as this will give you a good indication of the type of work they have previously carried out and the quality of work you can expect.

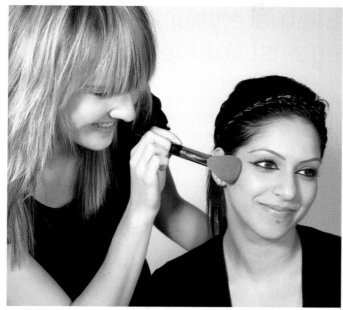

Use a qualified make-up artist to ensure the best results

If different models require identical make-up, use several make-up artists who can work on a conveyor belt system, for example, the first make-up artist applies the base to all the models, the second applies the eye make-up, and another applies the lip colour. As the same make-up artist is responsible for a specific part of the whole look, it should be much easier to recreate an identical image. Accessories may be anything that you would use to complement the image you are creating, for example, added hair, jewellery, etc.

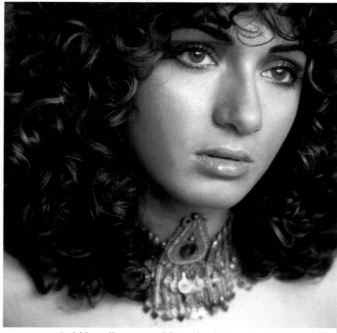

Bold jewellery can add emphasis to your creative style

Whatever image you want to create, you must consider the most suitable techniques to use to achieve the desired effect. You will probably use several of the techniques listed below.

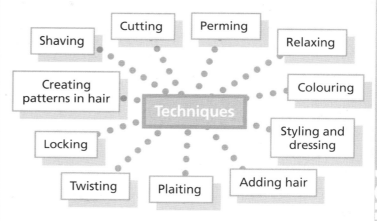

- Shaving
- Cutting
- Perming
- Relaxing
- Creating patterns in hair
- Colouring
- **Techniques**
- Styling and dressing
- Locking
- Twisting
- Plaiting
- Adding hair

How you choose to apply the techniques will be dependent on the results you wish to achieve.

Check it out

Make a list of all the products, tools and equipment available for the techniques you plan to use and the effects they can create. (This may help you choose the most appropriate ones to achieve your intended look.)

Be professional ★★★

Remember to follow the manufacturer's instructions when using any products, tools and equipment.

The use of added hair

Added hair has become very popular again over the last few years. However, for the type of work you will be carrying out, it has never really lost its appeal!

The main reasons for using added hair are:
- to add volume to fine hair
- to add length to the hair
- to add colour to the hair
- to blend or contrast giving maximum impact.

You should give considerable thought to the positioning of the added hair and how it may be incorporated most effectively into your styling. You also need to ensure that it blends effectively with the natural hair. The base or fixing of the added hair must be well hidden.

Most of the hairpieces available are made from synthetic fibres. The quality of these pieces is improving all the time.

They come in a variety of colours and may be used to match your client's natural hair colour or add contrast. However, although acrylic pieces come in a variety of colours and styles, there are limitations to their use.

Great care must be taken when using heated styling equipment on synthetic hairpieces, as they will melt. Some heated styling equipment has a very cool setting, which may be used on synthetic hair; however, you should test it first on an inconspicuous part of the piece. Specialist products are required for styling and finishing, therefore you must adhere to the manufacturer's instructions. Hairpieces made from real hair are more versatile as they may be styled and dressed in the conventional way using normal salon products. However, they are more expensive to buy.

> **Check it out**
>
> Discuss with colleagues / your tutor any non-conventional items that may be used when styling hair to give a variety of effects.

As with any hairstyling, the limitations of the piece will control your choice of styling, for example, if your chosen image necessitates a long pony-tail, the hairpiece you use must be long enough to create such an image. When using hairpieces, it is essential that they are properly secured. Your catwalk models must feel confident that the hairpieces are secure when showing your creative styling. If the models don't feel confident, this will be reflected in the way they walk and carry themselves.

Hairpieces are available in a variety of different forms, from a traditional postiche, for example, a chignon, to fun-coloured slices attached to small combs or pins. Hair extensions are a good idea as they add length and volume to the model's hair, thereby allowing a wider variety of images to be created. Natural or synthetic hair extensions are available depending on the look you wish to create.

When styling hair there are numerous non-conventional items that may be used to give a variety of different effects, for example, rolled or folded foil. African type hair may also be styled using alternative or unconventional items such as drinking straws and rolled up brown paper.

You must ensure that the final image meets your agreed design plan and any innovative features are clearly shown within the presentation of your work. Any work you produce should be of the highest standard if you wish to accurately reflect your creativity. The most effective way to do this is to practise your techniques until you are sure you could recreate the image under any circumstances and in any situation. Failure to do this may jeopardise your success.

Evaluate your results against the design plan

Once you have carried out your activity, you should be actively seeking feedback from a number of people on the impact of your image(s). This is essential if you are to evaluate your design plan effectively and make it better next time. An evaluation should be carried out both during and after any of the activities. During the activity, an evaluation should be carried out to consider the effectiveness of your proposed image(s) and seek ways to improve it. You should have this type of discussion with your colleagues and others who may be involved.

After the activity, an evaluation should be carried out to:

- ascertain whether you have met the objectives stated in your design plan
- gain constructive advice on your finished look(s)
- obtain advice on how to improve your creative skills
- gather any information as to how you can improve in any of the above areas
- assess the profitability of the event.

Feedback may be gathered from a number of different people including:

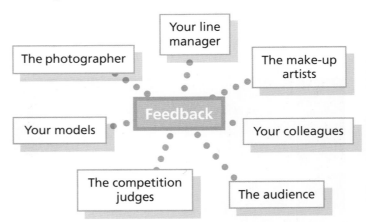

You should evaluate your own performance and try to be objective; in fact, you will probably be your own harshest critic, and therefore feedback should be sought from other sources.

You should try to gain feedback from as many different sources as possible. This will give you an insight into other people's perspectives. Most of the above are professional people who have great expertise in their own field of work and you should accept any criticism they give, so long as it is constructive. Any feedback given should be used as a learning tool that will enable you to develop and progress further in your chosen career. There are several areas on which you should actively seek feedback; most importantly, how your look was received. This should include information regarding:

- your interpretation of the image(s)
- the overall look you achieved
- the artistic quality of your work
- your technical expertise.

Most of the feedback you receive will be verbal. However, when putting on a show, you may wish to ask the audience for feedback. This would usually be in the form of an evaluation questionnaire, whereby several well thought-out questions are asked to the audience to gauge their responses, for example, questions relating to the length and pace of the show, appropriateness of the music, suitability of the venue, communication prior to the show, etc. This will also give you documentary evidence to use when assimilating your feedback and looking for ways to improve.

It is also useful to be able to read an audience by their body language. If they are bored, they will usually shuffle around in their seats. This can give you a good indication of whether things require speeding up, etc. If they are maintaining an interest and appear quite relaxed, this would indicate that they are enjoying the show.

You should look to evaluate your activity as soon as possible after the event while it is still fresh in your mind. In addition to the feedback received from other professionals, you should also evaluate your own performance against your objectives to enable you to identify how and where your design could be improved.

In addition, if the image(s) you created was avant-garde, you should evaluate the design image to see if it is possible for it to be adapted to make it more commercially viable.

Check your knowledge

The following questions will help you to check your understanding of this unit. The answers can be found on page 419. Take care, as there may be more than one correct answer for some questions.

1 Why is accurate planning important when carrying out a competition, hair show or photo shoot?
   a To make sure you don't go over budget
   b To make sure your model doesn't fall over
   c To make sure you don't get electrocuted
   d To make sure you have all the necessary resources

2 When researching a theme, you can use:
   a the Internet
   b the local library
   c TV
   d radio

3 You may present your design plans using:
   a photographs
   b sketches
   c TV
   d a library

4 You must always keep to the budget that has been set. This is to:
   a keep your boss happy
   b ensure that excessive spending doesn't occur
   c ensure that the activity doesn't end up costing too much
   d ensure that you have not made a profit at the end of the year

5 Clothing may be used as part of your final image to:
   a confirm the historical period
   b make the models look good
   c draw attention away from the styling
   d portray a futuristic image

6 You should always make sure the work you produce is of a excellent standard, since this will:
   a increase your professional profile
   b keep the models happy
   c create potential job opportunities
   d please the photographer

7 After the event, you should gain as much feedback as possible. This may be sought by:
   a questionnaire
   b telephone
   c the Internet
   d asking relevant people

8 You should always carry out an evaluation after any of the activities since this will indicate:
  a whether your objectives were met
  b your self worth
  c areas for improvement
  d how to increase your workload

9 Why is it important to make sure everyone understands what you have said to them?
  a To make sure every one concerned can see how important you are
  b To make sure your boss is suitably impressed
  c To make sure there are no misunderstandings
  d To make sure the model is happy

10 What types of hazards can occur when you are carrying out work away from the salon?
  a Spillages caused by using basins not designed for shampooing
  b Colleagues not carrying out their duties
  c Trailing wires and flexes
  d Retail stand falls over

Assessment guidance

You must demonstrate in your everyday work that you have met the standards for developing and enhancing your creative skills.

You must produce evidence of creating three different hair designs covering both types of image in the range. Your assessor must observe you on at least one occasion.

Simulated activity may not be used for any part of this unit.

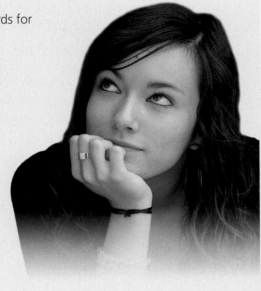

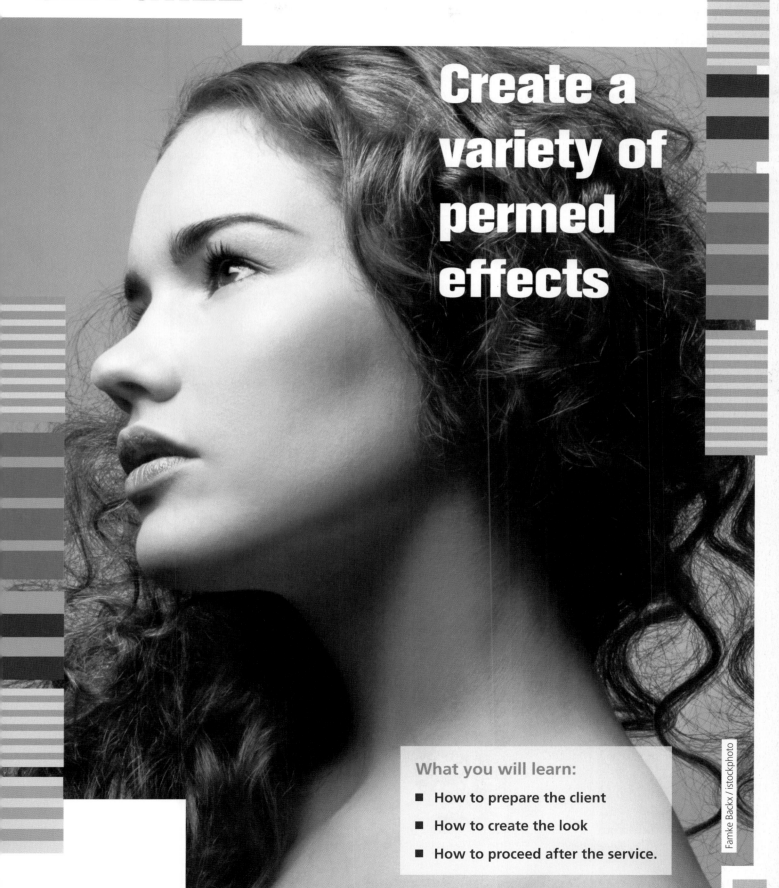

Unit GH22

Create a variety of permed effects

What you will learn:

- How to prepare the client
- How to create the look
- How to proceed after the service.

Introduction

This unit is concerned with providing fashion-related perming services to clients. You will need an understanding of how to create movement in the hair using a variety of advanced winding techniques or how to straighten hair to remove movement. The ability to personalise and adapt winding techniques to create the desired look is essential. Consideration must be given to the condition of the client's hair, especially when working with **sensitised hair**, and this should be reflected in the perming techniques and products used.

> **Sensitised hair**
>
> hair which is more porous due to chemical, heat or physical damage.

Over the last two decades, the popularity of perming hair has drastically reduced. However, both product manufacturers and the hairdressing industry have realised the enormous earning potential of perming becoming fashionable again. Every effort is now being made to educate the public in the benefits of permanently adding movement to the hair. Modern perm lotions are much gentler on the hair and most contain conditioning properties, allowing a more natural-looking curl or wave to be introduced. With straighter looks being predominantly fashionable, the need for permanent straightening has increased and the introduction of straightening products for hair that is not, African type has opened up a new market within the hairdressing industry.

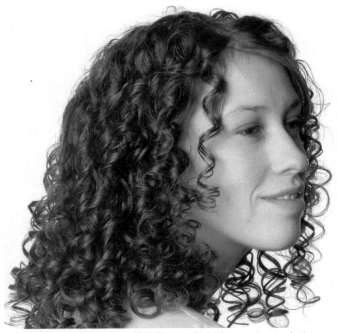

Create beautiful natural-looking curls with perming techniques

You the stylist

You have a responsibility as a hairdresser to be aware of the latest developments in perming techniques and products and sell the benefits of these to your clients.

Preparing the client

In this section you will learn about requirements for preparing both yourself and the client for the perming process.

Thorough consultation

The initial consultation with the client prior to any perming service should be carried out with rigour and accuracy. No detail should be left out; this will not only serve to fully inform you of the look the client requires, but allow you to thoroughly assess the client's hair. Establishing both the type of curl or wave required and the client's expectations of the new look will enable you to determine the correct winding technique and products to use on the hair.

You should be aware of your salon's expected service times and always work within them. It could help to let the client know how long the service might take, especially if it is a complicated wind or the hair is long, and you feel it may take longer than a regular perm. This will prevent any upset for the client if they are expecting to be finished by a certain time.

> **Be professional ★★★**
>
> The use of visual aids, such as style magazines, will help to clarify what look the client requires and also assist you to demonstrate the look you feel is achievable with the client's hair.

It is during the consultation that you should be deciding which tests need to be carried out on the hair in order to determine its condition and previous history. A record of the conversation and the outcomes of any tests should be recorded on a consultation sheet along with the client's record card. This would prove extremely useful if you were faced with legal action following a perming disaster. You cannot always trust a client to be completely truthful about what has previously been used on their hair. You must stress to the client the importance of having a good knowledge of the hair and how this affects the products you are using.

Salon life

A perming disaster

Natalie's story

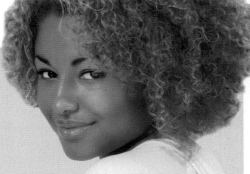

Mrs Hussein was one of my regulars although I had never permed her hair before. When she arrived I discussed exactly what she wanted and completed a record card. I checked whether she had used anything on her hair that I should know about, but she was sure she hadn't so I trusted her that I was treating virgin hair and continued to perm her hair without carrying out an incompatibility test.

When the perm had developed and I started to rinse the lotion off, Mrs Hussein's hair just broke off, with the perm rods still wound, until all the hair had completely broken off her head. I was horrified! I called over the manager immediately and we explained to Mrs Hussein what had just happened, she was in complete shock. The salon manager rushed out to buy her a wig and told me to keep hold of the hair for testing. Mrs Hussein was adamant that she hadn't put anything on her hair prior to it being permed, but I explained that there must have been something that was incompatible to cause such severe damage.

Later we heard from a solicitor representing Mrs Hussein in a case against the salon for neglect. On completion of tests on the hair samples by the product manufacturer, it appeared that Mrs Hussein had henna in her hair and this was incompatible with the perm solution. Even though Mrs Hussein hadn't told me about the henna at the time, I was still at fault for not carrying out an incompatibility test and this negligence meant the salon had to pay the client compensation. Now I always carry out all the necessary tests before any chemical services!

Be professional ★★★

- Always carry out all necessary tests before any chemical treatments.
- If you have any doubts about whether you can perm the hair successfully, then don't carry out the service. Talk the client into something else and make sure they understand that some damage is irreparable and not worth the risk.
- When you have permed a client's hair, always recommend both styling and care products for home use to keep their hair in maximum condition and looking its best.

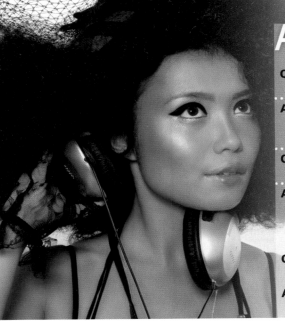

ASK THE PROFESSIONALS

Q *Is it more professional to trust what a client is telling you or should you carry out tests regardless of what they say?*

A You should always carry out all the necessary tests just to be sure, even if a client is adamant about what they have used, as your professional reputation is at stake.

Q *Even if the client had been somewhat at fault, what effect would this type of incident have on the salon's business?*

A As the hairdressing industry is very competitive, it is easy for clients to go elsewhere. This type of incident could have severe consequences for the salon's reputation and business. If the client base drops, then the salon may end up going out of business, with loss of jobs!

Q *What role would the client's consultation sheet and record card have played here?*

A These are important documents to prove whether the salon was negligent; the salon's whole reputation could rely on what has been recorded.

Unit GH22 Create a variety of permed effects

Contra-indications and influencing factors

Both **contra-indications** and **influencing factors** play a vital role in determining the perming process and outcome. Although contra-indications and influencing factors can be very similar, they are not exactly the same.

Contra-indications

these would prevent you from continuing with the service.

Influencing factors

these may not necessarily prevent you from continuing, but would need to be considered in all the decisions you make while the perming service is taking place.

Contra-indications

Contra-indications should never be overlooked. If this happens, you could be presented with problems that you did not foresee. Below is a table of contra-indications and how to detect their presence.

Contra-indication	How to detect its presence
Evident hair damage	Ask about previous treatment of the hair, elasticity and porosity test results
Previous history of allergic reaction to perming products	Ask the client during consultation and look at previous record card or consultation sheet information
Known allergies	Ask the client during consultation
Skin disorders	Thoroughly check the skin and scalp prior to commencing the perming service
Incompatible products	Carry out an incompatibility test on the hair
Specific medical advice or instructions	Ask the client during consultation about any medical advice or prescribed drug use and if you are unsure, then ask them to seek further guidance from their GP

Influencing factors

These are just as important as any contra-indications and will have an effect on the outcome of the perming process. By giving careful consideration to these, you can ensure perfect perming results.

Temperature

The temperature in the salon will affect the speed of the development of the perm. If the room is cold, then it will slow it down; alternatively, if the salon is hot, this will speed up development. If you are using heat to accelerate the development time, you must consider the hair's condition. If the hair is porous or sensitised, then the use of heat is likely to cause over-processing and irreparable damage to the hair's internal structure. Always follow the manufacturer's instructions as some perms require heat to develop.

Direction, degree and extent of movement required

The direction, degree and **extent of movement** required must be carefully considered. It will determine the choice of winding technique, the size and type of rod used and the type of perm solution. In fact, it is crucial to determine your client's exact requirements in order to achieve a successful result.

Extent of movement

how much curl or wave is added to the hair.

Hair condition

The hair's condition will need to be given great consideration to prevent any damage to the hair. The condition will affect the choice of perm rod, solution and development times. If the porosity of the hair is misjudged, this can lead to over-processing and either breakage or a frizzy result. Alternatively, if you do not assess the hair's resistance tendency correctly, you may find a weak curl result and the hair left with a dull appearance.

Hair texture

The hair's texture should be determined to assist you with the choice of rod size and perm solution. If the hair is fine, it may accept perm solution more readily and a weaker solution will be needed. However, if the hair is coarse, it can prove to be more resistant, which would necessitate the use of a stronger perm solution. Determining the texture correctly will prevent an unsatisfactory curl result.

Hair density

The hair's abundance will have to be taken into account when perming. If the hair is particularly thick and dense, it will affect the time taken to wind the hair and the amount of product used. It can also restrict the choice of winding technique for both finer and denser hair. With both of these extremes, consider the time and product used. This should be reflected in the price charged to the client.

Hair length

The length of the client's hair will not only affect the time spent and the amount of product used, but also the suitability of the winding technique and application of perm solution. If you are dealing with long hair and carrying out a spiral wind, then you may have to wind with solution to ensure that perm solution reaches to the ends of the hair.

> **Be professional ★★★**
>
> - Consider the time taken to wind and the effect the perm solution will have on the hair over a long period of time. This could be overcome by using a weak solution on the hair ends whilst winding.
> - You may want to set the price for perming services according to hair length in order to maximise your profitability.

Growth patterns

Any growth patterns over the head should be taken into consideration to prevent problems arising during winding. You must ensure that the growth pattern does not conflict with how you wish the hair to be wound. Conflicting growth patterns can prevent a suitable result from being achieved by preventing the hair from lying correctly.

Haircut

Perming the hair should enhance and personalise a haircut. You should always balance the hairstyle with your perm choice. On completion, the perm should accentuate the features of the haircut, working with the style and showing off the haircut's best features. The amount of movement added to the hair should improve the look of the haircut, not work against it. This should be considered in the direction, degree and extent of movement you add to the hair.

Degree of existing curl

If you are either curling or straightening the hair the **existing curl** will affect both the products used and the technique used. If the hair is very curly and you are straightening, then you will need to use a crème that is heavy and thicker in consistency to help hold the hair in a straight position whilst developing. Also, if you are perming to either reduce or increase curl, then the size of rod used will be important; a larger rod produces a larger curl and a smaller size rod a tighter curl.

> **Existing curl**
>
> the amount of curl already present in the hair, either naturally or artificially.

Tests and testing

The tests carried out on the hair both prior to and during the perming service are essential in order to preserve the hair's condition and reach a satisfactory result. The results of tests that are carried out may influence the decisions you make, especially if they reveal contra-indications. You will need to think carefully about the results and what your course of action will be in order to achieve success. Never underestimate the usefulness of testing the hair, as the potential consequences of failing to test can be catastrophic.

There are several tests that must be carried out and these are:

- elasticity
- porosity
- incompatibility
- skin test for clients with sensitive skin.

Each of these tests has been thoroughly covered in Unit G21 (see pages 40–2).

> **Check it out**
>
> For each of the tests listed, write down the purpose of the test, how the test is carried out, and what the potential consequences are of not carrying out the test. As these have been previously learnt whilst completing your initial training, you should now know the importance of each of the tests. However, if you need a reminder, refer back to Unit G21, pages 40–2.
>
> **Key Skills Links**: Level 2 Communication

> **Remember**
>
> You must accurately record the outcomes of any tests that you carry out. Not only could this prove to be useful if a problem occurs, but it will also serve to assist you with further hairdressing services that you provide for the client. Consideration should be given to your responsibility under the **Data Protection Act** – any information you store on a client must remain confidential.

> **Data Protection Act**
>
> under this law you have a duty not to misuse any data that you store on any client.

> **Check it out**
>
> Are you adopting and using the correct personal protective equipment when carrying out perming services in the salon?

Safe working practices

While completing perming services in the salon, adhering to safe working practices is crucial in order to prevent the risk of harm or injury to yourself or your client. You have responsibilities under certain legislation to maintain safe working practices. For example, the products you use are covered by COSHH Regulations and any electrical equipment must be used in line with the Electricity at Work Regulations (see Unit G22, pages 6–7).

Your own health is important and working while unwell is not recommended due to the risk of cross-infection. Keep yourself fresh and clean at all times — this will increase your stamina to work for long periods in the salon and will impress clients. Also, maintaining good posture while working will prevent the risk of long-term injury. As you will be standing for long periods of time whilst working in the salon, you will soon become fatigued and stressed if you adopt an unhealthy posture.

Always use the correct personal protective equipment whilst carrying out perming services. The gown, plastic cape, cotton wool and towel used on a client all serve to protect during the perming process. As the stylist, you should use an apron and gloves to protect yourself from the harmful effects of prolonged use of perm solution on the skin, which can cause contact dermatitis (see Unit G22, page 16); this condition could stop you from working in the salon!

Preparation of products, tools and equipment

Organising the preparation of everything required before the service begins will demonstrate your professionalism and save time. You must ensure that the products are available for you to use (via a regular stock check), and that the tools and equipment used are clean, safe for use and at hand. Correct sterilisation of the tools you are using will serve to prevent the spread of bacteria (see pages 13–14 of Unit G22 to recap on sterilisation methods used in the salon).

Your salon assistant, if trained correctly, should support you in preparation. Initially, observing you prepare for perming will educate the assistant in what is required. Once they are aware of how this is done, it will save you time if they prepare for you. It is crucial that you maintain clear and detailed communication with your assistant to prevent the misunderstanding of instructions. You may find it useful to ask the assistant to relay back any instructions given to allow you to clarify their understanding.

Remember

Leaving the client unattended while you find the items needed for the service wastes valuable time and will make you look unprepared. This can be avoided by being thoroughly prepared.

Creating the look

This section contains information on how to carry out the perming process and the chemical effects on the hair structure. The benefits of creating or reducing movement in the hair should be impressed upon your clients, especially given the fact that perming has been less popular in recent years.

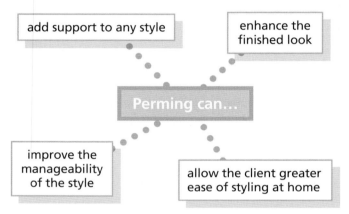

add support to any style

enhance the finished look

Perming can...

improve the manageability of the style

allow the client greater ease of styling at home

By stressing these important points, you may sway your client's decision on whether to proceed with a perming service.

Remember

It is essential that you read the manufacturer's instructions and ensure you fully understand them before proceeding with any perming services.

Perming science

In this section you will learn about the chemical processes and the effects of perm lotions, straightening creams and neutralisers on the molecular structure of hair. It is essential that you fully understand what is happening to the hair structure during the perming process in order to ensure accuracy and success when carrying out perms. If you are not fully aware of the effects of the chemicals you are using, serious problems may arise that could result in you facing legal action.

Structure of the hair

Although you will have learnt about the processes of perming during your initial training, it is easy to forget about the structure of the hair and how it is affected during perming. The illustration below shows the structure of polypeptide chains inside the cortex and the disulphide linkages that are affected during the perming process.

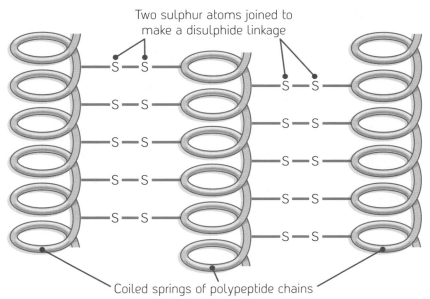

Two sulphur atoms joined to make a disulphide linkage

Coiled springs of polypeptide chains

The breakage of the linkages allows the hair to be moulded to the shape of the perm rod.

The disulphide linkages within the cortex are very strong and can be broken only by chemical intervention. As you can see from the illustration above, they link together the polypeptide chains within the hair's structure. A disulphide bond is also known as a molecule of cystine, which is a bond of two amino acids joined together, that is, two atoms of sulphur joining to form a disulphide bond.

During the reduction process when the disulphide bonds are broken by the addition of hydrogen, the one molecule of cystine becomes two molecules of cysteine, as indicated in the illustration below.

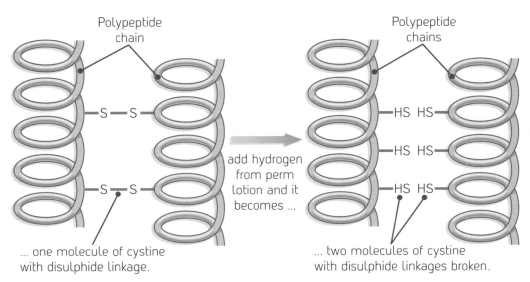

Polypeptide chain

add hydrogen from perm lotion and it becomes ...

Polypeptide chains

... one molecule of cystine with disulphide linkage.

... two molecules of cystine with disulphide linkages broken.

Unit GH22 create a variety of permed effects

There are three stages to the perming process.

1 Softening — when perm lotion or straightening cream is applied to wound hair, it will initially swell the cuticle scales allowing the chemicals to easily enter into the hair's cortex.

Diagram of the softening process.

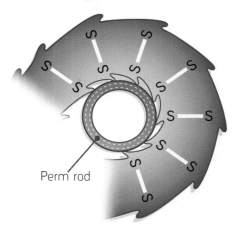

Perm rod

The cuticle scales have lifted slightly and the disulphide bonds are still intact.

2 Reduction — the reducing agent in perm lotion or straightening cream adds hydrogen to the hair, which breaks the disulphide linkages allowing the hair to mould into the new shape created by winding around a perm rod.

Diagram of the reduction process.

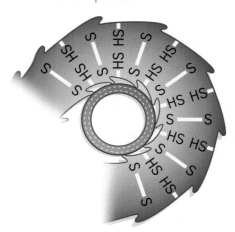

By the addition of hydrogen. 25%–30% of the disulphide linkages are broken during the reduction process.

3 Oxidation — the neutralising process adds oxygen to the hair that attracts the hydrogen, leaving the sulphur bonds to re-form into disulphide linkages. The new shape has now become fixed.

Diagram of the oxidation process.

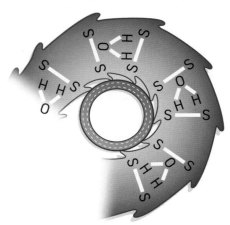

By the addition of oxygen the hydrogen is attracted away, allowing the sulphur bonds to reform into disulphide linkages.

When carrying out the perming process, accurate timing and thorough rinsing of products is crucial. If care is not taken on both these points, it may result in a weak curl or insufficient straightening due to either not enough sulphur bonds re-forming during the neutralising process or chemical damage to the hair if left on too long.

Remember

Only 25–30 per cent of the disulphide linkages should be broken during the perming process. If the lotion or cream is left on too long and more than 30 per cent are broken, this will result in irreparable damage to the hair's internal structure.

The importance of the hair's condition

Once you understand the way in which perm solution works within the hair's structure, it is easy to see why there are perm solutions of varying types and strengths. For example, a client with coarse, virgin hair is likely to require a stronger, alkaline solution to allow the chemicals to enter into the tightly packed cuticle scales. Alternatively, a client with sensitised hair will need a weaker, acid-type lotion to prevent further damage occurring.

If you consider the hair's condition carefully before you begin, then you can tailor your solution choice to the hair's needs. That is why pre-perm tests are crucial. If chemical processes or heat have previously weakened the hair, this will be detected by testing. You must give consideration to the condition of the cuticle layer and the structure within the cortex. If damage is apparent, then great caution must be taken, as the hair will accept the perm solution more readily, which can lead to irreparable damage or even breakage of the hair.

The effects of temperature

The perming process can be affected in two ways by temperature. Firstly, if the room is too cold, then this will slow down the process or even prevent the lotion or cream from working. Secondly, heat will speed up the process, which can serve to save time. However, you need to take care not to over-process the hair causing damage.

> **Remember**
>
> If the hair is already sensitised, the addition of heat is not advised, as the perming process will be quite speedy due to the weakened state of the hair.

Differing types and strengths of lotion or cream

There are many different types of lotions and creams available for use and you will probably have found your preferences. Try not to become narrow-minded and think that the only ones you use should be those you already know. New products are being developed all the time and you should regularly update your knowledge by attending training events or asking technical representatives for advice.

Due to the vast choice we have available to us, you need to be aware of the chemical composition of perm lotions and how they affect your choice for use on different hair types. The table below gives a summary.

Pre- and post-perm conditioners

The use of a conditioner before a perm may sound like a contradiction in terms because we always think of conditioners as creating a barrier to the perm lotion or cream by coating the cuticle scales. This is, in effect, true and if a surface conditioner were to be used prior to a perming service, then it would create a barrier to the lotion or cream entering the cortex. However, if the hair has been previously chemically treated or is sensitised, the use of a restructurant conditioner will help to prevent any further damage. The restructurant works by balancing out the porosity in the hair and allowing the perm lotion or cream to work evenly on the hair structure, thus preventing any further chemical damage by over-processing.

Following all perming services, irrespective of the type, it is essential to restore the hair to its natural pH balance. This can be done by the use of a pH balancing conditioner, which also serves to prevent creeping oxidation. These are known as anti-oxidant conditioners. When used, they not only help to stop the oxidation process, but they also add moisture to the hair and restore it to its natural acidic pH balance.

Type of perm lotion or cream	Composition	Additional information
Alkaline	Aqueous alkaline solution of reducing agents. Ammonium thioglycolate	Stronger and more likely to give a firmer curl. Useful on resistant hair
Acid	Thioglycolic acid activator and alkaline base lotion, ammonia or sodium hydroxide	Particularly useful on previously chemically treated or sensitised hair, due to its acidic nature
Exothermic	Aqueous alkaline solution of reducing agents. Ammonium thioglycolate	Needs additional heat to activate the buffer ingredient
Straightening cream	Aqueous alkaline solution of reducing agents. Ammonium thioglycolate	Lotion is thicker in consistency more like a gel to hold the hair in a straight position whilst developing

Create a variety of permed effects **Unit GH22**

Products, equipment and their use

This section is divided into two parts: products and equipment. There are many products and types of equipment available for use when perming and it would be impossible to have a working knowledge of every one. You will, however, be familiar with the ones you have chosen to work with in your salon. You should not let this familiarity become a barrier to you trying new products or equipment — you could be missing out on something extremely beneficial to you and your clients!

Products

When carrying out perming services in the salon, you must ensure that you are familiar with how to use all the products correctly. This will demonstrate your professionalism and reduce the risk of wastage. Using products economically will ensure cost effectiveness since throwing away waste products is throwing away money! Care should be taken when measuring out products and overuse should also be avoided. You have a responsibility to ensure that all staff, including junior staff, are trained in the correct use of the products.

The products you choose to use when carrying out perming services are likely to be the ones you have a good knowledge of, particularly if your salon uses only one product manufacturer. Do not let this familiarity cloud your judgement on other products available; you may try one that is not only more economical to use, but gives better results. In the table below you will see listed all the products you need to use when perming hair with a description of their uses. (A cross-section of product manufacturers has been represented.)

Product	Illustration	Uses
Barrier cream		Used to protect the client's skin from the harmful effects of perming chemicals
Pre-perm treatments		Used to even out the porosity of hair prior to a perm being carried out
Perm lotion / straightening cream		Used to break the disulphide linkages in order to mould the hair into a new shape
Neutraliser		Used to reform the disulphide linkages in order to fix the hair into a new shape
Post-perm treatments		Used to prevent creeping oxidation and to restore moisture and ph balance after the perming process

Types of perm lotions

When choosing the type of lotion or cream to use, you need to consider how much curl or curl reduction is required, the hair's condition, previous chemical treatments and the results of any tests you have carried out. This will help to determine which lotion will give you the best results.

Check it out

Look at the following case studies and decide which type of lotion you feel will give you the best results or whether you think the hair will be suitable for perming. Consider also the use of pre-perm treatments.

Case study 1
The client has below-shoulder-length hair in good condition; however, the last six centimetres still have the remnants of a previous perm. She would like a corkscrew perm that has a firm curl.

Case study 2
The client has above-shoulder-length, layered hair, with bleached highlights that were last touched up only two weeks ago. She would like a perm to add body and volume but not curl.

Case study 3
The client has a shoulder-length bob but has a quasi-permanent colour just to add tone and shine. She would like the natural wave taking out of her hair so that she won't have to use straightening irons as often.

Case study 4
The client has below-shoulder-length, layered hair and has recently had a full head of bleached and high-lift tinted highlights. She uses straightening irons daily, which has caused heat damage, and would like a perm to add movement and wave that she can straighten easily if required.

Types of neutraliser

You have read about the various types of perm lotions and straightening creams, but you will also find several types of neutralisers available for use. Some require you to dilute them with water on a 1:1 ratio and you must read the instructions carefully to ensure correct use. The neutraliser you use may be a foam-before-use type that is applied using a sponge and bowl, or the type that is applied straight from the bottle that it is supplied in.

Pre- and post-perm conditioners

Although these have been previously covered on page 251, it is important to consider the different types available for use. Pre-perm conditioners, also known as restructurants, are available in small bottles for individual use or larger bottles for bulk usage. Whichever you feel is more suitable for you will determine which one you buy. You need to consider that a large bottle will allow you the benefit of no wastage on shorter or finer hair, while an individual bottle can be sold to a client for use at home.

Restructurants can also be used to aid the hair's manageability following chemical or heat damage, or for use before and after colouring services, making it a versatile product. Post-perm treatments are essential to return the hair to its natural acidic pH balance and will also close the cuticle scales that have been lifted during the perming process, thereby restoring moisture to the hair. They are known as anti-oxidant conditioners and can also be used after colouring services, as this again is an oxidation process. A post-perm treatment will serve to prevent creeping oxidation; this is when the oxidation process continues working in the hair's structure and can cause chemical damage. They are usually bought in bulk for use at the back-wash area and are an essential part of the perming process.

Equipment

There are many different types of rod available for use when perming. You may be familiar with a wide range that is already used within your salon or you may be looking to expand your knowledge and experience.

The table overleaf shows a range of the types of rod available and their uses. Look at the photographs in this unit to see how they are used in the hair to create different effects.

Type of rod	Illustration of rod	Uses of rod
Traditional		This type of rod is the most commonly used and can be used in a variety of ways to produce many different effects
Spiral		This type of rod is used to create spiral curls on medium to longer length hair
Wella Formers		Used to create soft waves on medium length hair
L'Oreal Techni-wavers		Used to give volume or soft wave on shorter length hair
Bendies		Used to create various effects, spiral, curl or wave on most hair lengths
Pin-curl clips		Used to create volume and lift on shorter hair. Must be plastic as metal clips may react with chemicals used during perming processes

Sectioning and winding techniques and the permed effects they give

Goldwell

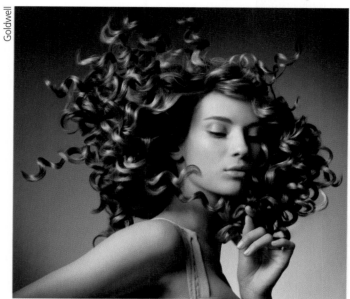

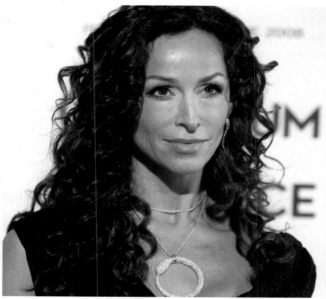

The types of permed effects you can achieve

The way in which you section and wind the hair will have been decided following a thorough and detailed consultation with your client. This section contains photographs of various winds, all of which you will have to carry out to complete the range. It also tells you about the effect you will achieve using the wind; the effects are in bold type to highlight their position.

Piggyback

This wind is carried out by taking fine sections with a section of hair between two rods left out, and wound on top of the two rods underneath. This will allow the rod to sit on top of the two underneath, as shown in the photograph below. They are usually wound from the nape up to the front. This wind is useful when you want to put plenty of volume and curl into the hair, particularly if the hair is abundant. You can alternate the size of rod used to create curls of varying tightness over the head, also giving **textured curls**.

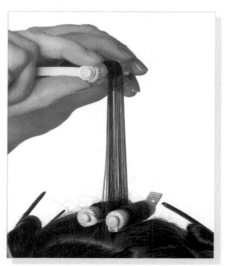

1

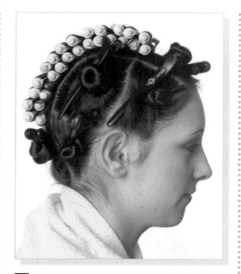

2

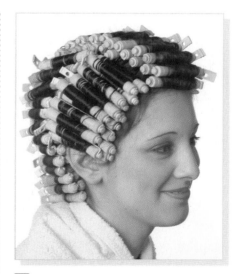

3

Spiral

This wind can be carried out using a variety of tools, for example, spiral rods, traditional rods, bendies or chopsticks. It is usually wound from the nape up to the front. It is used to create **corkscrew curls**, can be carried out on medium to shoulder-length hair and is best suited to a style with some layering.

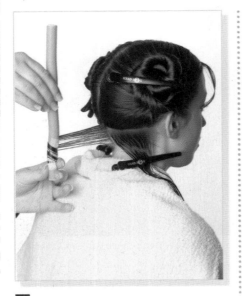

1

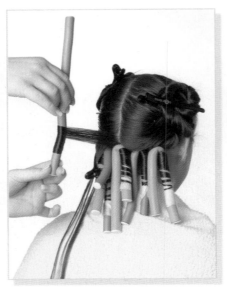

2

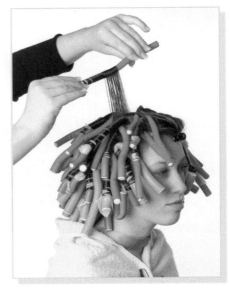

3

Weaving

This type of wind is carried out by winding the hair in any direction but weaving to leave out some as you go along. It can be used on hair of any length and is useful to achieve **textured curls**. Care must be taken when applying perm lotion and neutraliser to prevent it from touching the weaved-out sections, as this hair should remain un-permed. Using conditioner on the hair and wrapping it in packets or clingfilm will serve to protect the weaved-out sections.

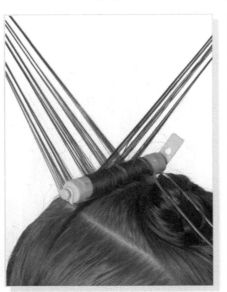

1

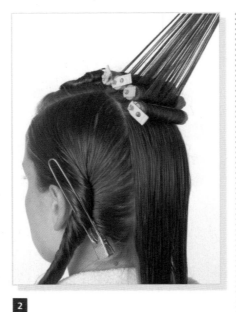

2

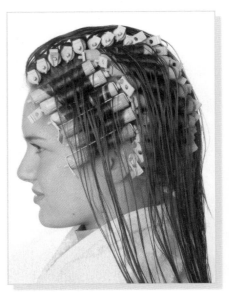

3

256

Root

This type of wind is used to give volume and style support at the root area, known as **root lift**. It is most commonly used on shorter styles, although if a client has very long hair and has a perm that is considerably grown out, you may just need to perm the root area to avoid over-perming the mid-lengths and ends. The ends of the hair can be blocked out by the use of conditioner and wrapping in clingfilm or packets or, alternatively, the hair can be wound leaving the ends out but protected. Great care must be taken to prevent any chemicals from touching the ends.

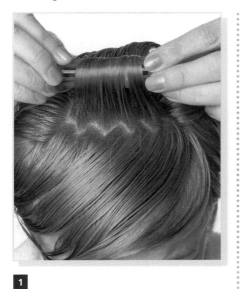
1

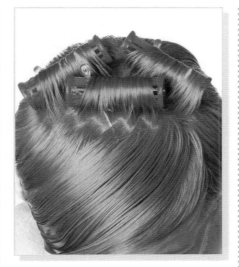
2

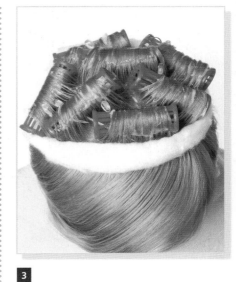
3

Hopscotch

This wind is carried out on any length of hair, except very short, and produces an extremely **textured look with curl or wave** going in various directions. The hair is wound, leaving out a fine section between each rod. The hair that is then left out is wound over the top of these rods in a conflicting direction, as demonstrated in the photograph. It is usually wound from the nape up to the front.

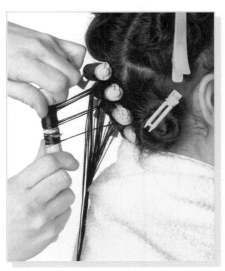
1

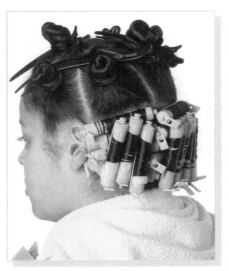
2

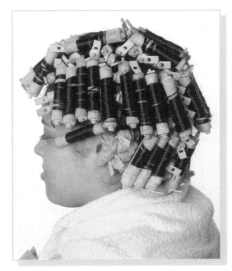
3

Create a variety of permed effects **Unit GH22**

257

Double wind

This type of wind is carried out by starting to wind the hair as normal and then introducing another rod along the section to give the effect of a tighter curl on the end and a looser curl at the root area. It is used on longer-length hair to create varying curl along the length of the hair. It is useful if a client requires a **loose wave** at the root area and tighter curl towards the ends of the hair, giving a **textured** effect. It is usually wound from the nape up to the front.

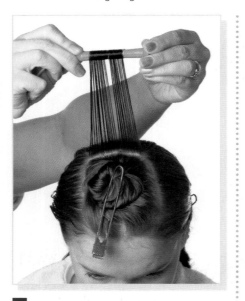

1

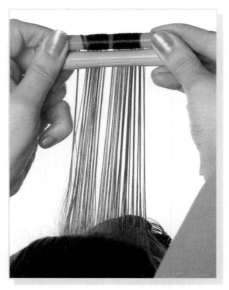

2

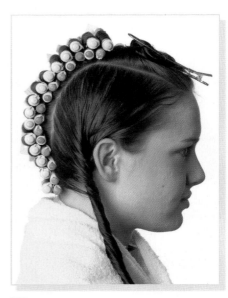

3

Consideration must be given to your application, development and neutralising of differing winds. You will need to judge the requirements of the product you are using and the outcomes of your consultation and tests to determine how to apply the lotion. It may be necessary to wind with solution; however, if the wind is complicated or the hair is sensitised, then application of the lotion after winding may be required. Whilst developing the perm, you may be required to carry out a development test curl and this must be done without disturbing the rest of the wind. Care should be taken not only to test hair in several places over the head, but also to prevent the pattern of the wind from being disrupted.

Once development is complete and the neutralising process is being carried out, you will again have to consider the wind used. It may be necessary to rinse the lotion at the front washbasin if the position of the rods prevents access at the nape or to prevent lotion from being rinsed over untreated hair. Care should be taken to ensure that all rods are both rinsed well and completely covered with neutraliser to prevent chemical damage or straight pieces. This will be more relevant with winds such as piggyback, hopscotch or double, where an extensive number of rods are used.

Straightening techniques and the effect they give

Although most straightening of hair will be carried out with a straightening cream and combed through the hair, you can still wind the hair and perm using a much larger rod. This will serve to reduce the curl and produce a straighter look for the client.

Straightening creams are obviously much thicker in consistency than perm lotion as the weight of the product on the hair helps to hold it in a straight position whilst developing. Great care should be taken as you are combing through as you can easily damage the hair whilst it is in this weakened state with the disulphide bonds broken. Comb using a wide-tooth comb and do not drag through the hair; you need to apply enough tension to keep the hair straight but without over-stretching and causing breakage. Using straightening techniques will create a **straighter effect** through the hair and reduce volume.

Solving perming problems

As perming is a detailed process, there are several problems that may arise. Even an experienced stylist can make mistakes, but if you are aware of how to deal with problems if and when they occur, you will never feel overwhelmed by them. Most importantly, any faults should be identified and dealt with as soon as possible. The table below identifies several faults and the possible causes and remedies of each.

Fault	Possible cause	Remedy
Fish hooks	Hair ends not wrapped around the rod correctly	Cut them off
Straight pieces	Perm lotion or neutraliser not applied evenly; an uneven wind	If hair condition allows, re-perm the straight pieces
Uneven result	Perm lotion / straightening cream or neutraliser not applied evenly; uneven winding technique; uneven tension on the wind	If the hair condition allows, re-perm the affected areas
Skin / scalp irritation	Chemicals used are too strong or have been left in contact with the skin	Rinse affected area immediately with cool water and seek medical advice if serious
Frizz	Lotion / cream used too strong; over processed or excessive tension used on winding / combing	Re-style to remove some of the frizz; apply restructurant or course of penetrating conditioning treatments
Hair too curly	Lotion too strong; over processed; rods used were too small	If hair condition allows, reduce curl by relaxing
Hair not curly enough	Lotion too weak; under processed; rods used where too large; poor neutralising	If hair condition allows, re-perm
Discoloration of hair	Metal tools allowed contact with the hair; presence of metallic dyes in hair	Colour over the affected areas
Pull burn	Tension on wind allows perm solution to enter follicle	Rinse immediately with cool water, and if serious, seek medical advice
Curl drops out or wave comes back	Poor neutralising; excessive tension used when drying hair	If hair condition allows, re-perm
Breakage	Over processed; lotion too strong; too much tension applied when winding or combing; bands placed incorrectly on rod	Use a restructurant or course of penetrating conditioning treatments
Band marks	Rubber bands placed incorrectly on rod	Use a restructurant or course of penetrating conditioning treatments

Although many difficulties may arise during perming, thorough consultation and preparation will help to prevent them. Most are easily remedied and worrying about what might happen should not put you off. You must, however, consider the role of your assistant and you should feel confident that you have fully prepared them to deal with their role in the process, making them aware of the consequences of not carrying out your instructions correctly.

Check it out

Look at the four case studies below and decide for yourself how each problem could have been avoided and what remedial action could be taken.

Case study 1
A client has had a straightening treatment a couple of days previously and has returned to the salon to complain, as he feels that his hair is just as curly as before.

Case study 2
On completion of a perm, while blow-drying, you are having difficulty curling the hair. The hair is frizzing and feels dry and brittle.

Case study 3
After neutralising a perm, you notice that the front section on the side of the head appears to have little or no curl in it.

Case study 4
While a perm is processing, a client complains that the lotion feels as if it is burning her scalp. On inspection you notice the scalp looks very red.

After the service

After the service you will need to dispose of any waste materials or products safely and complete an accurate record of the service carried out. You must also give your client advice on how to maintain and care for the perm at home.

Disposal of waste

On completion of the service, you must dispose of waste following your salon's policies and legislative requirements. Waste chemicals should be washed down the sink and not put into the general waste bin; this will prevent the risk of contact by an unsuspecting person. Any other waste, such as end papers or cotton wool, must be placed in a covered bin along with empty containers.

After-care advice

You have a duty to your clients to ensure they understand how to look after their new look, make sure they understand when they need to come back for further services and if possible book before they leave the salon to ensure their return. During your initial consultation you discussed lifestyle factors and whether a perming treatment is suitable for them. However, discuss it again during after-care advice and ensure they understand the time needed to style the hair and the physical effects that activities such as swimming will have; make sure they leave the salon with the correct products to care for their new look. How your clients maintain their hair on leaving the salon will advertise your work. Initially, the hair will be fragile after perming and care must be taken when styling not to apply too much tension. This might not only cause the hair to stretch and possibly break, but also runs the risk of pulling out the perm, leaving the hair straight again. Consider also advising on the use of heated appliances, as the hair is fragile and unnecessary added heat can cause breakage or irreparable damage. If heated appliances, such as straightening irons, are to be used, then advise against excessive use and tell your clients to always use a heat protection product first.

Check it out

Produce a table of products that you can use to summarise the uses of products in the salon, stating if they are to be used on wet or dry hair, on curly, wavy or straight looks, with or without use of heat.

 Key Skills Links: Level 2 Communication

Always thoroughly discuss with the client the effect a perming service has on future services in the salon. They must understand the need for regular trimming to maintain the curl or how often the root area will need re-perming or straightening. Most importantly, make sure you advise on what restrictions it puts on future chemical services, such as colouring.

Products for home use

You should be advising the client to use a suitable shampoo and conditioner for curly / permed hair and also recommending the correct styling products to use to create the finished look. Successful management of the permed look will depend on using the correct styling products and how the hair is styled into place. There are styling products available specifically for permed and curly hair such as mousses, curl-defining cream and anti-frizz serum. Explain how these work on the hair and tell the client the benefit of using them. If he or she has had a straightening treatment, then you should also advise on using anti-humidity type products to prevent the hair from starting to wave after styling.

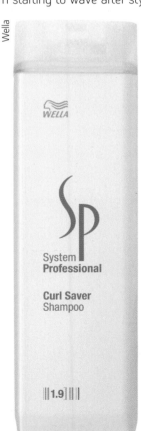

You should advise your client to use products specifically for permed hair

Completion of the record card

Completing the record card after the service is an essential requirement. It will keep a record of what has previously been used on a client's hair, providing you with a history, which is important when making further decisions on chemical processes. The diagram below indicates the minimum amount of information that should be stored on the card.

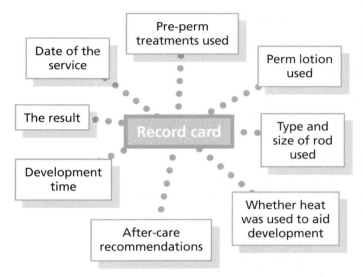

This information needs to be accurate, legible and up to date. Under the Data Protection Act, you are responsible for maintaining the information and ensuring its confidentiality. If any problems arise from the perming service, the information contained on the card will prove to be useful, especially if the client takes legal action against you. Accurate information could help to prove your competence.

Check your knowledge

The following questions will help you to check your understanding of this unit. The answers can be found on page 417. Take care, as there may be more than one correct answer for some questions.

1 Why should you record client responses to questioning during a consultation before a perming service?
  a To take up more of the client's time
  b So the client thinks you know what you are doing
  c To be sure that there is no misunderstanding
  d In case the information has to be reviewed at a later date

2 What important influencing factors must be taken into consideration before the perming service?
  a The hair's condition
  b If the client is going straight to work after the perming service
  c If the client has any unusual growth patterns
  d If the client has any open wounds on the scalp

3 What, if any, tests should be carried out on the hair before the perming service?
  a An elasticity test
  b No tests are required
  c A porosity test
  d A strand test

4 What type of personal protective equipment should you use during the perming service?
  a You don't really need any
  b A cutting collar
  c Gown
  d Cotton wool

5 Which strong bonds are broken during the reduction process?
  a Salt linkages
  b Fraternal bonds
  c Hydrogen bonds
  d Disulphide linkages

6 What factors might cause the hair to over-process during perming?
  a If the hair is already very porous
  b If the perm lotion is left on too long
  c If the perm lotion is not left on long enough
  d If the neutraliser is not left on long enough

7 Why would you use a pre-perm treatment?
  a To give the hair shine
  b So it is easier to wind
  c To even out porosity along the hair length
  d To help prevent damage to the hair

8 What is the effect on the hair of using an anti-oxidant conditioner?
  a It protects the hair from humidity
  b It prevents static in the hair
  c It makes the hair smell nice
  d It restores moisture and pH balance to the hair

9 Why would you recommend products specifically for permed hair following a perming service?
  a To ensure that the added curl or wave is maintained
  b To allow a colour to be applied soon after
  c To prevent the client from having to have the hair cut shorter
  d To keep the hair in the best condition possible

10 If a perm 'drops out' can you re-perm straight away?
  a Yes without delay
  b Only if the hair's condition allows
  c Not for at least three months
  d Not until you feel all the perm has grown out

Assessment guidance

This perming unit is all about providing fashion-related perming services for men and women. You will have to demonstrate on several clients how to personalise and adapt a variety of advanced perm-winding techniques across the range of permed effects to include:

- straightened
- root lifted
- waved
- corkscrewed
- textured curls.

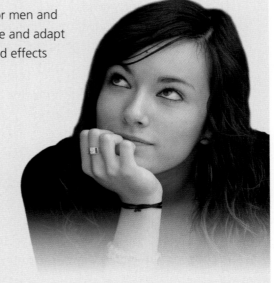

You will also need to demonstrate that you are able to successfully perm sensitised hair without causing any further damage to the hair.

Simulated activity is not allowed for any part of this unit.

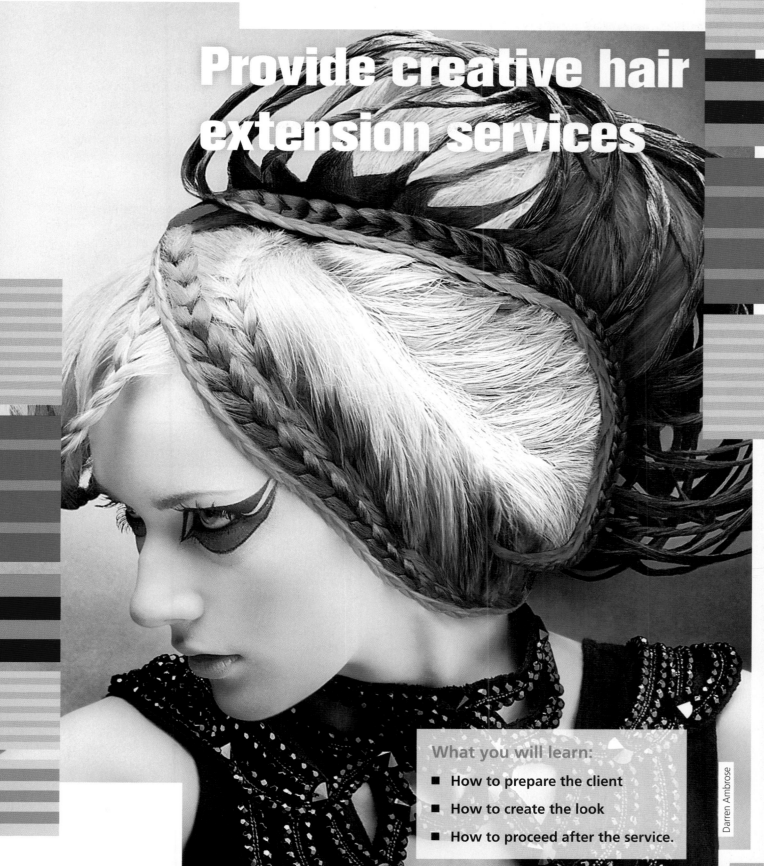

Unit GH23

Provide creative hair extension services

What you will learn:

- How to prepare the client
- How to create the look
- How to proceed after the service.

Introduction

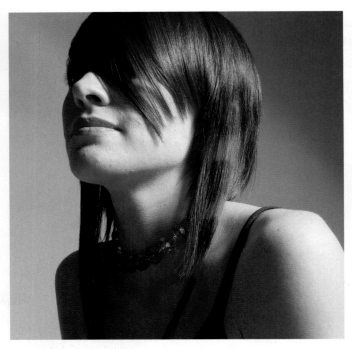

Throughout this unit we will be looking at how to provide creative hair-extension services. This service has become increasingly popular and requires a high level of skill and expertise.

Within the hair-extension service, you will be expected to:
● prepare the client's hair
● creatively select and blend the hair extensions
● place the hair extensions to add length, colour and / or volume
● cut the added hair effectively to blend with the natural hair
● innovatively style and finish the hair
● advise the client on the maintenance and removal of the new extensions.

You the stylist

You need to be skilled in using both hot and cold attachment systems, covering both full and partial head applications. You must be able to work effectively with both synthetic fibre and human hair and complete the look by creatively cutting, styling and finishing the service, ensuring a thorough blending of added and natural hair. The service you provide should be of an excellent standard, thus promoting yourself and the salon in a positive manner.

As this may be a lengthy service, you must always ensure that your clients are aware of the length of time required to perform the service and the cost.

Preparing the client

Thorough consultation

Prior to any hairdressing service a full and thorough consultation is essential. On completion of Unit G21 you will understand why this is a crucial part of the service that you must pay particular attention to. A number of things could go wrong without the consultation taking place that would leave you liable for legal proceedings and maybe even prosecution. Therefore you must pay it proper attention and ensure you record your discussion clearly and accurately so that any misunderstandings can be clarified should the need arise. You must explain in detail about how the procedure is carried out, proper maintenance and correct removal of the extensions, so that your client fully understands what they are taking on.

Be professional ★★★

Always inform a client of the expected length of service time, as with hair extensions this can be a particularly long time (sometimes a full day) and they may need to prepare for this. The type and number of extensions required will determine the time needed.

Check it out

What are the expected service times for the different attachment processes used in your salon?

Be professional ★★★

It is important to remember that some clients may experience some anxieties both before and during the extension service.
● You may need to explain the process to the client so they understand every step of the way.
● It may be that the client can't visualise the finished look, in which case it would be useful to have a portfolio of completed work that they can look through.
● The client may be experiencing some discomfort, in which case you should apply less tension and make sure you check the client is comfortable at regular intervals.

During consultation (remember that this continues throughout the service) the following tests may need to be carried out to determine the hair's suitability for hair extensions, and these must always be recorded on the client's record card for future reference:
● elasticity test
● skin test
● pull test.

Below is a table of the tests you may be required to carry out, their purposes and the consequences if you do not use them.

Type of test	Purpose of the test	How to carry out the test	When to carry out the test	Expected results	Potential consequences of not carrying out the test
Elasticity	Used to ensure the hair will withstand extensions being added	Hold a few strands of hair between the fingers and thumbs and pull gently. Best carried out when the hair is wet	Prior to the service	The hair should stretch and return to its original length. If the hair stretches and does not return to its original length, this indicates the presence of internal damage	The hair may overstretch and / or break. The extension service must not be carried out until the hair is in better condition
Skin	Used before the service to check for any allergic reaction to the products being used, for example glue	Cleanse a small area of skin behind the ear. Apply a small amount of the potential allergen (bonding glue) to the cleansed area	24–48 hours before the service	**A negative reaction** There has been no reaction at all. The skin looks as it did before the skin test took place **A positive reaction** This can vary from redness and mild irritation to severe swelling rendering the client unable to close their eyes, speak or breathe properly	The client may have an allergic reaction and should be referred to their GP. If the reaction has been to the bonding glue, then you could try either sewn in or plaited extensions. If the reaction has been to the added hair, then the service may not be possible
Pull	Carried out during the service to check if the hair extensions have the correct tension	Gently but with enough tension to pull at the hair, tug on the added hair to ensure it stays attached	At intervals throughout the extension service	The added hair should feel firmly attached and not become loose or come out upon tension being applied	The extensions could become loose or fall out within hours or days of the service being completed

It is important to follow the manufacturer's instructions relating to the above tests to ensure the well-being of the client and optimise the results of the service.

Checking for contra-indications and influencing factors

Contra-indications include things such as:

- skin sensitivities
- history of previous allergic reactions
- hair and scalp disorders
- medical advice or instructions.

To determine the presence of these you will have to visually check the hair and scalp and ask your client relevant questions. Some may be evident, for example, hair and scalp disorders such as psoriasis (see page 48 Unit G21) but others will rely on you questioning the client to determine their presence. You cannot visually check that a client has a history of allergic reactions to products!

Be professional ★★★

Always record the results of tests carried out on the hair and your clients' responses to questions relating to any contra-indications they may or may not have, as this will:

- promote a professional image
- ensure you have the necessary documentation should legal proceedings arise
- provide you with a history of your clients' treatment in your salon
- provide you with a history of your clients' previous allergies, skin sensitivities or medical treatment.

Remember

If you always follow the consultation sheet, you will never forget to ask the right questions.

Check it out

There are many different types of alopecia, all with different distinguishing characteristics. Make a list of the different types of alopecia and how you would recognise them. Refer back to Unit G21 pages 47–8 for help if necessary.

 Key Skills Links: Level 2 Communication

Influencing factors should be considered to ensure the best result possible. These are detailed in the following table.

Factor	Why it needs to be considered
Attachment method	Is the hair of suitable texture, density or length?
Direction and fall of the hair extensions	To ensure there is no unnecessary tension placed upon the hair
The quantity of added hair	To ensure you use the correct amount
The need to blend client's hair and hair extensions	So the finish is as natural as possible
Head and face shape	To suit the client
Hair growth pattern	So there is no conflict which could cause excessive tension and prevent the hair from lying correctly
Client's own hair length	To determine which technique to use and whether there is enough length to add hair
Hair texture	To ensure it matches the texture of the added hair so it looks as natural as possible
Hair density	To ensure the client has enough hair present to blend the extensions well or to take the weight
Hair elasticity	To prevent breakage
Evident hair damage	To prevent further damage
Traction alopecia	No extensions should be added
Lifestyle	To ensure they suit the client's lifestyle and have the time to maintain them. Some sports, such as high contact or swimming should be avoided as they could result in damage to the extended hair
Hairstyle	So the added hair and the current style blend well to look as natural as possible

There are several factors that need to be considered prior to the extension service that relate to the hair and skin. It's essential that you can recognise the signs of traction alopecia and what may cause this.

Traction alopecia may be recognised by hair loss at the point of tension, the hair becomes sparse and the follicles are raised. The client may also complain of a sensitive scalp. This is caused by excessive tension on the hair. If a client presents with any of these symptoms, you should not continue with the extension service but refer them to either a trichologist or their GP.

Safe working practices

In the salon there are several health and safety considerations that you must be aware of. Your own personal health and hygiene are important. If you are feeling unwell or run down, then it will be difficult for you to keep up the pace in the salon and you run the risk of passing an infection on to others. You should keep yourself clean and fresh at all times to avoid causing offence to your clients or colleagues.

Your posture while working in the salon is another important consideration. You will soon become fatigued and stressed if you adopt an unhealthy posture whilst working. Bear this in mind and it will prevent any long-term stress or injury to your body. You should avoid standing in the same position for too long and move about as much as you can. If you are finding it difficult to access certain parts of the head during the hair extension service, you must ask the client to assist you by moving their head. This will prevent you from working in an awkward position and help to maintain good posture. Take care though, as both you and your client may be holding a position for long periods of time during the extension service and you need to stop and stretch regularly and give the client a chance to do the same.

The personal protective equipment that you need to use is essential to prevent the risk of damage to clothing or accidents to both yourself and the client. As a minimum, your client should be wearing a gown and towel; you may also wish to use a cutting collar or cape during the cutting service to protect the client from hair clippings.

Certain chemicals are known to cause **contact dermatitis** and it is essential that you protect your hands when working. You can do this by wearing single-use gloves (vinyl or nitrile types) when working with irritants and ensure they are not re-used. Make sure you dry your hands thoroughly and regularly apply hand cream to prevent the hands from drying out.

> **Contact dermatitis**
>
> an inflammatory condition of the skin (most commonly affecting the hands of hairdressers). It can result in dryness, itching, redness, flaking, swelling and blistering.

> **Check it out**
>
> Are you aware of the 'Bad Hand Day' campaign? If not, log on to www.habia.org for more information. You may also refer back to page 16 of Unit G22 for more information.
>
> **Key Skills Links**: Level 2 Communication & Level 1 ICT

Preparation of hair, tools and equipment

The client's natural hair should be prepared before the hair extension service. For all systems the hair should be shampooed, conditioned and dried. When applying fusion or bonding systems, oil-type products shouldn't be used; however, when using sewing or plaited extensions, the use of oil is acceptable.

> **Remember**
>
> Always read the manufacturer's instructions relating to preparing the natural hair. This will ensure maximum results from the extension service.

Preparing the tools and work area

When preparing your work area, it is essential that all your tools are clean and sterilised. For more information regarding methods of sterilisation, refer to Unit G22 pages 13–14.

> **Check it out**
>
> Are you aware of your responsibilities relating to COSHH and the Electricity at Work Act? If you're not sure, refer to pages 6–7 of Unit G22.

Your work area should be kept clean and tidy throughout the service as this promotes a professional image and reduces the risk of cross-infection or infestation, thus maintaining good levels of hygiene.

All tools and equipment should be close to hand to ensure an efficient service takes place and to prevent you from over-stretching, which could result in injury. Working safely throughout the service will give the client confidence in the service you are providing.

> **Remember**
>
> Try to keep the hair for adding neat, as this will prevent it from falling on the floor. You should also consider hair cuttings from the cutting service as both of these will create a slippery surface. Ask your assistant to ensure the floor is swept at regular intervals.

Creating the look

You need to be a skilled hair extension specialist and have the necessary expertise to select, blend and place hair extensions to add length, colour and /or volume to your client's hair. You must also be able to cut and finish your client's hair ensuring that the extensions blend with the natural hair.

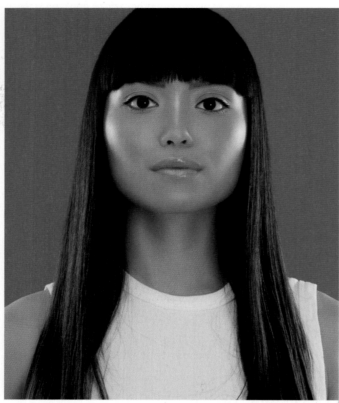

Hair extensions add length and a whole new dimension to the hair

Attachment systems

There are two types of attachment systems that you will need to be competent at using in this unit and they are hot and cold.

Hot attachment: any kind of system where heat is used to apply the extensions, such as using an applicator with hot glue, also known as fusion or bonding. Fusion uses a cold spirit-based gum that needs heat to hold the wefts in place.

Cold attachment: any kind of system where heat is not used, such as sewn-in wefts or plaited extensions.

Be professional ★★★

You must have full and thorough training in how to use any attachment system to prevent damage to the hair, but especially so with a hot system as there is the added risk of burning yourself or the client.

Hot attachment (bonding or fusion)

Different product companies may have different methods of attachment using glue that is already attached to the hair extensions, or separately that you need to apply yourself. Below is a description of how to apply hair extensions using separate glue and the step-by-step guide overleaf shows how to apply them using hair with the glue already attached.

The process

- If you are carrying out a full head, always start from the bottom and work up the head, take triangular sections without gaps.
- Draw the extension hair from the drawing boards (or mixing mats) and blend if necessary, then trim the ends so that you have a straight, clean edge to work with.
- Apply the glue to the trimmed ends (away from the client's own hair) and place under the receiving section, about 5mm away from the scalp to avoid unnecessary tension which could result in breakage.
- Using the silicone pad to protect your fingertips from the heat, push and roll the added hair into the section with your fingertips to ensure the glue bonds the two together. This creates a bead where the two are joined.
- Work across the row, always checking for any stray hairs that have been bonded into the wrong extension, as this would cause root drag and possible hair breakage.
- Ensure that you work to the shape of the head as you apply and leave a gap of 2–3 cms around the whole hairline, to prevent the extensions from being visible.

Remember

Carry out a pull test before your client leaves the salon to check that the extensions are firmly attached to the hair.

Racoon

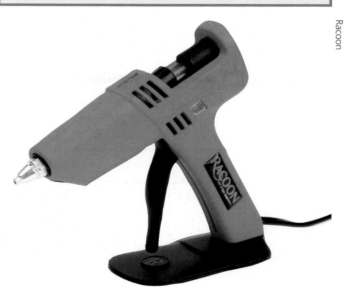

Hot attachment: a step-by-step guide

1 Before the hair is added.

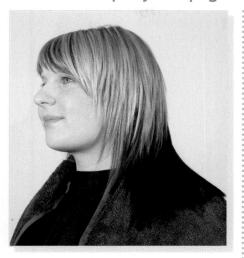

2 Section the hair in the nape and take a three-strand weave.

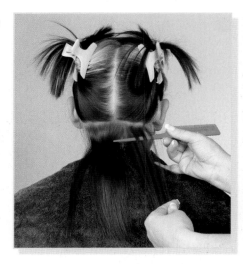

3 Apply the disc to the middle weave and twist, then secure with clips.

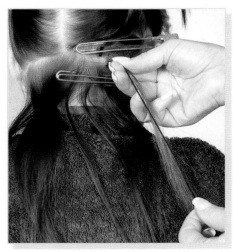

4 Attach the added hair to the twist using the glue gun.

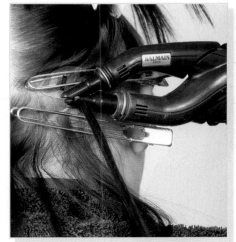

5 Once the glue has been applied, roll the softened glue between the fingers to secure the attached hair.

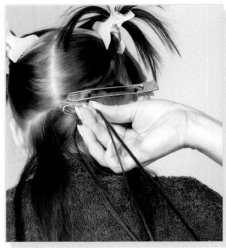

6 Continue until you have completed the extensions in the row.

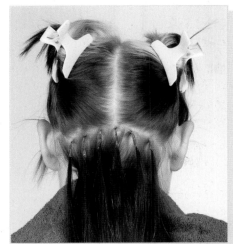

7 When enough hair has been added, razor cut the hair to blend the added and natural hair together.

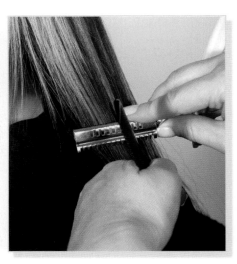

8 Straighten the hair to finish the look.

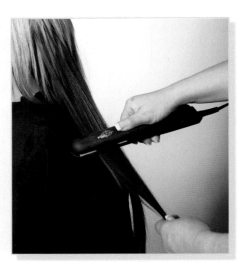

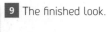

9 The finished look.

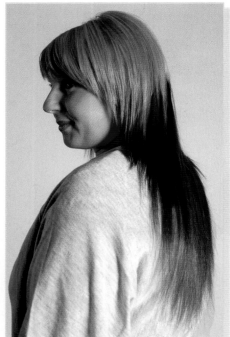

Cold attachment: a step-by-step guide

1 Take a one inch horizontal section in the nape, then take a small subsection.

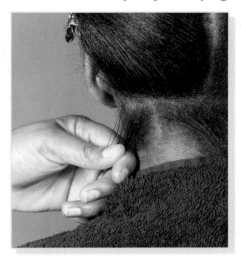

2 Add the extension hair by plaiting into the natural hair.

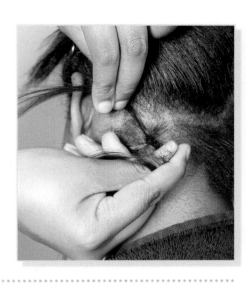

3 Start the cane row, keeping the tension even.

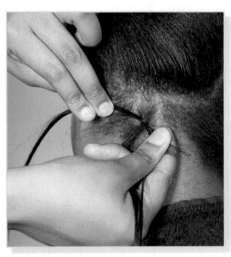

4 Work your way down the section until you run out of hair.

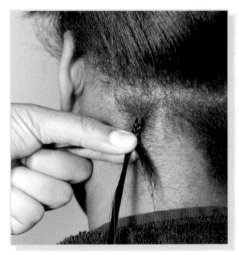

5 Secure the plaited extension by tying the ends with a couple of strands of hair.

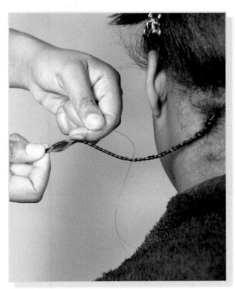

6 The first plaited extension is complete. Continue until the required number of extensions has been completed.

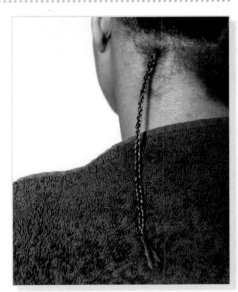

Check it out

Do you know what the manufacturers' instructions are relating to the attachment methods used in your salon? If you're not sure, then find out!

Advantages and disadvantages

The advantages and disadvantages of the different methods of attachment are shown in this table.

Attachment method	Advantages	Disadvantages
Fusion	• The scalp can be accessed to ensure thorough cleansing • Natural looking	• Maybe time-consuming to remove them • Can cause hair loss • Oil products can't be used
Bonding	• Quick and easy to apply • Easy to remove	• Doesn't last very long • Client may have allergic reaction to the adhesive • Oil products can't be used
Sewn in wefts	• The scalp can be accessed to ensure thorough cleansing • Damage to natural hair is minimal • Easy to remove	• They may be uncomfortable • Can appear lumpy if not done correctly
Plaited	• Damage to natural hair is minimal • No need to use heat on the hair • No chemicals are used on the hair e.g. glue	• May cause traction alopecia • Can reduce moisture levels in the natural hair • Time-consuming

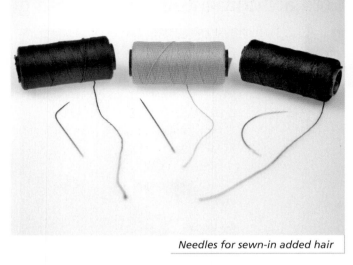

Needles for sewn-in added hair

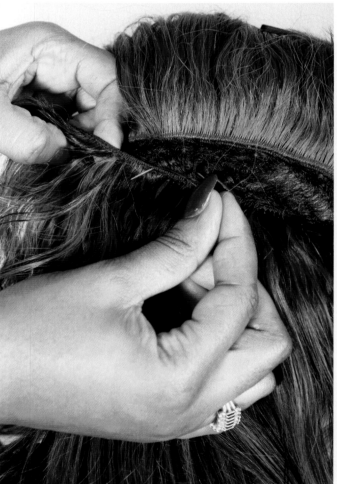

Sewn-in wefts

Types of added hair

You need to be proficient using both natural and synthetic fibre hair extensions and have an understanding of the pros and cons of each.

Human hair

This comes in a variety of lengths, colours, quality and movement. The best type of human hair to work with is 'cuticle hair' (or **Remy hair**), that is, hair that has been cut from the head and the cuticles are all lying in the same direction. This is expensive hair to buy but will last longer.

> **Remy hair**
>
> hair that has been cut from the head and the cuticles are all lying in the same direction.

Non-cuticle hair is collected from hairbrushes and hair that has fallen on the floor. This hair has to be treated before being sold to remove the cuticles to prevent the hair from becoming tangled. For this reason, it is cheaper to buy than cuticle hair.

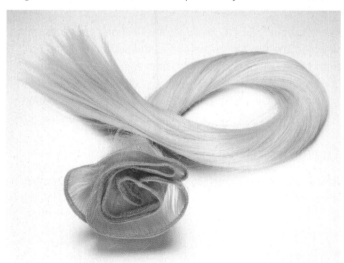

Human hair comes in a variety of lengths and colours

Synthetic fibre hair

There have been a lot of advancements in the production of **synthetic fibre hair** and generally speaking it is very easy to care for.

> **Synthetic fibre hair**
>
> hair which is not of natural origin.

Kanekalon is a good option, as the quality of the synthetic fibre is very good. Many stylists prefer to use kanekalon as it feels softer, tangles less and does not damage the natural hair.

Type of added hair	Advantages	Disadvantages
Human	• Can be styled using heat • Will be treated much the same as the client's own hair	• More expensive • Colour choice is more limited, if you want bold colours
Synthetic fibre	• Less expensive than human hair • Comes in a variety of colours which can be very bold	• Some cannot be styled using heat • Is more likely to look unnatural

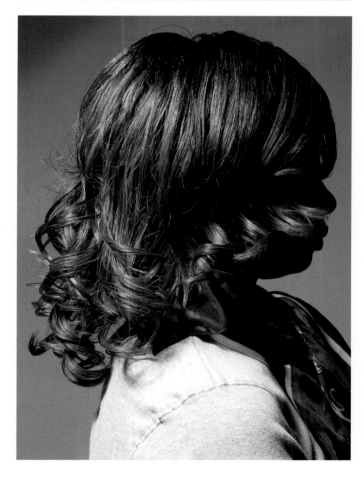

> **Check it out**
>
> Carry out some research using books and the Internet regarding the different types of both human and synthetic fibre hair that may be used for hair extensions.
>
> **KS** **Key Skills Links**: Level 2 Communication & ICT

Using added hair

It's essential that your finished result looks balanced and well proportioned. Therefore the amount of hair added will depend on the length and density of the client's hair, as if the client's hair is short, it is more likely to show the attachment point. You must also consider the hair's elasticity, to ensure the hair is strong enough to hold the hair extensions without causing damage to the hair, and, obviously, you will need to consider the finished look you are aiming for.

Coloured synthetic fibre extensions may be blended to give a personalised service for the client. This should enhance the total look and meet the client's requirements. You may add one colour to the client's hair or multiple colours to achieve a natural, multi-tonal effect.

Some clients may require extensions to give the effect of a block colour, others may want a highlighted result. In each instance, the placement of the extensions will vary. The block colour would be achieved by strategically placing the wefts or added hair to give the impression of a block colour. A highlighted effect can be created by adding the hair at intervals

Preparing added hair

In order to prepare the added hair for use you may need to use a hackle and mixing mats. The hackle is basically steel prongs protruding from a wooden board. It is used to disentangle the hair and blend colours by drawing the hair through the steel prongs. The mixing mats are wooden boards with short bristles coming out from the board. The pre-hackled hair is placed on top of one of the mixing mats and another mixing mat placed on top to hold the hair in place. This enables you to draw off small amounts of hair at a time without disturbing the remaining hair, which is held between the mixing mats. The hair may be cut to the desired length before, or after, using the hackle and mixing mats.

> **Remember**
>
> You must consider the overall look you are trying to achieve. Make sure it's suitable for the client's lifestyle and the positioning of the extensions are well thought through to ensure the final look meets the client's requirements.

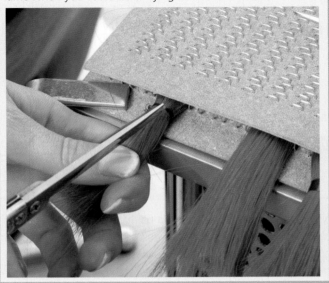

> **Be professional ★★★**
>
> It makes good financial sense to train your junior staff to prepare the hair for you as this can take a lot of your salon time when you could be carrying out other services.

It is important that you maintain a correct and even tension when adding the hair extensions as this will prevent the hair from being pulled and dragged, thus ensuring client comfort. You should also make sure you keep your sections clean to prevent any hair from other sections becoming incorporated by mistake, as this will undoubtedly cause the client discomfort!

Cutting tools

In this unit you will need to use the following cutting tools:

- scissors
- clippers
- thinning scissors
- razors.

Scissors

Scissors come in many different designs and several lengths of blades. They are used for a variety of cutting techniques such as club cutting, slicing, texturising or thinning. It is very important to find the right pair and to keep the blades sharp; remember that they need to feel comfortable to use, as they are really just an extension to your hand.

> **Remember**
>
> You should not be using your scissors to cut both human and synthetic hair as the blades will become dull when used on synthetic hair. Therefore you should have at least two pairs of scissors!

Thinning scissors

As well as straight-edged scissors, there are also thinning scissors with serrated edges. These can also be called **aesculap** or texturising scissors. They have one or more edges with serration. It is also possible to buy scissors with varying degrees of serration, which allow you to produce much more imaginative styles. Thinning scissors are used to remove bulk, not length, and must be used only on dry hair. You can also use them to thin the hair out and blend the join between natural and added hair.

> **Aesculap**
>
> initially a brand name of a company that developed thinning scissors; because of their popularity it became the most common name used for this type of scissors.

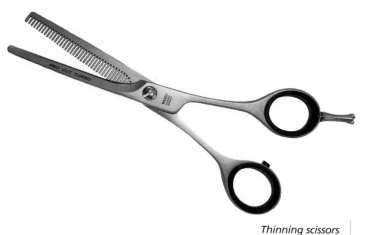

Thinning scissors

> **Remember**
>
> Your scissors must be handled with care and well maintained in order to prolong their working life and to ensure they give you the best possible results with each cut. Blunt scissors can cause damage to the hair ends by splitting them. Each time you use your scissors, wipe them when you have finished the cut to clean them. Use light oil on the hinge regularly, as this will prevent them from rusting or seizing up. You must sterilise them to prevent the passing on of infection or infestation. Because you are using them so close to the hair and skin, it is inevitable that they pick up bacteria from one client that could easily be passed on to another.

Clippers

Clippers are used to club cut the hair very short. You wouldn't use clippers anywhere on the head where you would cut the hair short enough to show where the added hair joins the natural hair. They must be maintained by removing the hair around the blades with a clipper brush with stiff bristles, often provided by the manufacturer. Use clipper oil on the blades regularly, but ensure they do not have oil on them whilst cutting or this will hinder their performance during the cut. In recent years, cordless clippers have become more popular and this type of clipper has the advantage of causing less of a hazard due to trailing wires. They are recharged when placed back in the base unit after use.

Razors

Razors can be used when cutting the hair to remove bulk or to thin out the ends. They are especially good for creating textured looks. You have the choice when using a razor for cutting hair of an open razor, a safety razor, or a shaper as shown below.

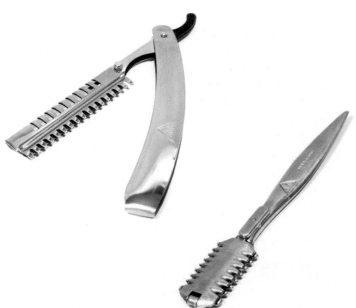

A safety razor and a shaper

It is essential that you hold and use a razor correctly, not only for your own and the client's safety, but also to prevent damage to the hair. You should ensure that your blade is extremely sharp.

Unit GH23 Provide creative hair extension services

Cutting techniques

The following list details the cutting techniques you must be competent at using in this unit:

- point cutting
- tapering
- freehand
- razoring
- texturising.

Point cutting

This can also be called chipping or point thinning. It can be carried out on wet or dry hair and is used to remove either length or bulk. The ends of the hair are cut into using the scissors, which gives a choppy, uneven finish, with soft broken edges. Because it texturises the hair it is particularly useful when blending. This method will help to prevent steps and blunt lines within the cut.

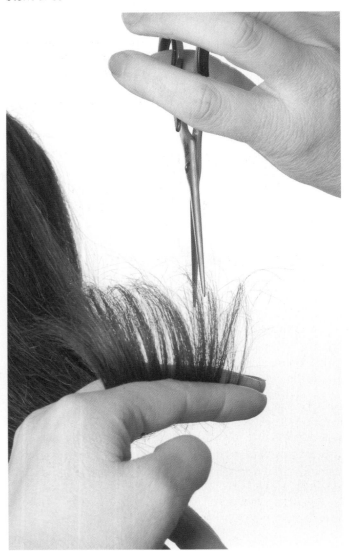

Tapering

This technique is used when you want to remove bulk or join together short layers with long layers. The scissors are allowed to slide into the hair, as you slightly open and close the blades, in a backcombing type of movement. With the razor method, you scoop into the hair sections and apply pressure according to the amount of hair you want to remove. This method requires a great deal of accuracy and skill so as not to cut off too much hair. However, it is a good method to use as it creates softer edges.

Freehand

This technique can be done on wet or dry hair and is carried out by cutting the hair without holding it between the fingers. The hair is just combed into place and the ends cut to allow it to fall in its natural lie. It is especially good when cutting a fringe, especially if a cowlick is present.

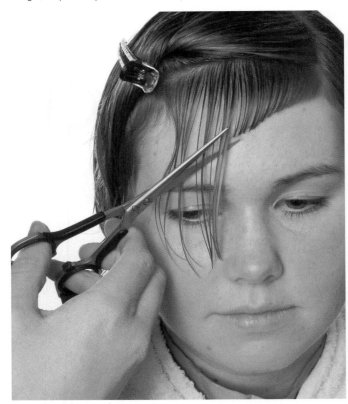

Razoring

This technique is commonly used as textured looks are very fashionable. Razors are often used on dry hair to reduce the length of the extensions and shape the hair. You must also make sure that your razor's edge is always sharp, to prevent dragging the added hair. Razor cutting can be done anywhere in a haircut and removes bulk and / or length, depending on where you use the technique.

With razor cutting, the hair is held between the fingers and can be cut either on top or below the section, with the razor held at a slight angle to the hair shaft. The amount of pressure you apply will determine the amount of hair removed, so take care – it is much safer to remove a little at a time than to take off too much. Razor cutting is especially good for creating very textured looks or for blending short layers into very long layers. This is a good method to use when cutting hair extensions, as it will produce softer lines.

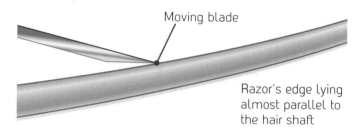

Moving blade

Razor's edge lying almost parallel to the hair shaft

Texturising

This technique can be used to remove both bulk and length and is especially good for blending between the natural and added hair. However, care should be taken not to cut hair too close to the root and leave added hair protruding, as this will show the area that the extensions have been placed. You can texturise anywhere in the haircut or along the hair length depending on style requirements and it can be carried out by both holding the hair and freehand. Again, by texturising the hair, you will produce softer lines than when club cutting.

Be professional ★★★

- You must establish and follow your guidelines to ensure you are working methodically through the haircut, as this will produce an even result!
- You will have to adapt your sectioning technique when cutting hair extensions by taking your sections away from the scalp to ensure you don't disturb or pull the extended hair.
- The preferred methods of cutting should include those that leave softer edges, for example, razoring, tapering, point cutting, etc.
- When checking the cut, again, make sure your sections aren't taken close to the scalp, to avoid disturbing the hair extensions.
- You should check the haircut to ensure the cut is even, well balanced and the completed look is as required.

Creative finishing

This applies to the completion of the style when the extensions have been added. You will need to apply product as required and then blow dry or set the hair, along with the use of heated styling appliances.

All attachment methods maybe finger dried, towel dried or dried naturally. Blow-drying using a brush with tension is not recommended as it may drag the extensions, causing them to become loose; however, blow-drying without tension may be carried out with care.

All systems may be set and plaits may be set using hot water.

Any of the attachment techniques may be tonged if human hair has been used; however, care must be taken with synthetic hair as it may melt. Great advancements have been made with synthetic hair and some do claim they can be tonged, but it would be wise to test this first!

Check it out

Are you aware of the correct methods for disposing of any waste at the end of the service? If not refer to Unit G22 page 260.

After the service

It is essential that you give your client clear and effective after-care advice as this will ensure the hair remains looking at its best for the longest possible time.

Maintenance / removal of hair extensions

It is important that the client is given the correct advice on how to maintain and remove (if applicable) their hair extensions. You need to check that the client has fully understood your advice to ensure the extensions remain in the best condition possible, for the longest period possible.

You should also advise your client to cover the hair with a silk scarf when sleeping to prevent disturbing the extensions, and to return to the salon for maintenance appointments once a week to ensure the extensions remain in optimum condition.

You must explain to your client how the hair should be disentangled – from point to root with the extended hair being supported at the point of attachment.

You should ensure that your client record cards are completed accurately, so the information is available for future reference. This is especially important if you need to record the shades of colour you have used. When the hair extensions are ready for removal you should advise your client to return to the salon for this service to ensure the client's natural hair is not damaged during the removal process. Most product manufacturers have their own removal solutions and it is highly recommended that you use the corresponding solution for the application system you have used.

The rate of hair growth will determine how long the extensions last. Hair grows about a centimetre a month, so after six weeks at the most the extensions would start to look loose and should be removed.

Plaited extensions may be removed at home. However, care must be taken to ensure that when cutting off the added hair, the natural hair is not cut. The plaits may then be unpicked. However, it should be recommended that the client returns to the salon for this process.

Sewn-in extensions should be removed by carefully cutting the thread used to sew the extensions in.

When the extensions have been removed, the hair should undergo a deep conditioning treatment to give the hair a chance to recover before the next extension service. You should be recommending that your client gives their hair a rest as they may experience scalp sensitivity, some hair loss, and a dry scalp and hair if the hair is worn with extensions over a long period of time.

Products for home use

You client must understand the correct products to use at home and those to avoid; this will be dependent on the type of extensions they have.

Most suppliers of hair extensions have their own brand of shampoos and conditioners. You should be promoting these as they will give the best results for your clients because they have been tried and tested by the manufacturer and will therefore give optimum results.

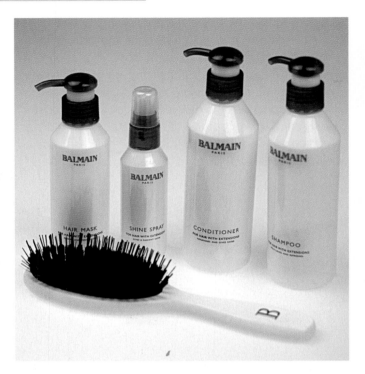

Oils and oil-based products should be recommended for clients that have sewn or plaited extensions as these will keep the hair and scalp lubricated, and also add sheen and lustre to the hair. However, oil-based products should not be recommended to clients with fused or bonded extensions as it will cause the glue to lose its adhesive properties and extensions may become lose and fall out.

Styling gel: good to use on sewn extensions but not great to use on other methods.

Wax: these are oil based so are good to use on sewn or plaited extensions but will need to be avoided where glue has been used.

Finishing spray: good for all types of extensions.

Serums: these are oil based so are good to use on sewn or plaited extensions but will need to be avoided where glue has been used.

Braid sprays: these types of sprays are oil based and have been designed for use on plaited hair. They serve to moisturise the scalp and keep the plaits in good condition.

Check it out

What guidance is given by the manufacturers of the attachment systems used in your salon for shampooing and conditioning the hair?

Check it out

What products are used in your salon to remove the different types of extensions?

Potential problems and how they can be remedied or treated

You need to be aware of the problems that could arise and make sure you know how to deal with them. If you work carefully and ensure you are following health and safety procedures, the possibility of them occurring will be greatly reduced.

Potential problems	How to remedy / treat the problems
The added hair is too tight and is causing the client discomfort	Remove the added hair, then re-apply with less tension / more care
The added hair becomes tangled	Disentangle from the points of the hair
The client complains of an itchy scalp	• Use appropriate after-care products (where applicable) • The client may be allergic to the added hair, in which case, remove the added hair and cleanse the scalp to remove any residue
The client has an allergic reaction to the bonding glue	Refer to GP for immediate attention
Too much bonding glue has been used and the excess is on the hair	Remove the excess glue with the correct removal solution
Long nails and rings may become caught in the client's hair causing discomfort	Remove jewellery prior to the service. If the hair does become caught in the stylist's nails or rings, it may have to be cut out
Traction alopecia	Do not carry out the hair extension service – refer the client to a trichologist and / or their GP
Reaction to removal solutions	Refer to GP for immediate attention
Carrying out sporting activities	These should be avoided if it is likely that the hair could be pulled at in any way, or exposed to harsh chemicals such as chlorine when swimming

Check your knowledge

The following questions will help you to check your understanding of this unit. The answers can be found on page 419. Take care, as there may be more than one correct answer for some questions.

1 Excessive tension on the hair may result in:
  a the hair growing quicker
  b the hair becoming lighter
  c traction alopecia
  d a sensitive scalp

2 Why is an elasticity test essential before carrying out any extension services?
  a To ensure the hair is of the correct length
  b To ensure the hair's internal structure is in good enough condition to carry out the process
  c To ensure the hair is dense enough to hide the joins from natural to extended hair
  d So the client thinks you know what you are doing

3 Why might it be necessary to cut the hair after applying hair extensions?
  a To ensure they blend correctly with the natural hair
  b To make sure the extensions are as natural as possible
  c So that the service takes longer and you can charge more
  d To prevent the ends from becoming split

4 Which of the following products are suitable for use with bonded extensions?
  a Braid spray
  b Serum
  c Wax
  d Finishing spray

5 Which of the following products are suitable for use with plaited extensions?
  a Braid spray
  b Serum
  c Wax
  d Styling gel

6 Traction alopecia may be recognised by:
  a the hair growing quicker than normal
  b the ends of the hair splitting
  c splits along the hair shaft
  d loss of hair at the root area

7 The advice given to clients on removal of hair extensions should be:
  a have a go at removing them yourself at home
  b always return to the salon for professional removal of the extensions
  c tell the client to ask a friend to remove them
  d leave them alone until they fall or grow out

8 What is the average rate of hair growth?
   a About 2 centimetres a month
   b About 4 centimetres a month
   c About 1 centimetre a month
   d About 3 centimetres a month

9 The most effective way to remove bonded extensions is to:
   a use the manufacturer's recommended removal solution
   b squeeze as hard as you can on the glue plug to crack it open and then unpick
   c wash the hair very harshly trying to rub out the extensions
   d brush the hair over and over to pull out the extensions

10 Remy hair is:
   a hair that has been cut from the head and the cuticles are all lying in the same direction
   b hair that has been collected from brushes or on the floor with cuticles lying in different directions
   c synthetic fibre hair
   d hair made up of many different colours

Assessment guidance

In order to prove your competence in this unit you must demonstrate your ability to provide hair extension services. You will be assessed on three different clients, which must include:

- a full head of extensions
- a partial head of extensions, covering at least 25 per cent of the head
- use of human hair and synthetic fibre extensions.

You will also be assessed cutting the client's hair to blend the hair extensions with the natural hair using a variety of cutting tools and techniques.

In addition, you will be assessed on your creative finishing techniques and the aftercare advice you give to your client.

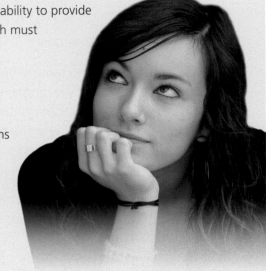

Unit H32

Contribute to the planning and implementation of promotional activities

What you will learn:

- How to contribute to the planning and preparation of promotional activities
- How to implement promotional activities
- How to participate in the evaluation of promotional activities.

Royston Blythe

Introduction

Promotional activities in the salon should serve to increase revenue, motivate staff and demonstrate your professionalism to clients. This unit is concerned with your contributions towards the salon's promotional activities. You will need to work with other people and be an active member of a team. You will work with others to plan, implement and evaluate hairdressing-related activities. You must be able to present information and interact with the public whilst competently demonstrating your hairdressing skills.

Promotional activity

any activity that is carried out to promote the salon in order to enhance salon image and increase salon business.

You the stylist

You will need to have a thorough knowledge of the range of services and products offered in your salon in order to fully sell their benefits. Recognising selling opportunities is important and in order to do this you will have to fine-tune your communication skills. Ensuring that you are always aware of your clients' needs and being able to advise them accordingly will also serve to assist you when carrying out a promotional event. You may need to support junior staff in their role, as you will have the benefit of experience when it comes to recognising client needs.

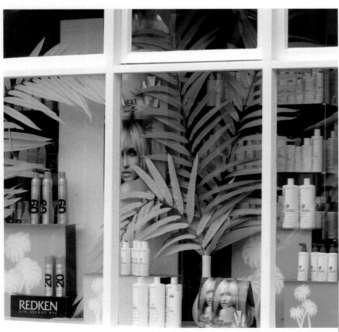

Your salon window is the ideal place to set up displays or advertising

Contributing to the planning and preparation

The promotional activities you must consider are:

- demonstrations (both in the salon and at other premises)
- displays (window displays / retail)
- advertising campaigns (media, newspaper, website, trade publications, leaflets and / or fliers, etc.).

In order to make an informed choice regarding the promotional activity you wish to undertake, there are several questions you should consider:

- How much money do you have to spend?
- What type of activity do you wish to undertake?
- How do you think it should be done?
- Who will you be aiming the activity at?
- What do you hope to achieve?
- Will you need the help of others?
- What resources will you need?
- When is the promotional activity to take place?
- Where will the promotional activity take place?
- How much time do you need to prepare for the event?
- What type of advertising are you thinking of using?
- How will you evaluate the activity?

Each of the above questions should be thoroughly thought out and your answers will enable you to produce an outline plan, highlighting your ideas. In addition to the above questions, it may be wise to check through the salon's past promotional events and their evaluations. This may prevent you from making mistakes or, better still, you may learn from other people's mistakes instead of your own!

The most important aspect of any promotional activity has to be the planning and preparation. These activities do not happen on their own; they require thorough planning followed by meticulous preparation.

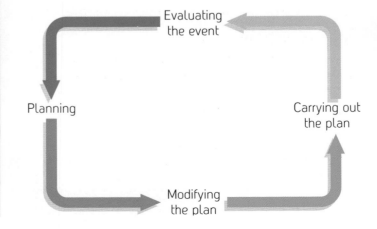

Make your initial recommendations / proposal

You should make an appointment with the relevant person, for example, the salon owner or manager, to discuss your ideas and recommendations for a promotional activity.

The meeting you have may be informal, where you can put forward several suggestions and discuss them on an unofficial basis. However, you will then need to prepare a more formal proposal which states the type of promotional activity you wish to carry out, your ideas as to how this may be done and the potential benefits for the salon. The most obvious benefit is to make money for the salon; therefore your ideas must be cost-effective, that is, they will make more money in the long term than the initial cost of the activity.

> **Remember**
>
> You must be prepared to justify your recommendations for promotional activities, as the salon will undoubtedly be paying for them and will expect a guaranteed return on its money!

The importance of working to a budget

You should be mindful that you will have a budget to adhere to and overspending may result in failure. Initially, when you are deciding on the budget for the promotion, and in order to safeguard your plan, you should allow for a pot of money to be put aside for emergency use. This will ensure that if problems are encountered you will have the money to provide a solution. Consider not only the money you will need to carry out the promotional activity, but also the money you may need for your contingency plans. If several people are involved in the financial side of the promotion, regular reports on spending will be needed to ensure no overspending in any areas. Remember that your main objectives are to increase revenue and to raise the salon's profile. If the promotion fails through overspending, then neither objective will be met.

Setting your objectives

There are many reasons for carrying out promotional activities, but the first questions you need to ask yourself are (a) what do you want to achieve?; and (b) what are your **objectives** for carrying out the activity?

> **Objectives**
>
> these are the aim or goal of your promotion, what you are trying to achieve by it.

Your main objectives should be to:
- increase the salon's business
- enhance the salon's image.

There are many ways that these objectives can be met, for example, launching the new season's looks should increase business and enhance the salon's image. You may want to promote new product lines, new services being offered by the salon or a new stylist joining the team, or your activity may be a means to shifting stock that is lying dormant in the stock room, especially after a product repackage.

Whatever your reasons, they should be thought through and then discussed and negotiated with your manager / salon owner. Any targets or objectives that are set should be mutually agreed.

When setting objectives for your promotional activity, you should ensure you follow the SMART principle, that is, you should make your objectives:
Specific – have you stated clearly what you intend to do?
Measurable – can you prove you have done it?
Achievable – do you have the potential to meet your target?
Realistic – are you planning something that is realistic?
Time bound – will you meet your target by a certain time or date?

You must also consider the target group at whom you are aiming your promotional activity, as this will undoubtedly have an impact on the type of activity you choose to undertake. For example, if you are aiming to bring in wealthy, young clientele with a good disposable income, then you will have to aim your promotion accordingly and ensure it has a hi-tech and vibrant feel to it!

Selecting the target group

> **Check it out**
>
> Make a list of the different target groups you could aim a promotional activity at. Which type of promotional activity would be best suited to each of the target groups?

You may decide to aim your promotional activity at a specific age group that reflects the type of clientele you are looking to attract, for example, 20–35 years. Alternatively, you may wish to open a section of the salon for men's hairdressing services if the salon doesn't already have one.

Once you have decided what you want to do, you need to think about how you are going to achieve it and which promotional activities will be best suited to your objectives and **target group**. You would not necessarily use the same activity aimed at a group of 16–20 year olds as perhaps the 50-plus age range, as their preferences may be very different. Time and consideration must be given to these factors if you wish your promotional activity to succeed.

Target group

the group at which you are aiming your promotional activity. It can be small or large depending on the objectives of your promotion.

Demonstrations

There are various ways of demonstrating the work of the salon. You may want to offer the public the chance to see your work at a showcase event in the salon. Alternatively, you might be involved in a large event where you carry out various hairdressing techniques on a stage to promote the salon's range of skills.

When carrying out any demonstration, consideration should be given to people's attention span. Most people have an attention span of only 20 minutes and if you are demonstrating something for longer, you need to think about whether it will be exciting enough to maintain interest. Demonstrations are an excellent way of advertising the talent of your salon. Remember, any stylist showcasing his or her work in this way must have the confidence and hairdressing experience to carry it off. If you can wow the crowd with your hairdressing ability and charm them with your line of banter, then you are likely to be successful. On the other hand, if you lack the skills and confidence to perform in front of a crowd, then it will not only be torture for you the stylist but it will also be professional suicide for the salon's reputation.

Displays

Displaying products for retail sale at reception is a subtle way of introducing your product range. You can then substantiate this by discussing the benefits of the products whilst using them on your clients. This type of promotion is commonly used; indeed, there are many ways of bringing products to your clients' attention, be they subtle or attention grabbing in their approach.

The cheapest and most cost-effective way of promoting products and services is to use the salon window. You don't necessarily need to employ a professional window dresser; use your imagination or find out if any members of staff have a flair for window dressing. You can change the display according to the seasons or when sales are down in order to target certain services. The only disadvantage is that it will reach only a limited audience, especially if your salon is not on a busy main road position. However, if used in conjunction with other promotional mediums, it can be extremely cost effective.

Your display may be at a larger promotional event, in which case consideration must be given to the audience it is designed for. You must decide the main objective of your display and ensure that you do not stray from this at any point. The design should be pleasing to the eye and not too fussy. The audience will be drawn to a focal point and this is where your main objective should be showcased. Unless you have an experienced designer on board, seek help from all the staff with themes and ideas. Bear in mind that different people have different concepts of what is and what is not attractive. To overcome this, seek advice and feedback from a wide range of people to enable you to produce a display that most people will appreciate.

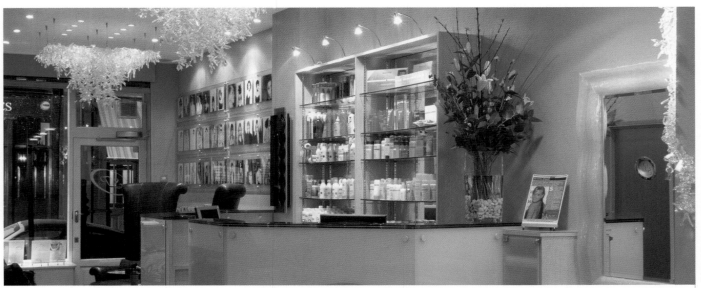

Displaying products at reception is a good way of attracting your clients' attention

Advertising campaigns

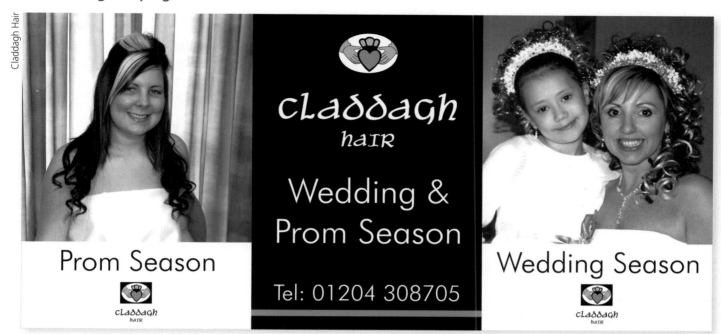

Claddagh Hair

claddagh hair

Wedding & Prom Season

Tel: 01204 308705

Prom Season

Wedding Season

Most salons use advertising in some form; however, for an advertising campaign to be successful you must have clearly defined objectives. Your objectives may be to:

● increase the clientele
● introduce new products or services
● increase retail sales
● promote a forthcoming event.

Whatever you decide, your objectives must be quantifiable and SMART. There are many different forms of advertising and the one you choose will be largely dependent on your budget, as some forms of advertising are more expensive than others. Some examples are shown below.

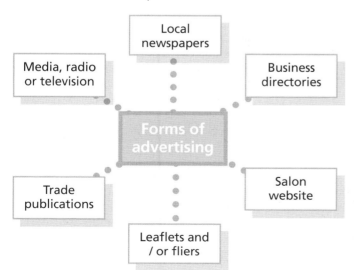

Local newspapers

Media, radio or television

Business directories

Forms of advertising

Trade publications

Salon website

Leaflets and / or fliers

Media, radio and television can be used to reach potential clients throughout the day. However, these can be expensive and often broadcast out of the vicinity of the salon. Using a local radio station may prove to be more successful, unless you are part of a nationwide chain and the advert can direct the audience to a salon in their area. You must consider this option very carefully as the high cost may outweigh the potential revenue gained.

Local newspapers may be a good medium for advertising, especially as most areas receive a free paper each week. The salon will have to pay for this type of advertising, so it is essential that the advert is both eye-catching and easily understood for the message to be successful. Newspapers like to run interesting stories, so if the salon is planning to carry out something 'newsworthy', for example, a percentage of the salon's takings is being donated to a charity, the paper may well send a photographer and run a story on the salon. This type of advertising is free, but it must impact on the audience.

Business directories such as Yellow Pages are good for long-term advertising, as they are usually distributed to every household in the area. An advertisement in such a directory must be carefully worded, as it will be listed alongside all the other salons in the area.

Salon websites are becoming more widespread as the Internet becomes more accessible to the general population. A salon website should be visually attractive to capture the eye of the user but easy to navigate with accessible information. The website may include photos of the salon and additional information regarding the services and products that are available. Websites are also a good medium to display this season's looks and update clients on current staff and the opening times of the salon but, be warned, you must have the time to update the website frequently as any out-of-date looks or information can be detrimental to your salon's reputation.

Remember

If you are developing your own website, it is recommended that the home page be fairly simple with few or no pictures. A potential user is likely to become bored if they have to wait more than a few seconds for a heavily image-based website to open. Keep the design of the home page to a minimum with links to the more detailed pages.

A trade publication is a good place to advertise because you know the people seeing your advertisement will be interested in hairdressing. This will help to enhance the image of the salon. However, if your objective is to increase the salon's business, this type of advertising may not be the most suitable method.

Leaflets and fliers are a good way to advertise, especially if you do not have a substantial budget for promotional activities. The leaflet must be eye-catching and the information easy to understand if your promotion is to impact on the public. Think about the amount of junk mail that you receive and never even read. If the leaflets / fliers are being hand delivered, you must ensure they are delivered to homes within the local vicinity of the salon. If you distribute the leaflets too far away from the salon, then the chance of anyone responding to the leaflet / flier is far less. You should also consider the person-hours required to carry out a leaflet drop and if the person responsible is trustworthy. How will you know if they have been delivered or not? Many beauty or nail salons will display leaflets for hairdressing salons, as long as the favour is reciprocated.

The team

For most promotional activities you will need the assistance of others. This may be to exchange thoughts and ideas that will enable you to gain another person's perspective. If your proposed activity is large, you will undoubtedly need the assistance of others to enable you to realise your goals.

It is very important that you consider who you will need to help you and what you want them to do. Allocate responsibilities according to individual's talents, for example, a good hairdresser should be given the role of demonstrator, or a good negotiator given the role of negotiating prices. They must be competent to carry out the roles you require. Failure to obtain competent assistance may lead to chaos. You should ensure that every member of the team wants to take part, as an unwilling member may cause problems later. If you suspect someone is losing interest or not fulfilling their role, then this must be challenged and not left to create a problem for you.

Regular meetings of the team will ensure that each individual is maintaining their role and not failing. It will also serve to communicate any changes if they arise and ensure that each person is coping with the workload.

Check it out

Make a list of all the roles that need to be covered, outlining the responsibilities connected to each role. Allocate members of the team to cover each role.

Produce a detailed plan

By now you should have a clear idea of the exact requirements for the promotional activity. You will now need to produce a detailed plan.

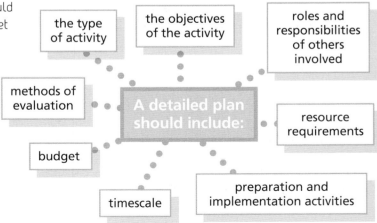

the type of activity

the objectives of the activity

roles and responsibilities of others involved

methods of evaluation

A detailed plan should include:

resource requirements

budget

timescale

preparation and implementation activities

Unit H32 Contribute to the planning and implementation of promotional activities

The type of activity you choose to promote your salon will be the one that allows you to best achieve your objectives. Also consider any constraints such as the budget and resources. You must be sure the activity you choose is realistically achievable and thoroughly planned.

The objectives of the activity must be made known to everyone involved to ensure that each person is working towards the same goals. You must ensure that the objectives remain the main focus – do not allow the activity to be sidetracked from their importance.

The roles and responsibilities of others involved should be clearly defined from the start. Make sure that everyone is sure of their role and is comfortable with what is expected of them. Each person must be informed of whom to go to when there is a problem. If problems do arise, it is important that they are dealt with quickly to prevent a more serious situation developing.

Resource requirements will need to be given careful consideration. It is crucial that detailed planning is carried out to ensure that no requirement is overlooked. Serious problems may arise if something of great importance is forgotten for the event. When making lists of what is required, involve all the team and brainstorm ideas to prevent any detail being missed.

Preparation and implementation activities will need to be attended by everyone concerned. If a member of the team does not attend at this stage, then something of importance may be overlooked, thereby creating a problem at a later stage. If the promotion is well planned, then implementation should run smoothly. However, if the planning stage is not given the serious consideration it deserves, problems will ensue.

Timescales need to be set to ensure that nothing is left to the last minute. A promotion should not be thrown together in a hurry. Each person involved must be aware of the timescales and the importance of working to them, otherwise problems will arise.

The budget will be set and agreed at the start and money put aside for any emergencies. If you feel at any time that the budgetary constraints are failing, then this must be discussed and a solution found to ensure the success of the promotion. The budget is set at the outset to guarantee there will be enough money for everything needed to implement the promotion. Therefore, careful consideration must be given to this initially, in order to achieve the objectives.

Methods of evaluation should be considered during the planning stages in order to allow you to prepare materials required in advance, for example, feedback questionnaires or business reply questionnaires. If your evaluation requires you to carry out some activity at the end of the event, then you must have materials ready for this. The methods of evaluation should gauge the effectiveness of the event, and must therefore be suited to the purpose. For example, if your promotion is an advertising campaign, then checking for increased revenue would be required; alternatively, if you give demonstrations at an event, a short questionnaire may be more successful.

Venue and legal requirements

The requirements and restrictions of any venue will differ depending upon many factors such as the size of the event, the location, and the need for electricity and water. The venue will need to be carefully considered, as there will be health and safety implications and other legal requirements that will be of great importance.

You have the responsibility to think about the requirements and restrictions of the venue.

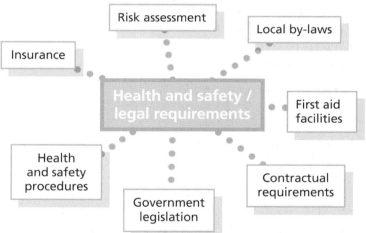

Insurance is an absolute must! You should look at the various types of insurance policies and check to be sure you are adequately covered. Most insurance companies will offer you free advice. Public liability insurance will most definitely be for a six-figure sum and, if you are using an external venue, you should check that the level of cover is adequate. You should also consider if an entertainment licence is required as your insurance could be void without one.

A risk assessment should be carried out prior to the event, in order to assess the steps needed to minimise any risk. All potential hazards will need to be considered and plans put into place to reduce exposure to these. Your risk assessment must take into account the safe use of utilities, for example, electricity, equipment, chemicals, exposure to extremes of temperature or risk to health from vibration, noise or radiation. In your assessment you must take into account whether staff are properly trained to fulfil their role and plan for any restrictions that need to be imposed due to lack of training.

CONTROL OF SUBSTANCES HAZARDOUTS TO HEALTH ASSESSMENT OF RISK

A risk assessment sheet used in a college salon

Local by-laws are specific laws written by your local authority. These laws may vary depending upon your locality. Therefore, it is a good idea to be aware of which area the venue for your promotional activity falls under. It is important that you are familiar with any restrictions under these laws and that you abide by them, not only to prevent the risk of prosecution but also to ensure that your insurance cover is valid.

First aid facilities are required by law. You must provide adequate first aid provision and it is important to check the facilities at any venue to ensure that you are fully prepared. You also need to be sure that you have designated personnel for the administering of first aid provision. It is crucial to check that these people have a current first aid qualification or else you are leaving yourself open to possible prosecution or litigation if a situation was to arise.

Contractual requirements are the terms of any contract that you have entered into. It is essential that you are fully aware of the specifics of the contract to prevent any misunderstanding which could result in an incident or accident; for example, checking to see who provides first aid provision. All aspects of the contract between yourself and another party must be thoroughly explored and, unless you are familiar with business law, you may want to consider employing the services of a business lawyer to check it over for you.

In the salon

Simon and Ed's promotional event

Simon and Ed were joint owners of a large city centre salon and were planning a promotional event to launch the salon's opening. After planning to showcase the work of the staff at a hair show event, they found a venue and signed a contract with the company, which required them to pay a substantial deposit upfront. As time went by, Simon and Ed realised that the venue they had originally booked would not be suitable to meet their requirements and they made a decision to change the venue. When they contacted the company to let them know, they were told that their deposit was not refundable after thirty days. Simon and Ed were both surprised and disappointed to discover they had lost a substantial amount of their budget. On checking the specifics of the contract they had signed, they discovered that these details were stated in print. They realised that they were unable to protest at the company's decision.

- In what area do you think Simon and Ed were negligent?
- How could they have avoided being in this situation?
- Do you think it would have been beneficial to seek legal advice before signing the contract?

Government legislation relating to your promotional activity should be given careful consideration. You need to be sure that you are familiar with all the laws affecting the activity and that you abide by these. This is to prevent the risk of exposure to litigation, prosecution or rendering your insurance invalid.

Unless you have been involved in the management of a business or promotional event previously, you will need to extend your knowledge of the laws that affect your activity. You should seek advice from government websites or your local business advice centre. However, the laws that are relevant to your needs will depend upon the activity you are undertaking. For example, if you are retailing, you will need to consider such legislation as the Sale of Goods Act 1994, The Supply of Goods and Services Act 1982, and the Consumer Protection Act 1987. Information regarding each of these laws can be found in Unit G11, pages 97–8.

Health and safety procedures, such as fire evacuation, must be explored thoroughly to ensure that everything is safe. The health and safety procedures applicable to your event will become apparent once you have planned the activity and booked the venue. Once you are aware of the use of electricity, gas, water, products, equipment and the size of the event, you can put into place any procedures to ensure safety. You should check that the venue has suitable fire fighting equipment and that the utilities you propose to use at the venue have been deemed suitable for purpose. All of this should be included during your risk assessment.

Check it out

In your work in the salon you will have become familiar with legislation that encompasses the needs of the hairdressing industry. Make a list of the relevant acts and regulations and decide which will need to be given consideration for your promotional activity. (See also Unit G22, pages 5–11.)

Resources

All the resources required need to be listed and given careful consideration. Planning should be about not only how much is needed but also how to obtain back-up if required. The type of resources you may need include:

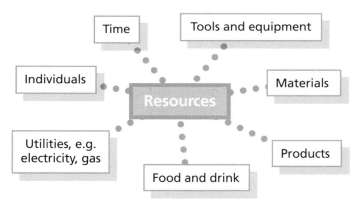

Time

Tools and equipment

Individuals

Resources

Materials

Utilities, e.g. electricity, gas

Products

Food and drink

Be professional ★★★

For each of your resources required, plan a back-up supply to prevent any serious problems from arising. For example, have an alternative supplier on standby.

The resources you use should be both accessible and affordable. Your promotional activity relies upon the resources needed to produce the results. During the planning stage, you must consider what will be required and ensure that you have enough of what is needed. Poor planning may lead to disappointment for all concerned if you run out of resources. Alternatively, it may be costly to be left with unused resources, which might render your promotion a financial failure.

Implementing promotional activities

This section is concerned with the practicalities of the promotional activity. In order to carry out the promotion successfully, all of the hard work completed in the planning stages must come to fruition. At this stage each person involved will be busy fulfilling their role but may still need a point of contact to discuss any problems as they arise. By maintaining communication throughout, not only will everyone be able to see how it is developing but if there is a problem, you can be united in putting into place any contingency plans.

Effective use of resources

As the event organiser you have the responsibility of making certain that the resources required are available for use. This is a very important task and should be given your full attention. Monitoring resource use is essential to prevent misuse and waste. You should also consider that the resources you are using might be governed by health and safety regulations. You must therefore ensure that everyone is aware of their responsibilities regarding safe use. You must also bear in mind any contractual agreement and whether or not there are any restrictions that prohibit use of certain equipment or materials. It is essential that any information regarding the use of resources be disseminated to each individual, to prevent problems arising later.

Be professional ★★★

List the resources and note at what point they will be needed. Check this with everyone involved to ensure accuracy. As the promotion is implemented, keep a close eye on the list to be certain that nothing is left to chance.

Features and benefits

Everyone involved in the promotional activity must understand the features and benefits of whatever you are promoting. These are your selling points and must reflect the best elements of the promotion. Features of a service or product are its attributes or characteristics, for example, using mousse will aid the styling process. The benefits of a service or product are the advantages that it will give to the client, for example, adding a colour to their hair to enhance the haircut. Whatever the objectives of your promotion, the products and services will have features and benefits, and a sound awareness of these is required in order to clearly understand the objectives of the exercise.

Selling skills

If you are to develop and use your selling skills to their best advantage, then it is important for you to recognise buying signals. A client will demonstrate buying signals if he or she is interested in your product or service. Failure to recognise these may lead to a missed selling opportunity.

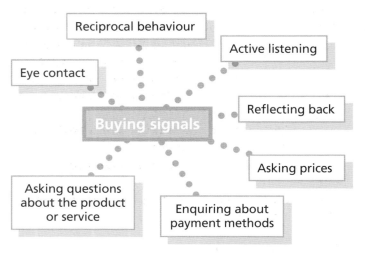

Once you have established an interest, you must tailor your presentation of the benefits of the product and / or service to meet the individual's needs. In order to carry this out successfully, you will need to have excellent communication skills. These will have been developed over time during your hairdressing career. It may, however, be required of you to support junior members of the team in their role, in order to enhance their selling and communication skills. You should already be aware of how to communicate effectively with people of various age groups and social and ethnic backgrounds. You must now use these skills to present your promotion at a level that is most suited to the audience.

Communication

The way in which you communicate with clients will play a crucial part in the success of the promotional activity. To make your communication effective you need to ensure that the information you are passing on is clear, legible (where necessary) and fully understood by the receiver. In your promotional work you will communicate with your clients and staff in many different ways.

Methods of communication

The methods of communication you choose to use must suit the type of promotional event that you are undertaking. For example, if you are showcasing your hairdressing work, invitations will need to be sent out, or if you are promoting a new product range, then a salon display may suffice. Remember that you also want to create a visual impact and this should substantiate the objectives of your promotion. It is of little use having your best stylist demonstrating his or her skills if you are in drab surroundings and the promotional materials you use are of a poor quality.

If you are conveying information via a presentation, it is important to remember that most people have an attention span of only 20 minutes, so keep it short. Make sure that you have planned the timing and pace and that your methods of presenting information suit the purpose. For example, if you are using presentation software such as Microsoft PowerPoint, are you fully conversant with how to use it and will it fully showcase what you want to demonstrate? You should judge how best to get the information across, for example, using pictures, graphics, music and varying your tone of voice.

You will also need to consider how information will be disseminated among the team. To ensure success, each person must be fully informed at every stage. You must decide how best to update the team, for example, via regular meetings, memos, bulletins or email. Ask the team how they would like to be updated – they may be able to offer alternative ideas.

Presenting and demonstrating

During the event, you need to look at which method of communication is likely to have the most impact on both the team and the target audience. Presenting information in logical steps will assist the listener in grasping the concept of what you are communicating. For example, if you are demonstrating a skill, carry out a skill analysis beforehand as this will allow you to break it down into easy-to-follow steps. Alternatively, if you are advertising, your advert needs to follow a step-by-step progression in order to help the reader or listener to understand your main selling points. You should encourage the target group to ask questions about the services and products you are promoting. This will not only give you an opportunity to sell the features and benefits, but it will also enthuse the audience and help them to understand why they need your product or services.

When you are presenting or demonstrating, ensure that you have informed the audience of when to ask questions, as interruptions during your presentation may be off-putting. As you begin discussing the products and services on offer, you must be able to respond to questions in a way that promotes goodwill and enhances the salon's image. It is of little use having an audience sending out buying signals if you proceed to put them off with your replies to their queries. Your manner should be confident and assertive; let them know you completely understand what you are offering. This is where your knowledge of the products and services on offer must be thorough and exact. If they are looking for an answer to their problems, then empathise by offering advice based on your experiences.

Problems and how to rectify them

During your planning of the promotional activity you should have set up contingency plans in case of problems arising. Although you can never plan for every eventuality, it will help if you have considered what might go wrong in order to pre-empt a situation with possible solutions. The table below lists some common problems and solutions.

Problem	Solution
Supplier lets you down	Have an alternative supplier ready and waiting
Venue is double-booked	Have an alternative venue planned
Models don't arrive	Have alternative models planned
Change of details, e.g. date of event	Set up ways of communicating changes to staff and audience
Staff are off sick	Ensure that staff are trained to cover other roles if required
Show / event is running over time	Plan for shortening demonstrations / presentation if needed
Show / event is running under time	Plan for extra activities if needed
Sound system malfunctions	Have a back-up system
Laptop crashes during PowerPoint presentation	Have a spare laptop available

After the event

When you have completed the promotional event, you must be sure to leave the venue as requested. All the products and equipment must be cleared away following both health and safety requirements and at the request of the venue. This will serve to prove your professionalism and assist you when negotiating future events. You should remember to include the clearing away in your initial plan. You must also allocate responsibilities for all resources used and the cleaning. This will not only prevent anything from being left behind or misplaced but will also look professional when you leave everything clean and tidy.

Participate in the evaluation of promotional activities

This section is concerned with the **evaluation** that takes place at the end of the promotional activity. When the promotional activity is over, you should collect all the evidence for your evaluation to enable you to gauge its effectiveness and success. This is the evidence you specified in your promotional plan. Once you have all the evidence, this should be collated and recorded in an easy-to-understand format. Charts and graphs are a good way to record the results, and may be used in conjunction with your evaluation presentation.

> **Evaluation**
>
> you will use evaluation activities to judge or assess the worth of the promotion both for future reference and to see if your objectives were achieved.

Methods of evaluation

The methods used to evaluate the promotion must suit the purpose. You will need to look at the elements that made up the event and decide what was promoted and how effective it was. It is of little use carrying out an evaluation if it does not give you the information you require. For example, asking for feedback on a questionnaire will be more successful if used immediately after the event. Not all evaluations can be carried out immediately. If your objective is to increase your client base, then this may have to be assessed over a period of time. You may have to complete several different methods at a time to ensure it suits the target group. For example, a telephone survey to the suppliers may be more appropriate, as it can be seen as a courtesy call.

A written questionnaire should ideally be given out at the end of an event. This will ensure that a person's perception of the event is still fresh in their minds and will give you a truer insight into their feelings. It is a valuable tool if used correctly. Consider keeping it anonymous to try to extract people's true feelings. If this is not possible, think of the implications of storing information under the Data Protection Act. You need to be clear about what you are trying to gain from the survey before you start. This will ensure you retrieve the information you require in order to make your evaluations. For anyone leaving the event early or forgetting to complete a survey, you could post it on the salon website allowing them to complete it at their leisure.

Business reply questionnaires are sent out along with a reply-paid envelope or on a reply-paid postcard. This will help to retrieve the same information as a written survey given out at the event, but there is more incentive to return it if the postage is free. However, you must consider that a couple of days later the audience may have forgotten some vital points they would have brought to your attention on the day. Consider also the need to pay for the postage to send and receive the questionnaires — this could prove to be a costly option.

Telephone questionnaires can be quick and easy to carry out but do you have the person-hours available to administer them? If people are busy at work in the day and do not have time to talk to you, then you might have to consider carrying it out in the evening. You will need to be sure that you have contact numbers for all the people you need to speak to.

Calculating sales may have to be done over a period of time, especially if your objective was to increase salon revenue. However, if the event was a one-off promotion, then this can be carried out immediately after the event. You must remember when calculating sales to deduct any VAT if necessary to give you a true figure.

Feedback from individuals involved can be gained in a number of ways, for example, a written survey or staff meeting. Whichever way you choose, it must suit the purpose and gain the most effective feedback. If you are chairing a staff meeting, then ensure your agenda reflects the feedback you wish to receive. You will need to produce a structured discussion plan and ensure you control it well, to prevent the discussion from straying off the track.

Increasing the client base will become evident over a period of time and you will have to structure a timetable of how and when the information will be collated. You will not only have to look at the number of clients coming into the salon but also the amount of money they are spending, particularly if the promotional event has targeted specific hairdressing services.

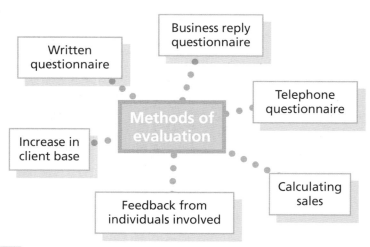

Collate, analyse and summarise feedback

You should next collate and analyse all the feedback from the activity and put it into an acceptable format. When collating your findings, it will make the process much easier if you store the information on a computer, especially if you have access to a spreadsheet and database program. This will allow you to manipulate the information and present it in different formats. Graphs and charts can be both colourful and interesting and are an excellent visual aid. You may also want to consider presenting your results in a PowerPoint presentation.

When analysing the information, you must check whether or not you have met the stated objectives. You will need to look at the elements that made up your promotional activity and decide which you are to assess. You must also consider if it was approached in the correct way and whether it could have been carried out differently. Finally, you should decide the best method to present your findings – this must be given careful consideration to ensure that the information is clear and concise.

Be professional ★★★

If you are storing information on a computer, you must keep back-up copies on disk. This will prevent you losing the information if you develop a system failure.

Check it out

Extend your computer skills by inputting information into a spreadsheet and then trying to present the information in different formats, for example, using pie, bar or flow charts. If you are unfamiliar with spreadsheet programs, seek advice from someone else, for example, your tutor, an ICT technician at college, or a friend.

 Key Skills Links: Level 2 Communication & Level 2 Application of Number

Presenting the evaluation report

When you have completed your evaluation, you may have to present your findings to other people. This may be your employer, business partner or other individuals that were involved with the event. Your results need to be clear and easy to understand; do not use too complex a method to present your findings or the group may lose interest.

The evaluation report should contain all the important information you gleaned from the evaluation methods used. The report will need to contain information to prove or disprove that you have met the objectives. You should consider including the following information:

- How much revenue has been gained or lost?
- Has the client base expanded?
- Was the venue suitable?
- What problems arose and how were they overcome?
- Did individuals fulfil their roles?
- Were the timescales set appropriate?

This list is not exhaustive and could be expanded depending on the particular areas you were promoting.

Once completed, discussing your evaluation report will allow you to present your summary in a clear and structured way. It will also allow the group to clarify any areas that they do not understand. You must be prepared for questions and be sure that you fully understand the information you are presenting, to allow you to elaborate if needed.

Check it out

When preparing your evaluation report for presenting, ensure you include an image and if you make this a type of graph that you can use to explain results, then not only will this provide evidence for your key skill communication but application of number skills too.

 Key Skills Links: Level 2 Communication & Level 2 Application of Number

Finally, consideration should be given to how improvements could be made. This should be discussed with everyone involved. You will need to look at how the activity can be improved in the future, and ensure that you learn from any mistakes made. All your records should be kept for future reference, as they will be extremely helpful when you are planning a promotional activity event in the future.

Unit H32 Contribute to the planning and implementation of promotional activities

Check your knowledge

The following questions will help you to check your understanding of this unit. The answers can be found on page 420. Take care, as there may be more than one correct answer for some questions.

1 The main objectives of a promotion should be to:
   a increase salon business and enhance salon image
   b make you popular with the staff
   c to decide which clients you can do without
   d to use up wasted time

2 Which of the following are acceptable forms of advertising?
   a Shouting through the salon window
   b Salon website
   c Visiting clients at home to sell products
   d Via media

3 Who might you ask permission from to implement a promotion?
   a The cleaner
   b Your junior
   c The salon owner
   d The technical representative

4 Which of the following might be a hazard at a hair show?
   a No fire exits
   b A qualified first-aider
   c Adequate lighting
   d Overloading electrical sockets

5 The acronym SMART stands for?
   a Sure, measurable, additional, retail, targets
   b Smart, moveable, achievable, realistic, time-bound
   c Smart, measurable, achievable, realistic, time-bound
   d Silly, moving, annoying, reachable, teams

6 Why is a risk assessment important?
   a To check everyone knows what to do
   b To show clients you know what your doing
   c To assess any hazards and minimise risk
   d To assess clients' ability to stand up at the event

7 What should you do if you discover a potential hazard when carrying out a risk assessment on the promotion event?

   a Ignore it

   b Tell the police

   c Put measures in place to deal with it

   d Make an announcement at the start of the event to draw attention to it

8 Why is it important to know the features and benefits of what you are promoting?

   a To ensure you look knowledgeable and professional

   b To show how clever you are

   c So that you feel important

   d To comply with consumer law

9 Identify buying signals from the following:

   a Client looking away while you're talking

   b Client asks for prices

   c Client wants to smell and feel the products

   d Client refuses an invitation to the promotional event

10 Why must a thorough evaluation be carried out at the end of the promotion?

   a To inform the manufacturer's sales representative

   b To use up any spare time

   c To prevent staff being bored

   d To determine whether or not you have achieved your stated objective

Unit H32 Contribute to the planning and implementation of promotional activities

Assessment guidance

For the practical element of this unit, evidence for your portfolio will be collected through observations of your promotional activities made by your assessor. To back this up you will also need to provide documents showing how you planned, implemented and evaluated your promotional activities. Your tutor or assessor will give you guidance on what documents are suitable for you to use as evidence.

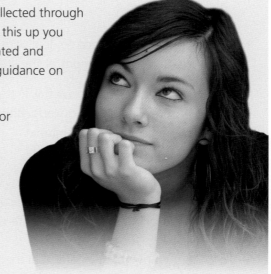

Examples are: minutes of planning meetings, photographs of your display or demonstrations, questionnaires used to obtain feedback.

You will need to provide evidence for three different types of promotional activity:

- displays
- demonstrations
- advertising campaigns.

The main objectives for carrying out each promotion must be:

- to enhance salon image
- to increase salon business.

3

Professional skills –
African
type hair

Unit AH28

Design and create intricate styles using plaiting techniques

What you will learn:

- How to prepare for the service
- How to plan and agree hair designs
- How to create the look
- How to proceed after the service.

Anne Veck, photographer: David Howard

Introduction

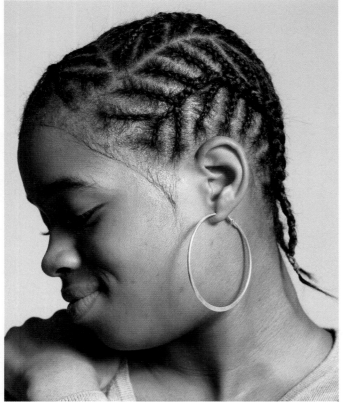

Use plaiting and styling techniques to add excitement to a client's look

This unit is about creating complex and innovative hairstyles using a variety of traditional African type hair plaiting techniques. You must be able to achieve the looks in a variety of ways, for example, designed cornrows, goddess braids and jumbo braids. Some of these you may already be familiar with and others you may know by another name. By studying the step-by-step photographs in this unit, you will develop a greater understanding of how to achieve some of the looks.

You the stylist

Before you begin to create intricate styles using plaiting styling techniques, you need to know about the correct products to use and how and why you will need to use them. It is also essential that you understand the importance of any influencing factors and the effect they may have on your client's chosen look. In order to plait the hair with skill, you will need to be dexterous, creative and conscious that the styling technique may take several hours to complete; patience is therefore the key to this unit. These skills will be developed over time, through practice and commitment.

Preparing for the service

In this section you will find all the information regarding the preparation of the client, yourself and your work area when carrying out plaiting techniques.

Thorough consultation and influencing factors

While completing your consultation you will be assessing the client's hair for the suitability of the chosen style. Looking at style books and discussing any pictures brought in by your client will be important in ascertaining your client's exact requirements. You should then be able to gauge the suitability of the style, taking into account all the influencing factors, and then select the appropriate products and tools required for you to carry out the requested service. You should discuss any implications for cost and length of service and make these clear to your client. You should also make sure you explain what is involved in the service, especially if the client is new to this type of service. The consultation you complete with the client must also take into account any influencing factors such as:

- the desired look
- hair elasticity
- head and face shape
- hair texture
- hair length
- hair density
- alopecia
- transition.

> **Remember**
>
> Make sure you confirm the look with the client before starting the service to make sure you are absolutely certain you understand their requirements.

The desired look

This should be thoroughly discussed with your client prior to starting the service. The use of visual aids, for example, stylebooks and / or other examples in the salon may assist your client in making their choice. You must be both honest and realistic when discussing styling possibilities with your client. If you know you can't achieve your client's choice of style, you must explain the reasons why and suggest a more suitable option.

You should also discuss the direction of the plaits. If your client has any strong hair growth patterns, this may influence the direction of the plaits. Plaits should follow the hair growth patterns as this will encourage the hair to lie flat to the scalp and therefore reduce the amount of tension placed at the root area.

Hair elasticity

This must be considered, as hair with poor elasticity may break if too much tension is applied. Hair that has recently had plaiting and or extensions, particularly with tension, for fairly long periods of time, is unlikely to have good elasticity.

> **Remember**
> Hair that has been chemically treated may have poorer elasticity.

Head and face shape

The style you wish to create must flatter your client's head and face shape. Refer to Unit G21 pages 52–4 for more information on head and face shapes.

Hair texture

The texture of the hair must be considered for several reasons.

- If the hair is very curly, it may require drying with a comb attachment on the hairdryer to elongate the curl prior to plaiting. This will stretch out the curl, leaving the hair easier to work with.
- The texture and curl pattern may vary across the head, for example, the hair at the frontal region is sometimes finer and therefore may have a tendency to break. It may be advisable to perform off-scalp plaiting in this area and avoid unnecessary tension. You may also choose to use added hair to give the illusion of thicker hair.
- The hair in the nape area often has a tighter curl and is more dehydrated and brittle.

> **Remember**
> The length of time the braids should remain in the hair will be dependent on:
> - the type of braid
> - the hair's texture
> - the client's ability to maintain the style.

Hair length

The length of the hair you will be working with should be considered. You must make sure the hair is long enough to achieve the desired results.

Hair density

The density of the hair will affect the size of the sections you take when plaiting the hair.

- If the hair is abundant, then smaller sectioning will be required.
- If the hair is less dense, then you may need to take thicker sections.

Alopecia

Traction alopecia is more prevalent among clients who wear their hair braided. This is due to the amount of tension used when braiding the hair. It usually occurs around the frontal and temporal areas of the scalp, due to the stylist starting the braids with too much tension.

It is important that you can identify the first signs of traction alopecia and begin a programme of correction before the condition deteriorates further. The first indications of traction alopecia include:

- thinning of the hair, usually in the frontal and temporal regions
- a sore and tender scalp
- evidence of raised follicles.

Traction alopecia may also occur in clients with hair extensions as a result of adding too much extension material, in proportion to the amount of natural hair within a section. The extension material becomes too heavy for the natural hair to support, thus putting undue stress on the natural hair.

Wearing the braids for too long may also cause traction alopecia. You should advise your clients to have their braids removed after six weeks (if not before) and allow their hair and scalp to recover before re-braiding the hair.

> **Be professional** ★★★
>
> If you have a client with traction alopecia, it is your responsibility to:
> - question them on their styling techniques to ascertain why the condition has happened
> - make notes on their record card of their responses and note all affected areas
> - make the client aware of all the affected areas and the potential consequences of ignoring the condition
> - ensure all tension is removed from the hair and treatments are applied to the hair and scalp
> - re-educate your clients so that the condition will not recur in the future
> - refer the client to a trichologist, if necessary.
>
> In the most severe cases, traction alopecia may never improve, due to the trauma caused to the follicle and surrounding tissue. This may ultimately result in **cicatricial alopecia**.

> **Cicatrical alopecia**
> alopecia caused by scarring.

Unit AH28 — Design and create intricate styles using plaiting techniques

In the event that you identify any adverse hair, skin or scalp conditions that may contra-indicate this service, it may be necessary to refer your clients to others for further treatment before you are able to carry out creating complex styling. Refer to Unit G21 pages 45–50 for more information on hair, skin and scalp conditions (including other types of alopecia).

Each of the influencing factors should be thoroughly explored and any areas for concern identified. For example, if a client is suffering from traction alopecia, then plaiting the hair and all the tension this places on the hair follicle is not advised.

In summary, when carrying out plaiting services it is essential that you have an understanding of the effects of these techniques on the hair. This will enable you to recognise any serious conditions, such as alopecia, and give advice accordingly.

Transition

Hair that is in transition – for example, where part of the hair has been relaxed while the remainder is natural – needs to be treated with care as the hair shaft has two different textures. At the point where the textures meet, the hair may be prone to breakage. Excessive tension is not advised.

Check it out

Write a short description on the influencing factors that would affect any plaiting services.

KS **Key Skills Links**: Level 2 Communication

Preparing the work area: checklist

What to do	Why / how?
All the necessary tools and equipment for the service should be ready	Saves time and conveys professional image to the client
Any products needed for the service should be available and ready to use	Regular and effective stocktaking will ensure that all products are available
Work area must be clean and tidy	Prevents accidents occurring, reduces risk of cross-infection and portrays a professional image
Instruct junior staff to prepare the work area correctly	Saves time. Make sure that you clearly communicate what is required – a short list of instructions may be given to junior staff
Tools and equipment should be clean, sterilised and fit for the purpose	The appropriate method of sterilisation should be used and equipment should be checked for defects

What to do	Why / how?
Electrical equipment should be used in compliance with health and safety legislation	Ensure that junior staff are complying with the safe use of electrical equipment (see Unit G22, page 16). This is your responsibility

Personal standards of hygiene: checklist

What to do	Why / how?
Make sure your body and clothes smell clean and fresh	The client will feel more comfortable in your presence. Daily washing and the use of a good deodorant are essential
Make sure your breath smells nice	Use a breath freshener. This will help to combat odours from strong-smelling foods or smoking
Do not work if you are feeling unwell	Infections can be spread in the salon. Keep yourself fit and healthy to ensure that you produce the best work possible
Maintain good posture while working. Think about whether your client is positioned correctly for your needs as well as their own comfort	This will minimise the risk of injury or fatigue. Make sure you keep your back straight and your balance evenly distributed. Having your tools and equipment close to hand will prevent you from over-stretching

Check it out

Think about the methods of sterilisation you currently use in the salon. Are they the most suitable options? Look at Unit G22 pages 13–14 and consider the various methods available to use, then decide if you need to change to a more suitable or economical method.

Personal protective equipment

The use of personal protective equipment benefits both you and your client. It is used to protect clothes and skin from the effects of any products that you are using and also to prevent the client from becoming covered in hair. The use of a gown and towel during plaiting services will protect your client both from stains from products being used and from hair. It is crucial that you use clean gowns and towels for each client to prevent cross-infection. Both items need to be boil-washed to ensure their cleanliness. You also need protection from products and hair and this can be achieved by wearing an apron.

Preparing the hair

It is essential to prepare the hair thoroughly prior to commencing the plaiting service. Depending on the look to be achieved you may have to shampoo, condition, blow-dry or wrap-dry the hair to thoroughly disentangle the hair and loosen the curl. Loosening the curl will enable you to achieve smoother results. This may be performed using the comb attachment on the hair dryer.

Remember

When using electrical equipment, you must consider your responsibilities under the Electricity at Work Regulations 1989.

However, before any plaiting takes place you should moisturise the hair and scalp with a dressing oil.

Avlon

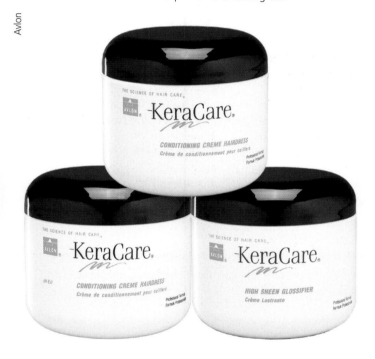

You may also need to apply a wax, gel or oil for dressing purposes as you continue with your styling. This, however, depends on the look you are creating. Accurate sectioning before you begin is essential and, as you continue with your styling, you must make sure your sections are neat and even as this will help you to control the hair. It will also determine the direction of the plait, create a strong base for the plait to ensure optimum results and the style will last longer. It will also reduce the risk of trauma to the scalp, if hair from one section is braided into another.

Creating the look

Once you are fully prepared and understand your client's requirements, you are ready to begin the service. As you are working towards the completion of the style you must be aware of how the style is to be achieved and which techniques, products and equipment you are using and why.

Correct positioning of self and client

Plaiting is a service that can take a long time to complete. Therefore, it is important that you remain aware of your personal stance and the positioning of the client's head throughout the service. These factors can have a dramatic effect on the outcome, as they can affect the angle of the plait. For your own safety you must stand and be working over your client in a position that allows you freedom of movement. Your position should not cause you any undue stretching or leaning, which may lead to fatigue, harm or injury.

As well as considering your own comfort, you must also think about the needs of your client. It is vital that the client's head is positioned to allow you to reach areas and achieve the degree of tension needed. However, you should not expect your client to feel discomfort during the service. You should check that your client is able to move their head into the position you require. Any prolonged bending of the head is likely to cause your client pain and discomfort.

Remember

As a stylist working in a salon, you cannot afford to ignore the potential long-term effects of incorrect posture. It may lead to repetitive strain injury, which could bring about an early end to your career as a hairdresser.

Be professional ★★★

As you will be concentrating and involved in what you are doing, it is easy to forget the needs of your client. To prevent this, ask a junior member of staff to check the client's welfare regularly and make sure that they are not experiencing any discomfort.

Products

Your salon may be loyal to only one product manufacturer. However, this is not always the best option — you could be missing an opportunity to use a styling product that is more suited to the needs of your clients. You can keep up to date with what is available on the market by:

- visiting the wholesaler and looking at other products
- talking to manufacturers' representatives visiting the salon
- looking through trade publications
- attending trade events, for example, competitions, trade fairs
- using websites.

However you choose to stay up to date is your own personal choice, but it is vitally important that you develop your product range in line with the needs of your clients. Failure to do so may result in you being left behind by the competition and your clients may choose to visit a salon with a more varied product range.

Features and benefits of products

Although there are a variety of products that you may use when plaiting, it is essential that you understand their particular features and benefits; the table below provides a quick reference to what's on offer.

Check it out

Take the time out to read the manufacturer's instructions on the styling and finishing products you use. You may find that you are misusing or wasting products by overuse, which is not cost-effective.

Remember

COSHH legislation governs any products that you use in the salon. Under these regulations you have a duty to store, handle, use and dispose of products according to salon policies, local by-laws and manufacturers' instructions. You must also ensure this information is relayed to the clients that purchase the products as retail.

All of the products should contain ingredients to protect the hair from the effects of humidity, by coating the hair with a protective film. They should also contain conditioning / moisturising agents to nourish and lubricate the hair and scalp. All products should be used economically to prevent unnecessary wastage and overloading the hair and scalp.

Product	Features	Benefits
Gel	Aids the styling process by holding the hair in place	Use of gel will aid with the styling process and hold the style in place for longer. It is also useful for keeping stray hairs smooth and tidy
Wax	Helps to soften the hair and make it more pliable. However, avoid overuse on fine hair	Wax will moisturise and help prevent damage to hair that is under stress. Helps to hold the style
Spray	Holds the hair in place both during and after styling	It will help to maintain the style for longer and hold the hair in place whilst carrying out the service
Sheen spray	Gives sheen to the hair	It adds moisture to the hair and helps prevent dehydration
Oil	Moisturises the hair and scalp. It is especially effective on dry, coarse hair	It will help to prevent the hair from becoming dehydrated and damaged

Tools and equipment

Tools and equipment	Uses
Blow dryer with comb attachment	To loosen the curl before plaiting the hair, and aids disentangling
Wide-tooth comb	To disentangle the hair prior to plaiting
Tail comb	For sectioning the hair to ensure even sections. May be used to help with the removal of plaits
Sectioning clips	To effectively secure any hair not being styled and to keep sections visible
Hackle	To disentangle the hair prior to use. May also be used to blend different colours of hair together
Mixing mats	To hold the disentangled hair until needed. They enable you to select a small amount of hair at a time without disturbing the rest
Hair grips and pins	To secure the hair into place
Scissors	To cut the added hair to the required length

Looks and styles

Designed cornrows

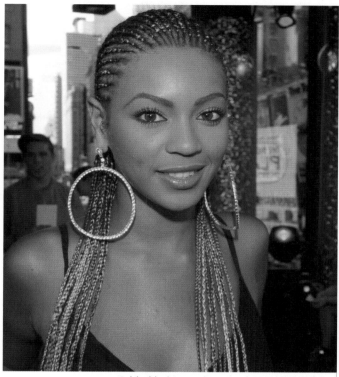

Added hair can give a multi-textured look

Jumbo braids

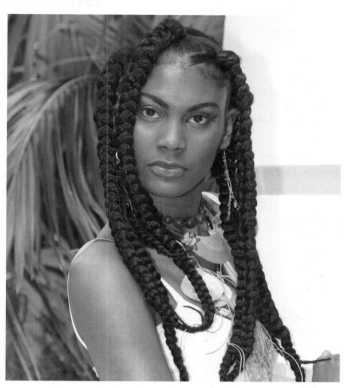

Goddess braids

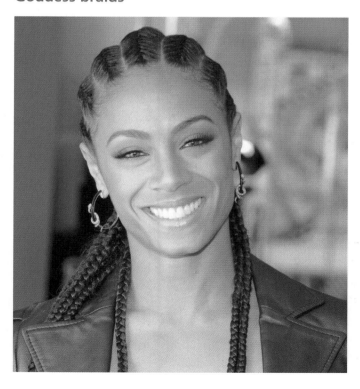

Added hair

The use of added hair when plaiting may be to:

- add volume to the hair
- give the style another dimension
- add colour
- extend the length of the style.

Types of added hair

There are many different types of added hair that may be used when creating styles using plaiting techniques. These include both natural and synthetic fibres that are available in a variety of lengths, textures and colours. The added hair may be purchased on a weft or as a bundle.

Nylon synthetic hair: this is the cheapest option to use. However, you must make sure that the quality of the hair is good as poor-quality nylon synthetic hair has been known to break the hair.

Kanekalon: this is a much better option, as the quality of the synthetic fibre is very good. Many stylists prefer to use kanekalon as it feels softer, tangles less and does not damage the natural hair.

Human hair: this is the most expensive option for added hair. The quality may vary quite considerably. You must ensure you use a reputable wholesaler who can guarantee the quality of the hair. This may be a good option if you have clients who are known to have allergies to synthetic products.

Yak: this is often used when adding hair, as it is relatively inexpensive. It is a natural fibre and when mixed with small quantities of human hair it loses the artificial shine.

How to divide and separate added hair

Experienced stylists will divide and separate added hair by picking it from the bundle as they work through the plaiting service. However, you may find it beneficial to prepare the hair prior to use. This necessitates the use of a hackle and mixing mats. The hackle is basically steel prongs protruding from a wooden board. It is used to disentangle the hair and blend colours by drawing the hair through the steel prongs. The mixing mats are wooden boards with short bristles coming out from the board. The pre-hackled hair is placed on top of one of the mixing mats, and another mixing mat placed on top to hold the hair in place. This enables you to draw off small amounts of hair at a time without disturbing the remaining hair, which is held in between the mixing mats. The hair may be cut to the desired length before, or after, using.

How much hair should be added?

The amount of added hair you use will depend on several factors. If the hair is very fine and you are using added hair to give the hair a thicker appearance, you must ensure the amount of hair you use will not put undue stress on the natural hair, as this may result in traction alopecia. It may be necessary to use only five or six strands of added hair.

Methods of securing the added hair

There are several different methods that may be used to secure added hair. The added hair may be:

- fed into the style during plaiting
- knotted onto a strand of the natural hair, then introduced into the plait or twist
- twisted around the natural hair and tied with a matching coloured thread.

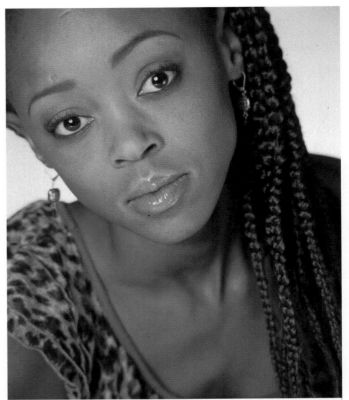

Braid extensions can help create an elegant, glamorous look

Check it out

Search the Internet (using search engines such as Google or Ask Jeeves) to find examples of the various plaits covered in this unit. Ask your tutor / trainer to demonstrate the looks.

 Key Skills Links: Level 1 ICT

Plaiting techniques

Plaiting the hair is a method of dividing the hair into sections and placing them over or under each other to achieve a variety of looks. As these techniques involve 'picking up' hair at the base, it is essential that the hair you pick up comes from underneath the area where you are plaiting. The picked-up hair must never come from another subsection or further down the plait, as this will create unnecessary tension on the roots of the hair, which may lead to breakage. Your plaiting should be carried out without undue tension being applied; however, the tension you use must remain even throughout the service if you are to create an even result.

The techniques you will use include **fishtail**, **cornrow** and **French plaiting**.

Fishtail

sometimes called a herringbone plait. The plait has four stems and the herringbone effect is achieved by crossing the hair strands over each other.

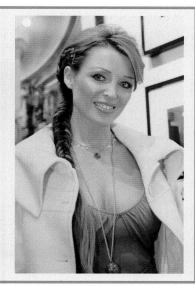

Cornrow

sometimes called canerow. It is a three-stem plait that sits on top of its own base.

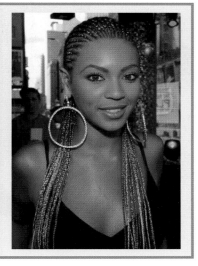

French plaiting

is a three-stem inverted plait.

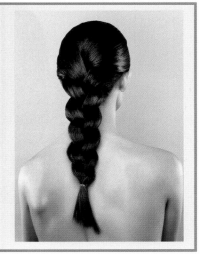

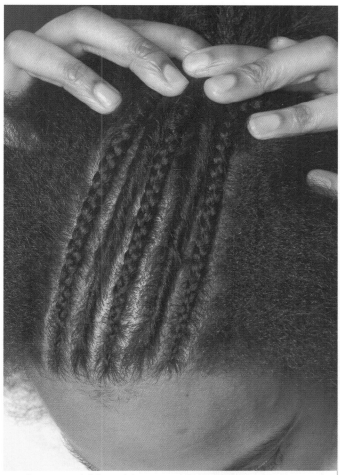

Carry out plaiting with even tension, to create an even result

Finishing off the plait

There are several different ways in which the plait may be finished, for example:

- Using covered elastics — these must be bands for professional use to prevent hair breakage.
- Knotting the ends of the hair and cutting off loose ends close to the knot.
- Using a braid sealer — this cuts and seals the ends of the hair at the same time.
- The ends may be dipped into hot water at the backwash. The hair must be long enough to reach the water. This method may be used if the clients like the ends of the plait to remain curly. Remember this method is only suitable for added hair, not natural hair!

Unit AH28 Design and create intricate styles using plaiting techniques

Cornrow plaits: a step-by-step guide

1 Before the service.

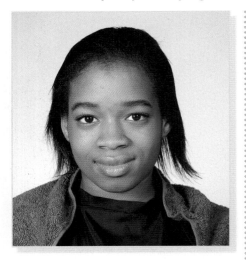

2 Moisturising products are applied to the scalp.

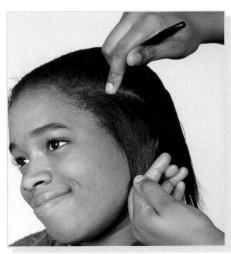

3 Section the hair into two parts — an upper and a lower section. Take a diagonal subsection from the upper section.

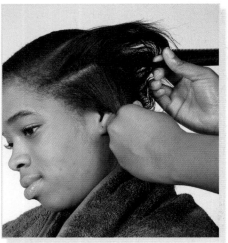

4 Begin the plait on the upper section.

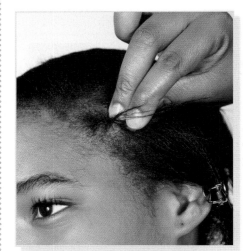

5 Plait the hair using diagonal sections. Complete the first plait but leave the ends out.

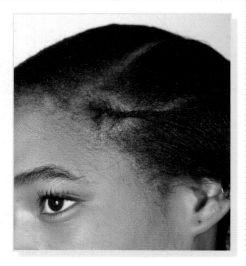

6 Complete the plaits in the upper section in a similar fashion.

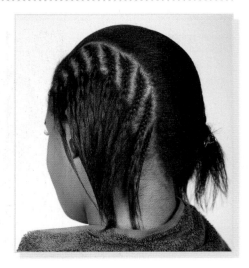

7 Plait the lower part of the section upwards, to meet the upper section.

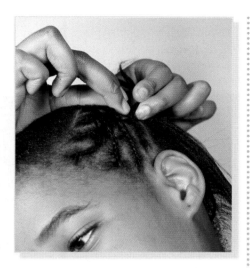

8 Plait the 'tails' of the plaits to form a cane row.

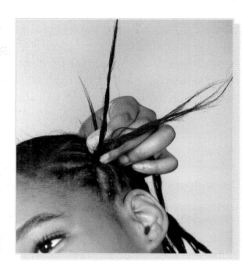

9 Plait the ends and secure.

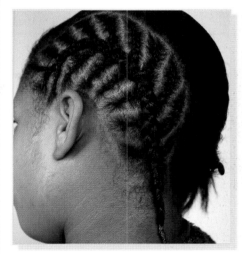

10 The first section is now complete. Continue in a similar fashion throughout the head.

11 The finished look from the back.

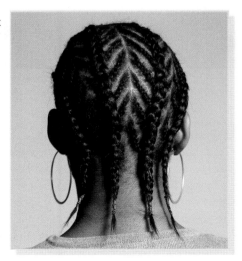

12 The finished look from the side.

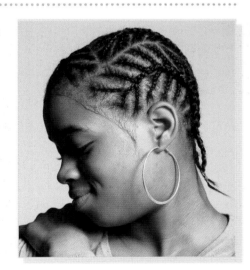

Unit AH28 Design and create intricate styles using plaiting techniques

313

After the service

Once you have achieved the finished look it is important that you complete the service professionally by ensuring the client is happy and understands how to maintain the look. You must advise the client on the products required to moisturise and nourish the hair and scalp. This also keeps the style in place longer. You must explain not only how to care for the style but the importance of correctly removing the plaits. Whether you advise a salon visit for this or advise on how to remove them at home depends on the complexity of the finished look and the client's requirements.

Check it out

List the different plaiting services that are available within your salon and find out the length of time given for each different styling technique.

KS **Key Skills Links**: Level 2 Communication

Confirmation of the finished look

On completion of the style you have created it is imperative that you check with your client to confirm their satisfaction. Discussing the finished look is all part of the professional service you are offering. You must show the client the new style from every angle using a back mirror, checking that they are happy with the finished effect. This will ensure your client does not leave the salon feeling disappointed with the finished look. It also gives your client an opportunity to discuss the outcome of the service and for you as a stylist to gain feedback on your work. This will help you to continually develop and improve your skills. The work you produce should be of a high standard that will enhance not only your own professional image, but also that of the salon.

Your work should be completed within a time that is deemed commercially viable for your salon.

After-care and home advice

You have a responsibility to your clients to make sure that they fully understand how to maintain the style and take care of their hair at home. Your clients are a walking advertisement for your salon, therefore you must ensure the work that you carry out reflects the kind of image you want to portray. Giving your clients expert advice on how to look after and maintain their hair will not only help them to feel confident about how they look, but will also enhance your reputation as a professional hairdresser.

Be professional ★★★

If a client shows signs of traction alopecia, you must advise immediate removal of all plaits. The hair must be given time to recover and no stress placed on the hair until it has grown back and is healthy once more.

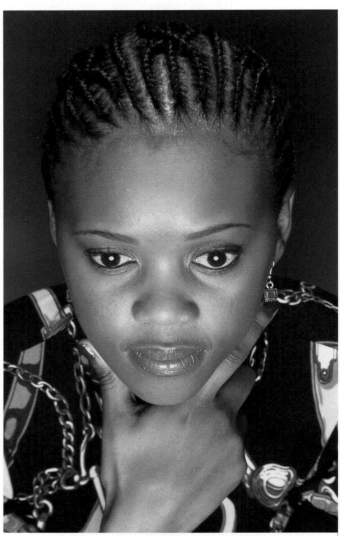

Your client will reflect the image you want to portray for your salon

Be professional ★★★

You should advise your clients to cover their hair when they sleep. The plaited hair should be covered with a silk scarf or a 'durag' as this will help to keep the oils in the hair, prevent the hair from matting and generally keep it tidy. Don't forget to advise your clients on the products they should be using at home to maintain their plaits in optimum condition, for example, a moisturising spray for braided hair will add moisture to the hair and scalp, and prevent dehydration.

The table below gives guidance on how to maintain the look and includes advice on shampooing and conditioning the hair.

Technique	Maintenance	Shampooing and conditioning
Plaiting	A light oil may be applied to the scalp to moisturise. A light oil-based spray may be used on the plaits to add shine and prevent the hair drying out	Use products specifically used for plaited hair, following the manufacturer's instructions. If shampooing the hair, apply the shampoo onto the palms and emulsify the shampoo in your hands. Apply the shampoo to the scalp using the fingertips and stroke the shampoo down the scalp between the plaits. Avoid vigorous massage techniques as this will matt the hair and the plaiting may become loose. Rinse the hair well to remove all the shampoo. However, advise clients to return to the salon for the removal service

Removal of plaits

Some clients will remove their plaits at home. However, you should be advising your client to return to the salon for this service, when a deep penetrating conditioning treatment may be carried out. This will help to maintain the hair's condition and prevent future services from becoming limited.

Plaits should be removed carefully by opening up the plait and, taking small sections at a time, undoing the plaited hair with your comb using a picking movement. When all the plaits have been removed, you should then disentangle the hair using a wide-toothed comb starting at the points of the hair and working up. This will also help to remove any braid debris. You must make sure that you support the root area whilst both unpicking and disentangling the hair. The hair can then be gently shampooed and a deep conditioning treatment should be carried out to add moisture to the hair.

Remember

When removing plaits, hair loss may be apparent. This may not necessarily be due to hair breakage, but the hairs that are normally shed on a daily basis have been contained within the plait and are now free to fall. It is essential that you reassure your client of this.

Be professional ★★★

If you are cutting off bands used to secure the plaits, care must be taken not to cut the hair.

In the salon

Itchy scalp dilemma

Sasha returned to the salon eight weeks after having cane row braiding in her hair. The braids looked slightly matted and she was complaining of an itchy scalp. Natalie, the stylist, questioned her regarding her home maintenance programme. It became obvious that Sasha had not been carrying out the maintenance programme that she was initially advised to follow. Natalie soon realised that Sasha's itchy scalp was caused by her not using the moisturising spray; therefore her scalp had become dehydrated. The matted hair was caused by her shampooing her hair too vigorously, and not wearing a scarf to bed.

1 As a stylist how can you ensure that the client fully understands the implications of not following your advised maintenance programme?
2 What should Natalie advise Sasha to do next?

Unit AH28 Design and create intricate styles using plaiting techniques

Check your knowledge

The following questions will help you to check your understanding of this unit. The answers can be found on page 420. Take care, as there may be more than one correct answer for some questions.

1 Why is important to section the hair accurately when plaiting the hair?
   a To ensure the client can see what you're doing
   b To make sure you can control the hair effectively
   c So you can achieve the required style
   d To make sure you can apply products effectively

2 What safety factors should be taken into consideration when plaiting hair?
   a Keep the floor clear of loose hair
   b Ensure the client is positioned correctly to ensure you are both comfortable throughout the service
   c If using bands to secure the ends of the braids, make sure you use professional bands
   d Use products following manufacturers' instructions

3 Why should products be used economically?
   a To make sure your employer remains happy
   b To set a good example to the other stylists
   c To avoid product build-up
   d To ensure the client will purchase retail products

4 How would you determine how much hair to add to the plaited look to ensure a well-balanced finish?
   a By the texture of the hair
   b By the thickness / thinness of the plaits
   c By visually checking the hair as you work
   d By the amount you have in your hand

5 How does the head and face shape of the client affect your styling choices?
   a It doesn't matter as long as the plaiting service is good
   b Added colour will help to detract from any imperfections, so it is not necessary to take it into consideration
   c You must make sure the style complements the head and face shape
   d It determines the styling products to be used

6 How would you recognise traction alopecia?
   a The hair becomes less dense
   b Small round patches of baldness
   c A receding hairline
   d Red, weeping areas with pus

7 What advice would you give to a client with early signs of traction alopecia?
  a It's ok to continue with the plaiting service as long as you don't apply too much tension
  b Keep away from the braiding service until normal hair growth resumes
  c To avoid added hair in the plaiting service
  d To see a trichologist

8 What types of added hair may be used when plaiting the hair?
  a Kanekalon
  b Human hair
  c Yak
  d Lin

9 What are the potential effects of wearing added hair over a long period of time?
  a Headaches
  b The hair becomes dry
  c The scalp becomes itchy
  d The natural hair may become damaged

10 What retail products would you recommend to a client after a plaiting service?
  a Braid spray
  b Wax
  c Oil
  d Sheen spray

Assessment guidance

You must practically demonstrate in your everyday work that you have met the standards for designing and creating intricate plaited styles.

You will be assessed on at least three occasions. One of the observations must be a look consisting of jumbo braids created with added hair using the French plaiting technique.

Simulated activity is not allowed for any part of this unit.

Unit AH28 Design and create intricate styles using plaiting techniques

Style African type hair using thermal styling techniques

What you will learn:

- How to prepare the client
- How to prepare the hair for thermal styling
- How to create a variety of fashion looks using thermal styling techniques
- How to proceed after the service.

Anne Veck, photographer: David Howard

Introduction

Throughout this unit you will be looking at how to style African type hair using a variety of thermal techniques. You will need to be aware of the different characteristics of hair and how these affect your choice of thermal styling technique. You must also consider the risk of using hot tools on the client's hair and the likelihood of them feeling some heat near the scalp. There are several **thermal styling** techniques that you will have to become familiar with and they are: curling, waving, straightening and blending in.

> **Thermal styling**
>
> is a method of using heat to mould the hair into a new shape temporarily.

Hair contains weak hydrogen bonds that are easily broken — the heat you apply will break the bonds and allow you to mould hair into a variety of shapes and styles.

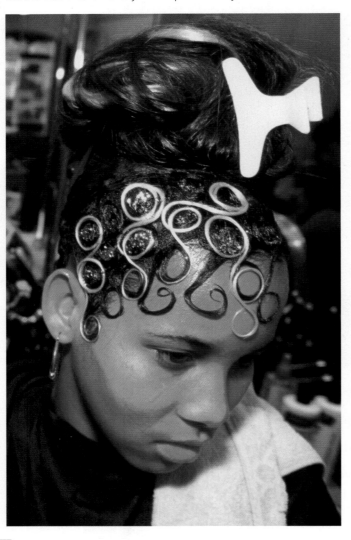

You the stylist

As you become more confident in thermal styling, develop your skills by mixing and matching techniques to create individual and personalised styling for your clients. This will help to increase your client base and improve your employability.

Preparing the client

This section looks at everything that is important when preparing the client for thermal styling. You will need to take into account the health and safety considerations that apply when using thermal styling tools and equipment. The most obvious of these is the risk of burning the client, therefore you must remain alert to this hazard at all times.

Thorough consultation

Your initial consultation with your client is a major factor in determining the finished outcome (see Unit G21, pages 29–32 for more detailed information). It is essential that at this stage you get it right to allow you to style the client's hair using the correct method. Choosing the incorrect thermal styling technique at this stage can lead to burning of the client's hair, skin or scalp. This could lead to irreversible damage. You must begin by talking to your client about their requirements. This is best carried out before the gown is placed on the client to enable you to see the way the client dresses, as this may influence the styling technique you choose. A client may have a picture of the look they require or your salon may have some stylebooks. This will help to give a clearer picture of the client's requirements. It also allows you as the stylist to show your ideas and to advise on what is realistically achievable.

> **Remember**
>
> During the consultation, be sure to inform your client of any discomfort that they may feel during the service. This may include the feeling of heat close to the scalp, but it is essential that the client maintains their position as any sudden movements may cause burning.
>
> If the client is experienced at having thermal styling treatments, then this should not be a problem. However, it may be the first time and you must be sure you have explained thoroughly the implications of using hot tools.

Checking for contra-indications

An essential part of your consultation will be checking for any contra-indications. These are the factors that might prevent you from continuing with the service or cause you to change the techniques you use.

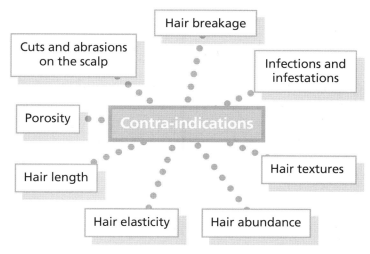

- Hair breakage
- Cuts and abrasions on the scalp
- Infections and infestations
- Porosity
- **Contra-indications**
- Hair length
- Hair textures
- Hair elasticity
- Hair abundance

It is your responsibility as the stylist to determine if the client's hair is suitable for the service. If the hair is **porous**, broken or highly bleached, then you must advise against thermal styling. This is due to the extreme heat used on the hair, which can cause the hair to become dehydrated, porous and brittle. You can advise on a course of conditioning treatments to improve the condition of the hair, which may allow thermal styling in the future. When styling hair that has previously been permed, care must be taken as the hair is more fragile and therefore more likely to be damaged.

Porous hair

hair that has cuticle damage.

Personal health and hygiene

As the stylist, it is important for your own personal health and hygiene to be of a high standard to ensure you maintain a high level of professionalism. You will be working in close proximity with your client and you need to smell fresh and clean to avoid offence. Make sure your breath is fresh, especially after lunch or a cigarette break. Clients and colleagues may be offended by unpleasant odours, therefore it is essential you maintain good levels of personal hygiene. Ensure that your hands and nails are clean and presentable as they are constantly on show. If you wear make-up, touch it up throughout the day to ensure you always look your best.

Remember

You own health is very important when you are working in the salon. If you do not feel one hundred per cent, the quality of your work may reflect this. If you are suffering from an infectious illness, you run the risk of infecting your clients and colleagues.

Check it out

- Does your salon have a specific policy for gowning clients?
- Do you feel the salon should have its own gowning policy?

Personal protective equipment

It is an essential requirement when thermally styling hair that your client is adequately protected, not only from the heated appliances that you are using, but also from any products that you are using on their hair.

Your client must be wearing a protective gown and a towel around the shoulders. If you accidentally over-saturate the hair with product, the gown and towel will help to protect the client's clothing. When you are thermally styling, many of the products that you are using are cream- and oil-based, therefore if they were to be spilled onto your client's clothing, they would cause staining and there is always the possibility that stains cannot be removed. You would then be liable for the cost of any cleaning or replacement of your client's clothing. It is much safer and more professional to make sure your client is adequately protected with a gown at all times. During thermal styling the equipment that you use is extremely hot. Thermal heat pads are available to protect your fingers and hands from the heat.

> **Remember**
>
> Keep checking throughout the service that the client is still appropriately protected and make any adjustments necessary to ensure the client's skin and / or clothing is covered.

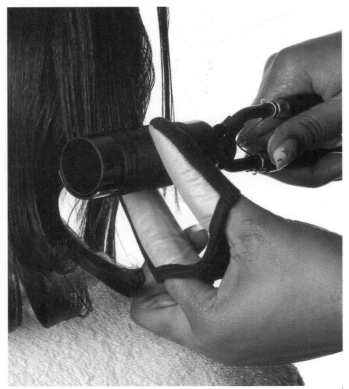

Using thermal heat pads

Preparing your work area

It is vital that you have all the necessary products, tools and equipment ready for the start of the service and they are positioned to ensure everything is within easy reach; this will prevent you from over-stretching and possibly pulling a muscle. It also enables you to provide an efficient service. Being organised in this way will show your client that you are a professional and help to instil confidence in your ability as a stylist. It does not create a good impression if you have to keep leaving your client whilst you find something essential to the service.

> **Remember**
>
> If using an oven to heat your styling tools, this should be switched on early enough to ensure the tools have heated to the correct temperature by the time they are needed.

The tools and equipment you use should always be maintained correctly and checked before use for any faults. For example, thermal irons should be kept clean and well oiled at the joints as this will help to prolong their working life. All tools and equipment must be fit for purpose to prevent the risk of harm or injury to yourself or your client.

If you are using electrical equipment, it should be used following the requirements of the Electricity at Work Regulations (see Unit G22, page 6). This applies to the thermal styling tools you use and also the electric oven.

> **Check it out**
>
> What other items used during thermal styling are covered under the Electricity at Work Regulations?

You must consider the regulations regarding the use of products (for example, COSHH) and ensure you are fulfilling any legal requirements on storage, handling, usage and disposal. Read the manufacturer's instructions if you have any doubt about a product's ability. The manufacturers have tried and tested their products in a variety of different ways and their instructions will ensure optimum results.

Below are the items you should have ready on your trolley prior to the service.

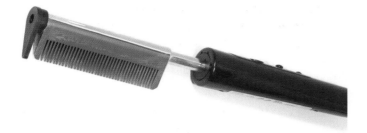

Electric pressing comb

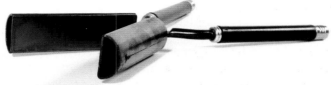

Curling irons of various sizes

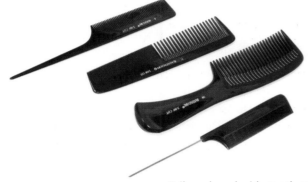

Tail comb and wide-tooth comb

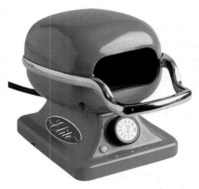

Electric or gas heater

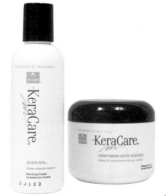

White tissue paper

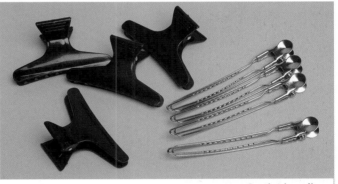

Sectioning clips

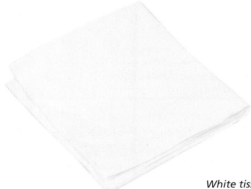

Protective cream / oil

Style African type hair using thermal styling techniques **Unit AH30**

In addition, you must be aware of the potential problems that may occur during the thermal styling process. The table below lists some common problems and the remedial action that should be taken.

Problems	Caused by	Remedial action
Burning the skin or scalp	Lack of due care. Not placing vulcanite comb underneath irons to protect the skin, especially around the ears. Not positioning the client correctly when using tools around the ears and neck	Apply cold water immediately. If serious, seek medical advice
Overly dehydrated or damaged hair	Tools are too hot for the hair. Not using protective products on the hair prior to thermal styling. Hair in poor condition before service commenced	A course of intensive conditioning treatments. No further heat or chemical treatments to be used until the hair's condition has improved
Alopecia	Cicatrical Alopecia, caused by scarring from a heat burn. Traction Alopecia, caused by excessive tension when pressing the hair	No treatment available, permanent scarring. Cease applying tension to the hair and it should grow back
Indentations	Incorrect use of thermal styling tools, or incorrect sectioning techniques	Re-style the hair using the tools correctly and sectioning accurately

When using thermal styling tools in an oven, the temperature of the tools should be tested prior to each use and regularly throughout the service. Placing the thermal styling tool onto a piece of white tissue will show if the tools are the correct temperature. If the tools are too hot, the tissue will discolour and scorch.

Test your thermal styling tools on white tissue

Be professional ★★★

The practice of testing the temperature of thermal styling tools on the ends of the hair should not be undertaken whilst you are learning these new skills. Many experienced African type hair stylists use this method in the salon. However, this practice should be discouraged, as the risk of burning the hair is high.

Stock levels must be checked regularly in order to prevent the embarrassment of running out of a particular product; it is not always possible to substitute one product for another. This would create an unprofessional image, as the finished result might not be satisfactory.

Check it out

- How often are stock checks carried out in your salon?
- What systems are in place for reporting low levels of stock and is this system efficient? If not, design a new one that will save time on stock checks.

 Key Skills Links: Level 2 Communication & Level 2 Application of Number

Your work area must remain clean and tidy at all times. This will not only look good to your clients, but will prevent the risk of cross-infection. If you regularly clean and sterilise your tools, there will be less chance of any bacteria being spread. Your combs should be kept in a chemical jar to prevent the growth of bacteria, and brushes can be sterilised in an ultra-violet cabinet. The heated equipment that is used during pressing should always be wiped over immediately after use. This will prevent build-up of product and carbon on the equipment, which will affect its efficiency. Should product build-up occur, you must use the product manufacturer's recommended cleaning aids.

Check it out

Does your salon have a specific policy for storing, handling and cleaning thermal styling equipment? If not, why not write one yourself that can be used for staff training?

 Key Skills Links: Level 2 Communication

Unit AH30 style African type hair using thermal styling techniques

Preparing the hair for thermal styling

This section looks at preparing the hair and the tools and equipment you would use for thermal styling. It is also important that you understand the effects this type of styling will have on the hair structure. As with all hairdressing services, problems may occur and you need to know how to overcome them. With practice and dedication, you can develop skills that will allow you to create a variety of effects on hair. However, in order to create wonderful looks, it is vital that you understand the underlying principles relating to thermal styling.

The science of thermal styling

When you are thermal styling or pressing the hair, the internal structure is undergoing some changes of which you need to be aware. As you already know, within the cortex lie a number of polypeptide chains, which run along the length of the hair. The chains are spiral-shaped (called an alpha (α) helix) and have cross-linkages that join them to their neighbouring polypeptide chains. Some of these linkages are permanent and others are temporary. The hydrogen bonds, which are one of the temporary linkages, are the ones that enable us to style the hair. The hydrogen bonds are not only joined to their neighbouring polypeptide chain, but are also connected to the same polypeptide chain between the coils of the alpha helix. It is these hydrogen bonds that enable the hair to be stretched during styling, giving the hair its elasticity.

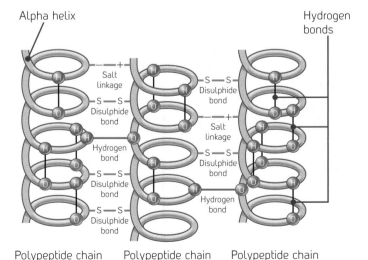

The hair in its natural state – alpha keratin

Prior to styling, when the hair is in its natural state, this is known as alpha (α) keratin. Once the hair has been styled using thermal styling equipment, many of the hydrogen bonds are broken, allowing the hair to be stretched into a new shape. Once the hair has been heated, moulded and allowed to cool into this new shape, the hair is said to be in beta (β) keratin state. It is essential that the hair be allowed to cool before styling and finishing as, if the hair is still warm, some of the new shape may be lost.

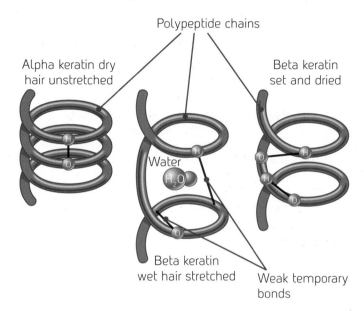

Alpha and beta keratin

The hair will stay in this new position until the hair is made wet or it absorbs atmospheric moisture. This is because the hair is hygroscopic — it has the ability to absorb moisture from the atmosphere. **Humidity levels** will affect the length of time the style will last. The level of humidity in some salons may be quite high due to the evaporation of water from the hair, towels and so on. This is also true during damp weather, therefore it is essential that good styling products are used as this will help to prevent the atmospheric moisture entering the hair quickly, prolonging the life of your styling.

Humidity levels

the degree of moisture in the atmosphere.

When using heated styling equipment on dry hair, the hair's internal moisture breaks some of the hydrogen bonds; however, you must heat the equipment sufficiently to turn the internal moisture into steam. This breaks the hydrogen bonds and allows us to shape hair into a variety of styles.

As temporary setting utilises the natural moisture that is present in hair, overuse of heated styling equipment will cause the hair to dehydrate. Leaving the hair to cool down before dressing is important. If you disturb the hair before it has cooled and set into the new shape, then you will have undone the work you have achieved.

Be professional ★★★

If you are forcing moisture out of the hair with heat styling, you must replace this moisture by using moisturising and conditioning products on the hair.

Check it out

What factors about a client's hair do you think might influence the thermal styling process? Make a list of these and state how you think each may affect the process

 Key Skills Links: Level 2 Communication

The hydrogen bonds within the hair structure are easily broken by moisture. If you have styled a client's hair and they enter a moist atmosphere, then the style will easily 'drop' out. You must advise your clients of this to enable them to prolong the life of the style.

Styling products

There are a variety of styling products that you can use to help you overcome the effects of humidity on hair.

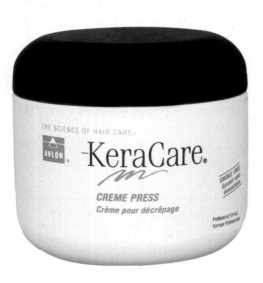
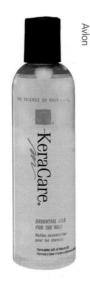

Avlon

The thermal styling products used coat the hair shaft and help prevent any moisture from being absorbed. Some of the products contain ingredients that repel any moisture. Any product that you put on the client's hair will usually have an effect for a few days but will gradually wear off. The client can maintain the style at home by adding more products to the hair; this will help to extend the life of the style. It is important to remember that despite the amount of product used to combat the effects of the hair's hygroscopic nature, some moisture will penetrate the hair shaft, affecting the style. If the client is caught in a rain shower or sweats heavily, then you cannot guarantee the style will hold.

Thermal styling on white hair

When you are thermal styling on white hair, there are several factors that you must consider:

1 Take care not to discolour the hair through scorching or over-heating. You should always test the temperature of the tools you are using before using them on the hair. Think of the way hot tools will scorch white tissue paper – the effects on white hair will be exactly the same.
2 Take care not to discolour the hair with product usage. If you apply excessive amounts of styling or moisturising products to the hair, then you run the risk of staining any white hair. Ensure that you apply only the correct amount of product and always follow the manufacturer's instructions.
3 The texture of white hair must be taken into consideration. White hair tends to be coarser and more resistant, so take care not to apply too much heat to combat this. It will lead only to irreparable damage.
4 Watch out for discoloration due to prolonged use of heated appliances. When you are thermally styling white hair, although you are aware of the amount of heat you are using at the time, over a longer period continued heat application may cause damage to the hair. If this occurs, you should be advising your client to give the hair a rest from heat and trying alternative styling methods.

If you take note of the above points, then thermally styling white hair should not present any problems to you.

Influencing factors

There are several influencing factors that you need to consider when styling hair using thermal styling tools. Each of the factors may present problems to you during the process if you have not taken time to consider their relevance.

The haircut and length

You will need to consider the client's haircut, as you must ensure the styling technique you choose is suitable for the length and style of the client's hair. For example, if the client's hair is very long, you would not choose to create a head of barrel curls but would perhaps choose spiral curls.

Shorter hair is ideal for barrel curls. If the hair is too short though, there is a greater risk of burning when pressing and it may just not be possible.

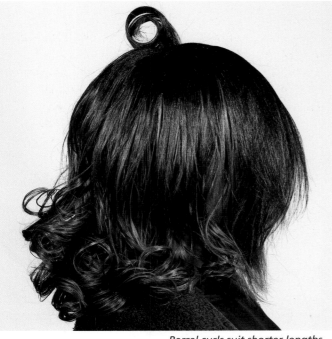

Barrel curls suit shorter lengths

The hair re-growth of chemically relaxed hair

You will need to ensure there is enough re-growth for you to work with. You should be able to judge your level of skill with the pressing comb and know your limitations. Care must be taken when pressing short hair, especially around the front hairline, as the hair tends to be finer and the likelihood of burning the client becomes greater. Another important factor to consider is that if the hair has been chemically relaxed, then it will be more fragile than the root area that you are pressing. Take care not to overlap as breakage may occur on the previously relaxed hair.

Hair elasticity

You will need to carry out an elasticity test on the hair (see Unit G21, page 41). Hair with poor elasticity is usually due to internal damage, in which case you must reconsider the hair's suitability for thermal styling. If the hair is chemically treated, then it is most likely that the elasticity will be poor. The addition of heat is likely to further weaken the hair's condition, and may cause breakage.

> **Remember**
>
> If you feel the hair's elasticity is too poor for thermal styling, recommend conditioning treatments until such a time as the hair's condition improves sufficiently to carry out the desired service.

Hair density

> **Hair density**
>
> how much hair a client has, e.g. abundant or sparse.

The amount of hair a client has will determine the size of the sections you take. Your sections will need to be finer if the hair is thicker. This will allow better penetration of heat through the hair and will ensure an even result. For example, if you are tonging the hair, make sure that the section you take is no larger than the barrel of the tongs. Alternatively, if you are crimping, take a finer section to ensure a good indentation is left in the hair.

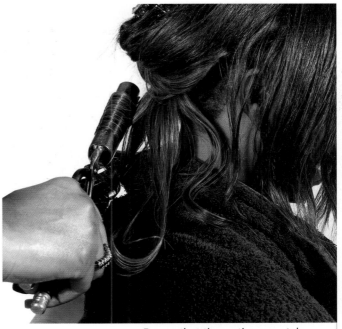

Ensure that the sections you take are appropriate to the hair's density

Hair texture

> **Hair texture**
>
> thickness of each individual strand of hair.

In hairdressing the different textures are known as fine, medium or coarse. The finer the hair, the less heat it will require to style. Alternatively, the coarser it is, the more heat will be needed. An example of this is when you are pressing the hair; if it is coarse, it will require hard pressing and if it is fine, a softer press.

Curl pattern

Our genes will predetermine the curl pattern of our hair. There are several types of curl pattern ranging from tightly curled to wavy and they will affect the techniques that you carry out. For example, a client with curly hair will require more tension and heat to straighten the hair than a client with wavy hair. You will need to consider the implications on the hair's condition of using more heat and tension. Over the whole of the head there can be several different curl patterns, and you should be looking at all the different areas to assess how resistant the curl formation will be.

Head and face shape

> **Check it out**
>
> What effect will extremes of heat and tension have on the hair?

As with all hair styling, this is an influencing factor that cannot be overlooked. You must ensure that the finished look will suit the client's head and face shape. This is carried out at the initial consultation and you will by now be familiar with the many different face shapes and which styles are best suited to them (you should have learned about this in Unit G21, pages 52–4).

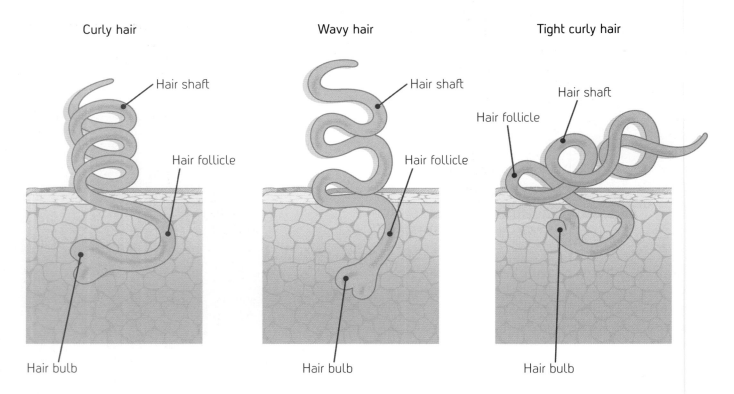

Types of curl patterns

Unit AH30 Style African type hair using thermal styling techniques

Creating a variety of fashion looks using thermal styling techniques

Check it out

When using thermal styling techniques, remember you can mix and match the techniques to create individual and personalised styling for your clients. Keep your camera handy so you can photograph the work you produce; this may be used as evidence in your portfolio.

KS **Key Skills Links**: Level 2 Communication

There are several different techniques that you need to perfect within this unit. Below is a table showing each of the techniques, with examples of the tools used and the effects they produce.

Technique	Tools used	Effect produced
Soft or hard pressing	A pressing comb can be heated in a stove or electrically	Straightening. Hair can be prepared by blow drying (or wrap-drying) to smooth it out first
Curling	Tongs or irons can be heated in a stove or electrically	Barrel curls, flicks or smoothed hair
Crimping	Crimping irons	Zigzag indentations
Smoothing / straightening	Flat irons	Flattens and smoothes the hair
Blending in	Small flat irons or pencil tongs	Smooth with a slight bend

You need to be familiar with each of the techniques and be able to decide which one is correct for your client's hair. This will depend on the client's requirements, the hair's condition and its texture. You should have determined the outcome of the service during the consultation.

Before starting work with the thermal styling equipment, the hair should be shampooed, conditioned, blow-dried or **wrap-dried**. A wide-tooth comb attachment may be used when blow-drying the hair straight; this helps to prepare the hair for subsequent treatments as it smoothes and disentangles the hair, making it much easier to work with. You also need to make your client aware of the need for correct positioning whilst the treatment is being carried out. Working on the hair in confined areas, such as in the nape or around the ear, will require you to move the client's head to an appropriate position. You must then keep the head positioned where it is to prevent any contact between the hot tools and the skin.

Wrap-dry

the hair is wound either clockwise or anti-clockwise so the contours of the head form the finished shape to the hair.

Be professional ★★★

Check with your client that they are comfortable throughout the process. Do not exert too much pressure when moving their head into the correct position, as this can cause discomfort or even injury to the client.

Unit AH30 style African type hair using thermal styling techniques

Styling hair using thermal techniques: a step-by-step guide

1 Before the service.

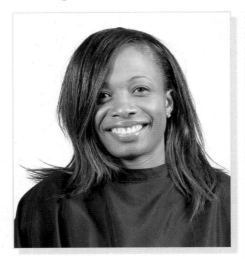

2 Apply moisturising products to the hair.

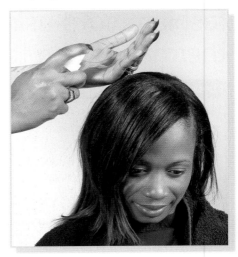

3 Check the temperature of the irons before using.

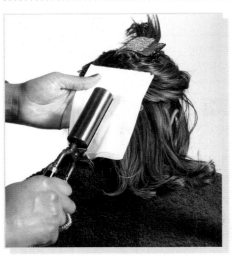

4 Smooth the hair with the irons.

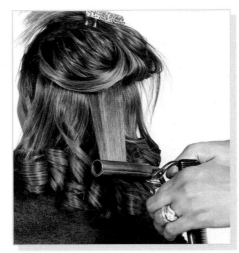

5 Start to curl the hair, making sure the ends are tucked in.

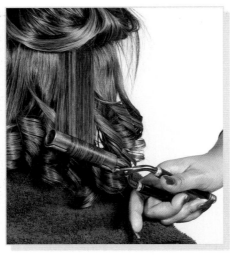

6 Curl the hair upwards towards the scalp.

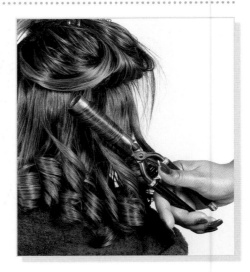

7 Gently release the hair and unwind.

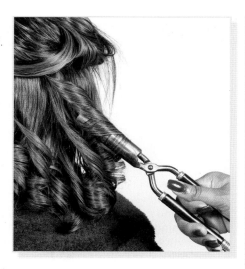

8 The completed curl. Continue in this way throughout the hair.

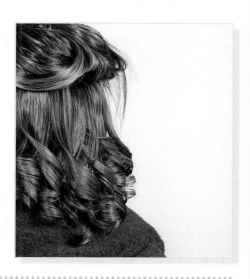

9 Apply finishing products.

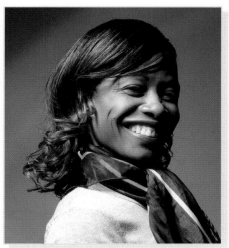

10 Apply styling gel to smooth down any stray hairs.

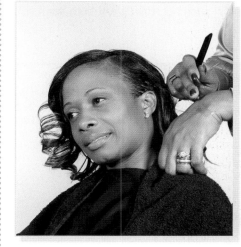

11 The finished look from the front.

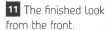

12 The finished look from the side.

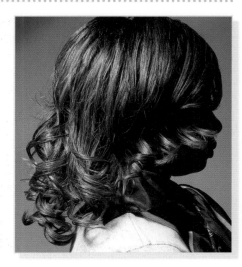

Hair pressing

This technique uses a hot comb to straighten and smooth the hair. It is a good technique to use on a client with a re-growth requiring relaxing, or on a full head to be straightened. Pressing combs can be heated electrically or by using a hot oven. The advantage of electrical combs is that they are thermostatically controlled. Some electrical combs have a temperature dial so you can select the correct temperature for your client's hair (for example, a client with fine, tinted or bleached hair would need a lower temperature to achieve the desired result). This means that they will not overheat and burn or damage the hair. If you are using a pressing comb that you heat in an oven, then, as the operator, you must determine if the comb is at the right temperature. You need to use a piece of white tissue paper, press the comb against it and look for signs of scorching or burning. This tells you whether or not the comb is too hot. If you put the pressing comb into the hair and it is too hot, then it will burn the hair, causing irreparable damage.

> **Remember**
>
> Checking the temperature of your tools at the start of the service is not enough. Your thermal styling tools should be checked each time they are removed from the oven.

Using the pressing comb with an oven takes a lot of practice; with experience you will find it much easier to judge. You must, however, always remain alert to the hazard of burning the hair or skin.

> **Be professional ★★★**
>
> The teeth of the comb and the back of the comb have two different functions when pressing hair. The teeth of the comb separate the hair, allowing the comb to glide through the hair more easily. Combs have different-sized teeth, with different spacing between them. As a general rule, the smaller the teeth and the more tension you use, the straighter the results. Most importantly, it is the back of the comb that actually straightens the hair.

You must keep your tension even while pressing to ensure that your finished result is of an even straightness. The pressure and angle that you hold the comb at must also remain even throughout, for the same reason.

The effects of pressing oils and creams are shown below.

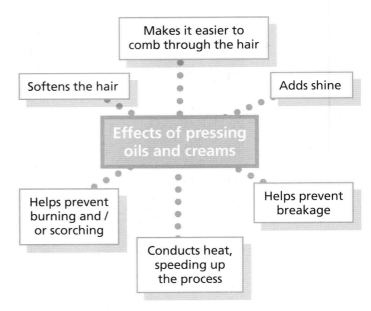

These products should be used sparingly before pressing, as overuse may cause the hair to smoke, which may be a little disconcerting to the client!

Sectioning guide when pressing hair

The texture and density of the hair must be taken into consideration when sectioning the hair for pressing. A general guide is shown in the table below.

Hair type	Size of section
Fine, sparse	2–3 cm
Medium	1.5–2.5 cm
Coarse, dense	1–2 cm

There will always be exceptions to every rule, but practice and experience will enable you to make these decisions based on your knowledge of African type hair.

Styling the hair using curling irons

Curling irons or tongs are available with different-sized barrels, weights and styles and give a variety of different effects, from large curls through to waves in the hair. They may be heated electrically or by using a gas or electric oven.

> **Remember**
>
> When placing the irons in the heater, make sure they are placed correctly as a serious burn could result if they fell out onto somebody.

Conventional curling irons

These are available in different sizes and weights and get much hotter than electrically heated irons; this makes them more versatile, as they may be used on all African type hair. Great care must be taken when using the irons as they may easily burn the hair and skin.

Electrically heated irons

These are the safer option, as they do not get as hot as the conventional irons. They are thermostatically controlled; therefore the risk of burning the hair or skin is less. They are available as cordless appliances that are heated on a base unit, alleviating the problem of the flex wearing away due to continued use. However, this makes them less durable as they may not be hot enough for very coarse hair.

The temperature of the irons should be tested in the same way as the pressing comb, that is, by placing the barrel onto white tissue paper for five seconds. If the tissue discolours or burns, the irons are too hot and will need to be placed onto a cooling pad until they reach the required temperature.

The desired temperature of the irons is dependent on the hair texture and condition. As a general rule, coarse hair can withstand more heat; if the hair is fine or has been lightened or tinted, the temperature should be lower. Hair in poor condition may break if thermal styling is carried out, therefore it is important to test the hair's elasticity prior to the service. If the hair shows signs of damage, thermal styling should not be carried out, as once the hair has been scorched the damage is irreversible.

Remember

- Excessive or continual use of heat can cause the hair to become dehydrated, brittle and prone to breakage.
- Switch off the irons at the socket when you have finished using them – this will help to prolong their working life and prevent accidents.

Holding the irons

Holding the irons correctly will ensure you have control of them when working. Hold the irons in the right hand (not too close to the joint to avoid the heat), place the first three fingers on the lower handle, with the little finger on top. The thumb gives support and balance whilst using the irons.

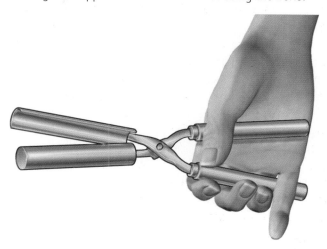

Holding irons correctly

Practise opening and closing the barrel using your fingers to control the movement; this should produce a clicking sound as the barrel closes.

Now practise turning the irons: move your hand forwards, towards your body. This is the technique you will use to create curls. You will need to learn both of these techniques, as the two combined will enable you to create movement in the hair. When first using curling irons, practise with cold irons until you have mastered the art of turning or rolling them.

Creating barrel curls

Barrel curls are usually used on short or medium-length hair to create lift, curl and movement. The hair should be prepared prior to curling. The size of irons you use will depend on the texture and length of the hair and the amount of curl you wish to achieve.

Remember

The angle at which you comb the hair will determine the direction of the curl.

Salon life

Working with hot irons

Rechelle's story

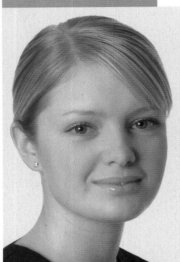

It was a very busy Friday afternoon and I was tonging a client's hair. The client was a regular client to the salon and I usually carried out the client's styling session. I looked up as the door to the salon opened and saw a rep come in that I needed to speak to regarding a training event that I wanted details of. I turned away from my client to try to attract the rep's attention, when I turned back to my client and opened the tongs to remove them from the client's hair, I discovered that the client's hair had stuck to the tongs. I couldn't believe that I had let my attention slip in this way and had to explain to my client what had happened. Obviously she was unhappy and I offered a service for free to try to help repair some of the damage.

Be professional ★★★

- When placing the irons in the heater, make sure they are in correctly as a serious burn could result if they fell out onto somebody.
- Switch off the irons at the socket when you have finished using them – this will help to prolong their working life and prevent accidents.
- Test the heat of the equipment you are using both before you put it on the hair and during the service.
- Make sure your thermal styling equipment is kept clean and free from product residue to ensure they work effectively. Failure to do this may result in the hair becoming discoloured and the equipment may 'smoke', which could be alarming to the client.

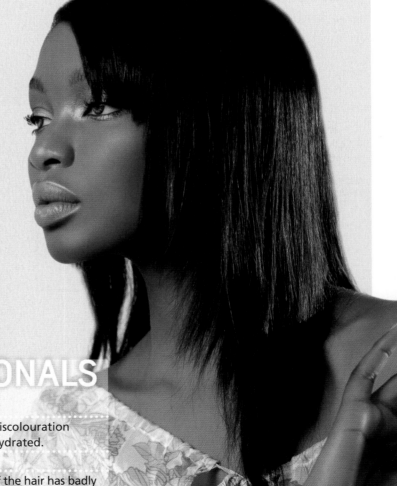

ASK THE PROFESSIONALS

Q *What type of damage had the client's hair suffered?*

A Heat damage. Possible signs of burning / singeing, discolouration and / or hair breakage. The hair will be severely dehydrated.

Q *What could be done to correct it?*

A Intensive conditioning / restructuring treatments but if the hair has badly burnt, then you may have to cut it to remove the damaged hair.

The irons should be placed about 1 cm from the scalp. You must ensure you apply a little tension here to prepare the base. After sliding the irons along the hair shaft, make sure the ends are tucked in properly to prevent **fish hooks**, then wind the hair down so the irons sit on their own base. As with roller setting, you can curl the hair to add volume or to minimise it when necessary.

Fish hooks

when the ends of the hair become bent over, which doesn't give a smooth finish.

Curling to add volume

Comb the section of hair at an obtuse angle to the base (over-directed) and place the irons approximately 1 cm from the scalp. Begin to wrap the hair around the barrel of the irons. Hold the hair in this position for a few seconds to form a strong base. Then rotate the irons until they reach the root area. The curl will sit off base. This method of curling will create maximum lift and volume.

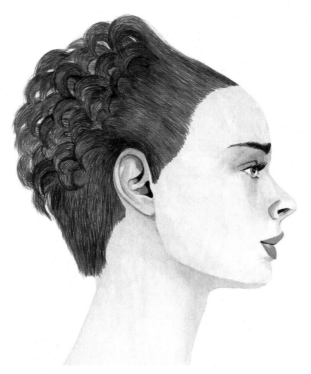

Curling to add volume

Remember

Place a vulcanite comb between the irons and the scalp to prevent burning the client's scalp.

Curling to reduce volume

Comb the section of hair at an acute angle to the base (dragging the roots) and place the irons approximately 1 cm from the scalp. Begin to wrap the hair around the barrel of the irons; you should not need to hold this position, as a strong base is not required. Rotate the irons to complete the curl. Again, the curl will sit off base. This method of curling will produce very little curl or volume and is generally used to blend the hair between the style lines or when the finished result requires just the ends to curl, for example, a bob.

Spiral curling

Spiral curling is carried out on longer hair. The hair should be cleansed and prepared for the service and the correct products used following the manufacturer's instructions. The hair should be sectioned off before you start to curl the hair, as this will help you to work in a methodical manner. The hair should then be divided into vertical sub-sections for you to curl.

Place the irons into the section, close to the root (about 1 cm away), then open and close the irons whilst you turn them and feed the hair into the irons. You must ensure the ends are tucked in properly to prevent fish hooks.

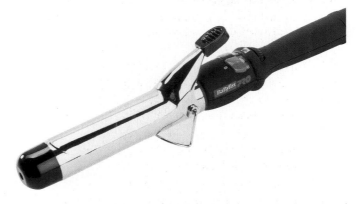

Curling irons: these can be used to wave the hair

Waving the hair using irons

This procedure would usually be carried out on hair that has been chemically relaxed. This effect may also be achieved using waving irons. The hair should be prepared as for thermal pressing.

The irons should be placed into the hair about 1 cm from the roots, with the rod at the top. As you close the irons, comb the hair to the left and move the irons to the right, then turn the irons towards you for half a turn. Allow the hair to heat, then open the irons and move them down the section of hair a little until the groove of the irons is slightly below the wave you have just produced and turn the irons upwards. Allow the hair to heat, then continue until you have completed the waving.

Flat irons and crimping irons

Both of these types of irons, although producing a different look, are used on the hair in a similar way. To prepare the hair, you would always shampoo, condition, blow-dry or wrap-dry first. Starting in the nape and working up the head, small sections are taken and the irons are used along the length of the hair from root to point. The flat irons are taken along the hair length in order to straighten and smooth the hair. The finished look should be even and without indentations.

The crimping irons are placed along the hair length at even intervals to produce the crimped look. It is important to apply the crimping irons evenly otherwise the finished result will have an uneven crimp.

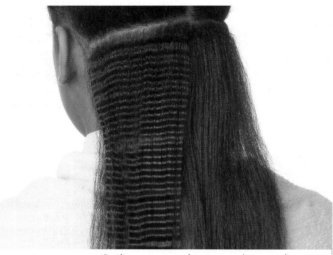

Both an even and uneven crimp can be seen

> **Remember**
>
> You can use a combination of thermal styling tools to create innovative looks.

> **Check it out**
>
> What are your salon's expected service times for the thermal styling techniques you carry out? Are the senior staff times different from those for the junior staff?

After the service

After the service is complete, ensure you fill in / update the client's record card. You should give the client any necessary advice and ensure that you dispose of any waste materials as soon as possible.

Completing client records

You should record details of the treatment and also the information extracted from the client during consultation, for example, hair colourants used, whether these are professional or home colours, how the client cares for their hair between visits, and so on. A record card provides you with essential information about the client. This information is vital to you the stylist and will influence any decisions you make about their hair treatments.

> **Remember**
>
> The information stored on a record card needs to be accurate, up to date and legible. Not only is this a requirement of law but if legal action was brought against you, it could be used as evidence in court.

Confirmation of the finished look

When you have finished styling the hair, you will need to check the balance, overall shape and volume of the finished style, and confirm with the client that they like the end result. Always look in the mirror and check the overall balance from every angle around the head, as this is what everyone will see of your client's look. Show the client the back, making sure that she can actually see through the back mirror. A good rule of thumb is if you can see the back or sides through the mirror, then your client will also.

After-care advice

It is an essential part of the service to provide your client with after-care advice. This advice should cover things such as products for home use, maintenance of the style and potential for style change. Not only is it a fantastic selling opportunity, but it also presents a professional image. You must have thorough product knowledge and ensure that you always have the full product range in stock. The products that you use on your clients whilst carrying out the service should always be offered to the client to buy and use at home. This will help the client to maintain the style with the correct products; oil-based products are used as they help to prevent the hair reverting back to its alpha keratin state.

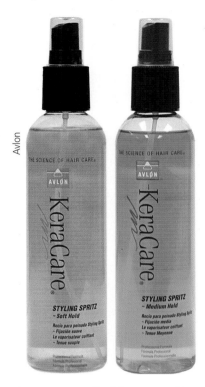

Avlon

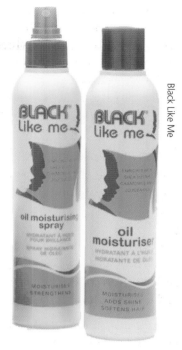

Black Like Me

Get to know the full range of products in your salon

You must make sure your client is aware of how often to cleanse their hair, this will depend on their hairstyle, hair and scalp condition and life-style, but generally you should be advising them to cleanse their hair once a week.

Encourage your client to cover their hair with a silk scarf or **durag** when sleeping as this will cause less friction and help to maintain the style.

> **Durag**
>
> silk-like material wrapped around the head to protect the hair.

> **Remember**
>
> Always advise your client on how moisture will affect the hair and the types of environment to avoid, for example, steamy conditions and sports that are associated with damp conditions, such as swimming, as this can cause the hair to revert back to alpha keratin more quickly.

Spending a little time offering the client some advice on how to style and maintain the look will be time well spent. It will show the client that you are interested in how they look after their hair, which ultimately reflects on your salon. This should include when their hair will require cutting to maintain the shape.

Ensure they fully understand the products they should be using and those to avoid, for example, products that are wet sprays / water-based products will reverse the thermal styling process. Also, be certain you have explained the possibility for style change. If they have had their hair styled for a special occasion and need to wear it less dramatically for work, will they need to return to the salon or can they re-dress it at home themselves?

Disposal of waste

Any waste produced by the service, for example, used tissue, should be removed and your work area cleaned in preparation for your next client. You must dispose of any waste in line with your salon's policy and following the requirements of law. However, if you are using products correctly and following the manufacturer's instructions, then there should be no need for waste. Product wastage can be costly for the salon and should be discouraged.

> **Check it out**
>
> Are you fully aware of all the salon's rules regarding disposal of waste? Is your salon environmentally friendly and adopting a waste recycling policy? For example, is there a paper recycling collection point in your area? Maybe this is something that you could recommend.

Check your knowledge

The following questions will help you to check your understanding of this unit. The answers can be found on page 420. Take care, as there may be more than one correct answer for some questions.

1 What responsibilities do stylists have when using styling and finishing products as stated under the Control of Substances Hazardous to Health Regulations?
   a Store, handle, use and dispose
   b Store, mishandle, use and dispose
   c Show, handle, use and dispose
   d Store, handle, misuse and discolour

2 During thermal styling, why should white hair be treated differently?
   a To prevent it from scorching
   b Because it is older than non-white hair
   c To prevent it from discolouring
   d Because it retains heat

3 What remedial action could you take if you burnt the skin or scalp during a thermal styling service?
   a Leave it to cool down
   b Carry on but avoid the area
   c Stop and administer first aid immediately
   d Apologise to the client

4 Why should thermal styling tools be kept free of excess oils and dirt?
   a So your tools always look good
   b To prevent the build-up of product and carbon on the equipment
   c To give your junior a job to do
   d To ensure they run at optimum efficiency

5 What is meant by the term hygroscopic?
   a Able to displace moisture
   b Able to absorb moisture from the atmosphere
   c Able to expel moisture easily
   d Able to absorb moisture with the aid of styling products

6 Why is it essential that you consider the elasticity of the hair prior to thermal styling?
   a So that the client will think you are professional
   b To prevent hair breakage
   c To weaken the hair's condition
   d Because thermal styling changes the internal structure of the hair permanently

7 Following thermal styling, what are the benefits of giving the client effective after-care advice?

   a To present a professional image of your salon

   b To ensure your client's hair stays in optimum condition

   c To improve your retail sales income

   d To ensure the new style lasts as long as possible for the client

8 What after-care advice would you give a thermal styling client?

   a Make sure you go out in the rain

   b Avoid getting the hair wet or damp

   c Use correct products to maintain the style

   d Cover the hair with a silk scarf or durag when sleeping

9 Under what circumstances would you repeat pressing and add pressure?

   a If the client asked for it to be repeated

   b If the hair is very thick

   c If the hair is very fine

   d When the client wants a hard press

10 If the client requires a lot of volume in the hair, when curling the hair using irons it should be:

   a wound off base

   b wound on base

   c wound using the largest irons

   d wound using the smallest irons

Unit AH30 Style African type hair using thermal styling techniques

Assessment guidance

You must practically demonstrate in your everyday work that you have met the standards for thermal styling African type hair.

You will be assessed on at least three occasions and you will have to prove that you can competently carry out:

- a short graduation which includes the use of pencil irons
- thermal styling on a client with some white hair.

Simulated activity is not allowed for any part of this unit.

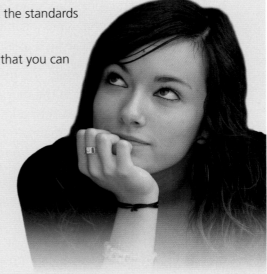

Unit AH30 Style African type hair using thermal styling techniques

4

Professional skills –

barbering

Unit GB6

Provide shaving services

What you will learn:

- How to prepare the client
- What the different shaving tools and equipment are
- How to create the look
- How to proceed after the service.

Guy Kremer

Introduction

This unit is about providing a professional **shaving service** to clients. In order to deliver a service professionally, a good knowledge of the tools for use is required along with a high level of skill when using an open blade razor. With the widespread use of safety razors and electric razors, the majority of men take care of their shaving needs at home. However, since most men require daily shaving to feel clean and look presentable, there is a great need for this service. As a stylist offering shaving services, you should be making every effort to attract clients into the salon.

Shaving services

this relates to any type of shaving service that you offer, for example, full face, beard outline or neckline.

You the stylist

When carrying out shaving, you are removing the visible part of the hair over the face and neck with minimum irritation to the skin. Shaving can take place over the whole face or just in certain areas to tidy up the outline of a beard or moustache. There are factors that must be considered during the shave, for example, hair density, facial contour and direction of growth, each of which will affect the way in which shaving is carried out. You must also consider your own position and that of the client during the service, as ease of access to the areas to be shaved is important to ensure accuracy.

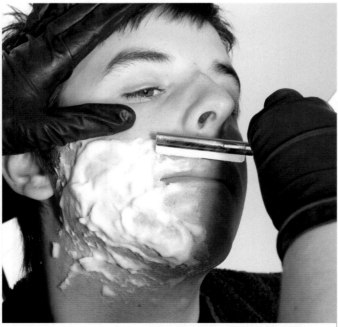

Daily shaving is a must for most men

Preparing the client

This section looks at everything that is important when preparing the client for the shaving service. Being prepared and ready with everything to hand reflects not only your own level of professionalism, but also that of the salon. It will also serve to save you time and increase your client's confidence in your ability.

You will cover:
- thorough consultation
- influencing factors
- safe working practices
- preparing yourself and the client for a service.

Thorough consultation

Determining your client's requirements accurately is essential in order to provide a service that the client is happy with. You must be able to communicate well with your client, not only to extract the right information from him, but also to ensure he fully understands your perceptions of this. It is during this initial process that you will determine the service to be provided, for example, will the client need a beard trim before a full face shave or is just the outlining of the beard required?

You must appear confident and knowledgeable in order for the client to feel confident in your ability. Remember that you are using an open blade directly on the face and a high level of trust between yourself and the client is required. Discuss your client's shave in detail, ensuring that he is made aware of the full process and knows what to expect at each stage.

All the information taken during consultation and regarding the service given and products and equipment used / recommended should be written down on the client's record card. This keeps an accurate and up-to-date account of exactly what the client wants and what you offered / carried out. This would be especially useful if you need to refer back to clear up any discrepancies. For more detailed information on record keeping refer to page 31, in Unit G21.

- During the shave, most clients will close their eyes and relax, knowing that moving or talking could result in cutting the skin. However, it is always wise to have discussed this during consultation and make it known to the client that, although you may continue to communicate, the client needs to remain still.
- You need to inform the client of the expected length of the service and this should fall within the expected service times for your salon. Remember that these will differ according to the type of service required, for example, full or partial shave.

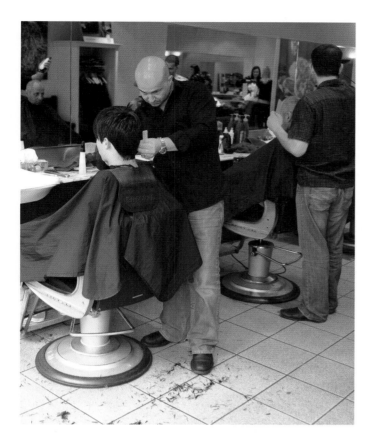

Factors

Factors are all the points that must be considered during the consultation; you must ask appropriate questions to determine these, in order to discover any contra-indications. These may affect the service you provide or even prevent you from continuing!

> **Check it out**
>
> List the types of skin and scalp disorders likely to affect the shaving service and state the reasons why they might prevent you from continuing with the shave. Present the information in a table, using images of the skin and scalp disorders. This can be used as a quick reference guide in the salon both when training staff or to determine what disorder you suspect a client has.
>
> **KS** **Key Skills Links**: Level 2 Communication

It is very important for you to know the structure of the skin in order to understand how it functions and what effect shaving has on the skin. Look at page 34 of Unit G21, where there is a clear and detailed diagram of how the skin is made up.

Hair growth patterns

The way in which the hair grows over the neck or face must be looked at in great detail prior to commencing the shave. Once you have applied the lather, you can no longer see the pattern of growth, therefore it must be considered initially. You should look for deviance in patterns, for example, whorls or bald patches, as again this will affect the shave. The razor should be used over the hair in the pattern of growth to prevent any discomfort or skin irritation. Shaving over the hair against the pattern of growth is advised only on a client with coarse, stubborn hair, as it is more likely to cause irritation and in-growing hairs.

Adverse skin conditions

Skin and scalp disorders may prevent you from carrying out the service and should be given careful consideration. If the client is suffering from an infection or infestation, you must not continue with the service, as there is a high risk of cross-infection. It is crucial that these are found on initial consultation and not during the service.

Unusual features and facial contours

Looking for unusual features and checking the facial contours is important as they may affect the shaving process. Care should be taken in sensitive areas such as over the Adam's apple; if it is larger than average, extra care will be needed. Dimples in the cheeks or chin will also need to be catered for by stretching the skin to pull out the fold, allowing you access with the razor. Look at the area below the lower lip to see if the bottom lip rolls over the skin, hiding any hair in this area. This is a sensitive area and you should take extra care when shaving there. Also, the style of the facial hair, if not all is being removed, will play a role as unusual facial contours can be balanced by facial hair, for example. sharp jaw-lines can be softened by softer more rounded facial hair shapes.

Hair density

The density of the client's facial hair, that is, how thick the hair is on the face, will determine how you complete the shaving service. If a client's facial hair is sparse, then you will be able to begin the shave with the hair at a longer length. However, if a client has a dense beard growth, then you will have to remove as much length as possible (using the clippers) before you begin shaving. This will provide you with a smoother shaving surface, enabling you to glide over the skin with ease and reduce the risk of skin injury. Also, on very dense hair, particularly Asian type hair, you may have to carry out a second over-shave to ensure that all the hair has been removed; this will of course depend on the client's skin sensitivity.

Client's wishes

During the consultation, you will have determined your client's wishes and will know if they affect the service in any way. For example, the client may have long or thick sideburns that he does not want shaving, or a beard or moustache that he requires outlining. You may need to advise the client on another option if you feel what they require is not suitable, but remember to do this with tact and professionalism.

Facial piercing

Any piercing worn in the face must be removed prior to the shaving service being carried out. It will hinder the use of the razor over the skin and could lead to a severe cut. If your client does have any facial piercing, take note of when it was carried out and if it looks inflamed or infected. It may be that if it is relatively new, the skin may still be inflamed, in which case you would advise the client to leave the service and re-book at a later date.

Safe working practices

While working in the salon, it is a requirement of law that you comply with health and safety legislation. The tools you use must always be thoroughly cleaned, disinfected, sterilised and fit for purpose. The methods of cleaning, disinfection and sterilisation you use will depend upon what is available in the salon; however, it may be that you have other options to consider. (Refer back to G22, pages 13–14 to refresh your memory.)

Check it out

List the tools and equipment that you use in the salon while shaving and write next to each one the method of sterilisation that you currently use. You should check that what you are using is sufficient by looking in Unit G22, pages 13–14. Could your methods be adapted to improve your sterilisation routine?

KS **Key Skills Links**: Level 2 Communication

Be professional ★★★

- Before sterilising any tools or equipment you should thoroughly clean them with soap and water, and if they are electrical, a suitable cleaning lotion.
- You also need to consider your responsibilities under the Electricity at Work Regulations. Do you visually check any electrical equipment before use? Is all the electrical equipment tested regularly for faults? You must be sure that both you and the staff for whom you have responsibility are complying with the safe use of electrical equipment.

Check it out

Go to your local council offices and look up any local by-laws that affect the work you do in the salon, particularly regarding the use of open blade razors. You have a duty to follow these, and remember that if you move to another salon in a different area, the relevant by-laws may change.

Preparation of self and client

Preparing yourself for the shaving service is crucial to presenting a professional approach. You must use the correct personal protective equipment. Wearing an apron and gloves will not only protect your clothes from spillage, but also your hands from becoming irritated through regular use of detergent. You should be wearing gloves when applying lather and during the shave. Your client should be gowned correctly following salon policy.

The positioning of the client prior to commencing the service is important. You must adjust your chair for both your own comfort and that of the client. The client needs to feel comfortable and relaxed and you need to adopt good posture whilst working to prevent fatigue. If either you or the client moves to find a comfortable position during the shave, this could result in an accident, causing injury. Ensuring that all your equipment and products are close at hand and fit for purpose is also important. Regular stock checks will avoid the problem of running out of products and equipment.

Remember

Wearing gloves during the shaving service will help to reduce the risk of cross-infection. If you were to cut the client's skin, you may become exposed to body fluids, which can lead to you contracting very serious illnesses such as hepatitis or HIV.

Be professional ★★★

Preparing the client for the shave may involve some facial hair trimming prior to lathering and care must be taken to prevent any loose hair cuttings from falling onto the client's clothing.

Shaving tools and equipment

This section covers the process of the shaving service. You will need to be aware of the types of razors for use, the different techniques employed during the shave, and how to use them safely. Your greatest concern when shaving is damage to the skin and this can be prevented only by taking care while performing the shave and by using sterile, sharp tools. Your success in shaving will become apparent through attention to detail and experience.

You will cover:
- tools and equipment
- lathering products and techniques.

Tools and equipment

Several of the tools you use during the shaving process will already be familiar to you in your haircutting work, such as the clippers and razor. Although you will have gained plenty of experience with clippers, using the razor with an open blade is likely to be less familiar. You must use it with great care and give it the respect it demands.

Clippers

Before you commence the shave, you need to assess the length of the facial hair. If it is too long, then you must remove some. Clippers may be used to remove a dense growth of facial hair. Cutting close to the skin, leaving only short facial hair, will help you enormously in your task. However, care must be taken to ensure the skin is not irritated by close clipper work, as this could lead to damage to the skin during the shaving process.

Open blade razor

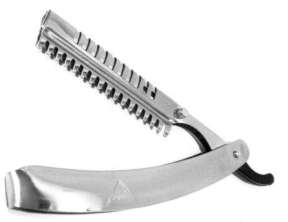

A safety razor

An open blade razor is a razor that has a blade with the sharp edge exposed. You can purchase them with a removable guard that can also be used for cutting hair, as in the photo below left. It is imperative for the blade to be extremely sharp, as a blunt edge will cause grazing or even cutting of the skin. The use of open blade razors is governed not only by government regulation, but also local by-laws. Some local areas prevent the use of fixed blade razors and will permit use only of razors with disposable blades.

When using a razor with a detachable blade, a new one must be used for each client to prevent the risk of cross-infection. It should be disposed of immediately after use. Always remove or fit a new blade with the razor edge facing away from your body to prevent accidents, and when in use ensure that the handle has been fully opened allowing your little finger to rest on the tang, as in the example below.

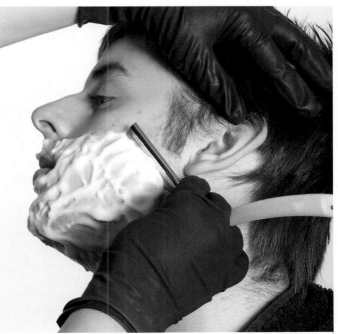

The razor must be held correctly

Remember

If your salon does not have a sharps box, then you are not abiding by the rules of safe disposal of used sharps. There is a high risk of cross-infection or injury when disposing of used sharps and the correct use of a sharps box is essential.

Be professional ★★★

Before the shave, let the client see you fitting the new blade. This will prove your professionalism to the client and serve to increase his confidence in your skills.

Lathering tools

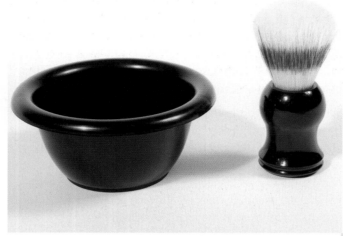

A bowl and lather brush

Most lather is applied to the face using a bowl and lather brush. There are, however, lather dispensers that serve not only to dispense the right amount of lather, but also to pre-heat the lather, making it more comfortable for the client.

Sponges

Sponges are used during a sponge shave. They are soaked in hot water and drawn over the face just before the blade to open the follicle and lift the hair, allowing coarse hair to be more easily removed.

> **Remember**
>
> Sponge shaving must be carried out only following a second over-shave on a coarse beard. Care should be taken as damage may be caused to the skin by using such an aggressive technique.

> **Be professional ★★★**
>
> It is most important to sterilise the lathering brush and sponges after each client to prevent the risk of cross-infection.

Lathering products and techniques

There are many products now available to use whilst shaving, such as the traditional creams, and also oils that can be massaged over the skin. Shaving oil can be used either alone or under your usual lathering product, and provides exceptional cushion and glide. A shaving oil massaged into the beard will swell and soften the hair allowing a closer, more comfortable, shave. This is particularly important for strong bristles, which really benefit from the softening action. Initially you will have to use a variety to try to find a product that you prefer using but with experience you will find which ones work best for your client's skin type.

It is necessary before lathering the face to apply hot towels, as lather should be applied to warm skin. This will serve to:

- soften the hair
- cleanse the face
- open the follicle and lift the hair
- prepare the skin for the lather.

A few towels used one at a time over the face will suffice and the lather should be applied directly following the removal of the last towel. This will ensure the lather is applied to a warm face. Towels can be heated via a warming cabinet or by running under hot water and ringing out thoroughly. The towels should be moist and warm but never dripping wet or very hot.

> **Remember**
>
> You should check that the heat is comfortable on the client's face before applying the towel. This will prevent you from burning the client's skin. The towel is then unrolled and placed on the face as in the photo below, leaving the nose exposed, and allowing the client to breathe.

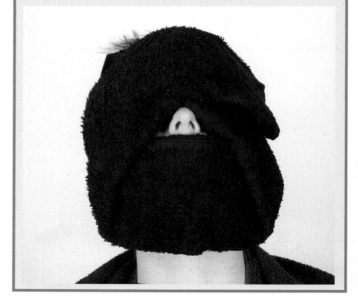

348

Be professional ★★★

Hot towels should never be used on a client with sensitive or irritated skin, as they could cause further irritation, which would prevent you from shaving the face.

Use of hot towels should be adapted to suit the needs of your client. Your client may not like the feel of the towels over the whole face and you should discuss this with him beforehand to determine how you will proceed with this part of the service.

Traditionally, lather was made up beforehand from soap and applied with a brush. However, we now have the benefit of various creams available for use. These can be applied by the traditional brush method but, as a time saver, you can apply using a gloved hand. The brush serves to lift the hairs ready for shaving when brushed over the skin, so you must emulate this action when massaging the lather over the face. Oils should be massaged over the skin and this action lifts the facial hair in preparation for the shave, allowing them to be removed much more easily.

Be professional ★★★

Oils do not cover the facial hair in the same way that lather does, therefore you can clearly see any unusual facial features or beard outlines that you need to watch out for, reducing the risk of taking off a mole or shaving into an outline. Never cover with lather any areas you will not be shaving. You need to leave these exposed to give you a clear indication of any outlines or contra-indicated areas.

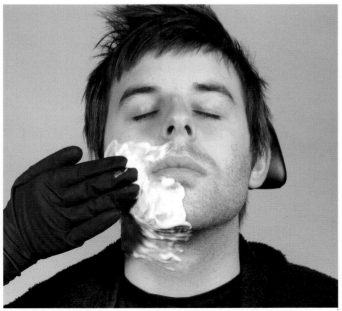

To save time, you can apply lather by hand, wearing a glove

Lathering products should be applied quickly, taking care not to cover the nose and mouth, or getting it into the ears or eyes. Most contain conditioners and a lubricant to help the razor glide over the surface of the skin. However, while you are carrying out the shave, if you feel the lathering product drying, you must re-apply to prevent any damage to the skin. As with all products you use in the salon, take care not to dispense more than necessary to prevent waste, as this costs the salon money and takes away from the profits.

In the salon

Stella's busy day

Stella was having a very busy day in the salon and, as it reached late afternoon, she was feeling tired and anxious. Like any other busy day, she soldiered on without complaining. Her next client wanted a full-face shave so she carried out her consultation and then began the service. As she applied the hot towels, she forgot to ask the client if the towels felt comfortable. As the client was a regular and trusted Stella, he did not raise any objection when the towels felt uncomfortably hot. On removing the last towel, Stella did not pay enough attention to detail and carried on lathering the client's face. What she had not noticed was that on the sensitive area around the lip, the skin had blistered slightly and she had now covered it with lather.

The client felt relief at the towels being removed and the lather had somewhat cooled the face so he did not raise any objections. As Stella was shaving over the blistered area, the client felt sharp pain and stopped Stella, asking her to check if he was cut. Stella was surprised, as she had not felt the skin pull anywhere and felt sure everything was okay. Just to reassure the client, she wiped off the lather to take a look. When the skin was exposed, she could see that there were several small blisters around the lip that she had taken the top off. Stella explained to the client what had happened and he said he felt the towels were uncomfortably hot at the time and this must have caused the blistering. Stella was extremely apologetic and offered to finish the rest of the shave free of charge. However, the client had lost trust in her professionalism and decided to leave.

- What should Stella have done when she felt tired and anxious?
- Not checking with the client regarding the heat of the towels was Stella's first mistake, but what was her second?
- Do you think the client was justified in leaving the salon and how could she ensure his return?

Creating the look

The practice of shaving the skin with an open blade requires a great deal of skill and accuracy. The shaving strokes need to be fluent and methodical and this will only be achieved through practice. It is a good idea to begin by practising shaving on fine facial hair that is less stubborn to remove. You should also consider that mature skin, having lost its elasticity, drags more easily and requires greater tensioning. Therefore, practise first on younger clients. Once you become more experienced and build up your confidence, you will find the skill becomes much easier to carry out. You will become more aware of the influencing factors and what problems may arise and how to overcome them. For example, continued use of close shaving on dark skin can cause darkening and thickening of the skin. With experience, you will recognise the signs and advise **remedial action** accordingly.

> **Remedial action**
>
> positive steps that must be taken to correct any problems arising from the shaving service.

You will cover:

- backhand and forehand shaving
- skin tensioning
- sponge shaving
- shaving outlines
- cooling the skin
- finishing products
- problem solving.

Backhand and forehand shaving

The razor may be held in the forehand or backhand position. Whilst working in forehand, the razor is used working towards yourself and when using backhand, the razor is drawn away from you. You should follow a methodical pattern throughout the shave to ensure that your work is accurate. Look at the example below and use it as a guide.

Position during the shave

During the shave, if you are right-handed, you must stand on the right of the client and if you are left-handed, you must stand to the left. This will ensure smooth operating. You should begin with the side closest to you and work over to the side of the face furthest away to allow you ease of access to the lathered face.

Skin tensioning

While carrying out the shave, you must keep tension on the skin in the area you are drawing the blade across. The hand you use to pull the skin with should be kept dry and free from lather to prevent slipping. Tensioning the skin will help to prevent cuts, allowing the razor to glide over the skin with ease. The older we are, the less elasticity our skin has, therefore more tension is required as the skin will be more likely to fold.

The pattern to follow when shaving

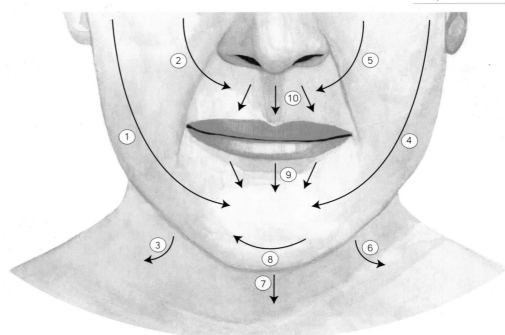

Shaving techniques: a step-by-step guide

1 Before the shave.

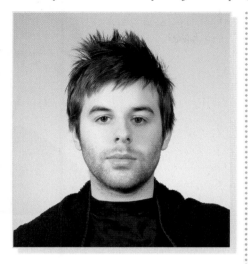

2 A hot towel is applied.

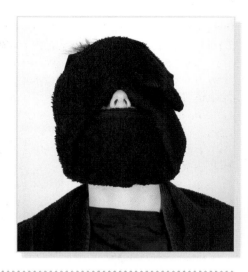

3 The lather is applied.

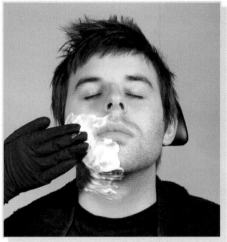

4 The face is fully lathered ready for the shave.

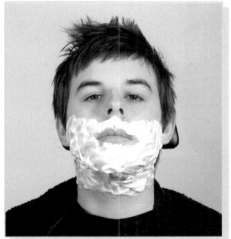

5 Begin the first stroke from the ear sweeping across the face, while the skin is tensioned with the free hand.

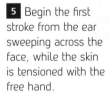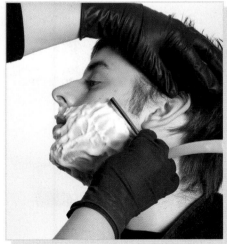

6 Keeping good tension, this stroke is continued down the face and across the cheek.

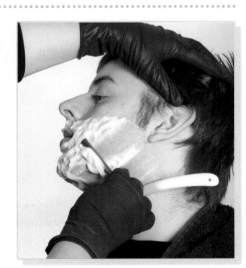

7 Shaving is continued down the neck area.

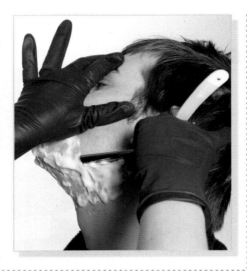

8 Again, tensioning the skin, sweep across the chin area.

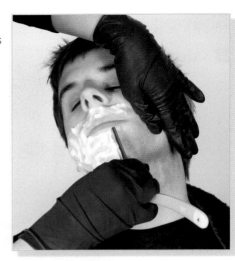

9 Once the shave is completed, the excess lather is removed by patting the face with a damp towel. Never rub the skin.

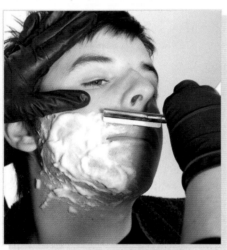

10 A cool towel is then applied.

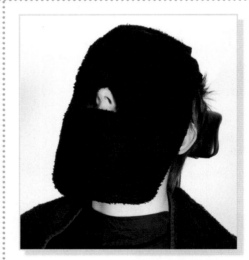

11 Moisturising after-shave balm is applied.

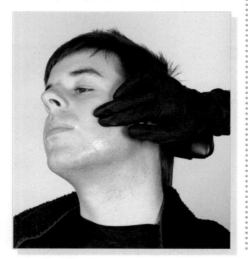

12 The finished look.

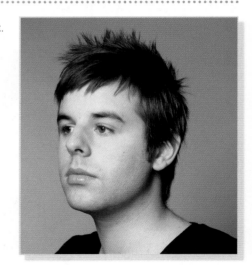

Be professional ★★★

During the shaving process you will need to remove the lather from the blade. To prevent any damage to the blade or cutting of skin, you must wipe the blade away from yourself and the client. Keep the blade flat and wipe with the blade drawn away.

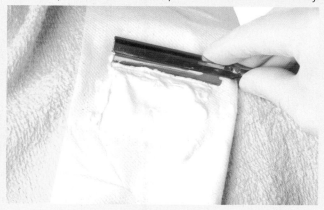

A second over-shave may be required if the hair was not removed first time. This is carried out by shaving against the grain of the beard and should be done only on coarse, stubborn hair and never on fine or sensitive skin. Second over-shaving can cause **irritation** to the skin and in-growing hairs, so should be done only if completely necessary.

Irritation

tenderness of the skin resulting from excessive contact.

Sponge shaving

Sponge shaving is carried out only on a coarse, stubborn beard when a second over-shave was not enough. It involves dipping a sterilised sponge in hot water and wiping over the skin directly before the razor is drawn over. This will serve to open the follicle and lift the hair, allowing the blade to remove any stubborn hairs. Great care must be taken, as shaving so closely can damage the skin or cause in-growing hairs. This type of aggressive shaving should never be carried out unless absolutely necessary and never on fine or sensitive skin.

Shaving outlines

You will need to thoroughly assess the look the client wants and take great care not to shave into the shape required. Tensioning is still required and shaving outlines calls for you to be both precise and **dexterous** in your work, as a large degree of accuracy is needed. When shaving the outline of facial hair or a neckline, care should be taken not to apply too much lather. Blocking your view of the outline could lead to an unsatisfactory result.

Dexterous

ability to use your hands with a high level of skill.

Remember

As soon as the shave service is completed, the razor blade must be disposed of safely in a sharps box.

Cooling the skin

The final stage of the shaving process is to cool the skin. If a client is proceeding to a facial massage, this is not required, therefore you must be sure of your client's requirements. Once all the lather has been removed with a damp towel or sponge, you must pat dry the face, taking care not to drag or pull the skin, as it may feel sensitive. You can now apply a cool towel but be sure to ask the client how cool they would like the towel to be. Some clients prefer only a cool towel and others prefer the fresh feel of a cold towel. The towel is applied in the same way the hot towels were applied at the beginning and this serves to cool the skin and close the follicles.

Finishing products

These are used to leave the skin feeling fresh, dry and to help prevent irritation. Nowadays there are various products available other than aftershave, which is an astringent, such as balms and moisturisers that will both moisturise and soothe the skin, helping to prevent irritation following a shave. These are ideal to use if the client does not like the feel of aftershave on the skin. You can also apply talcum powder to dry off the face and prevent chapping.

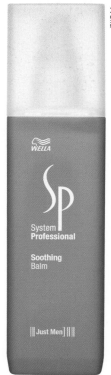

Wella

There is a wide range of products available to moisturise and soothe the skin following the shaving service

Always check with your client at the end of the service that the finished look is to his satisfaction. This ensures an all-round professional service.

Problem solving

There are several problems that you may encounter during the shaving service, the most obvious being cutting the skin. However, no matter how serious the cut is, you must not feel overawed and, with the correct training, you should feel in control at all times.

The table below shows the kinds of problems that you may experience, along with the cause and action or remedy you may use.

Problem	Possible cause	Possible action / remedy
Cuts to the skin	Incorrect skin tensioning, using a razor with a dull edge	Stop shaving, apply pressure and only continue if bleeding stops
Uneven skin surface	Dimples, acne, moles or scar tissue	Take greater care and omit areas of concern
Patchy shave result	Dull edge on blade, uneven pressure applied whilst shaving	Use a new blade. Ensure steady pressure is used all over the face
Folliculitis	Inflammation of the hair follicle or in-growing hair	Do not proceed with shave and advise client to seek medical advice
Shave is not close enough	Coarse facial hair	Carry out a second over-shave and possibly a sponge shave
	Lather has dried out	Re-apply lather as required
	Poor tensioning of skin or holding razor incorrectly	Ensure good tensioning whilst shaving and check the angle of razor
Discomfort during shave	Blade has a dull edge	Use a new blade
	Shaving dry skin	Lather efficiently
	Shaving against the hair growth pattern	Always shave with the grain of the beard unless second over-shave
Shaving rash	Blade has a dull edge	Use a new blade
	Shaving dry skin	Lather efficiently
	Shaving against the hair growth pattern	Always shave with the grain of the beard unless second over-shave
	Shaving too close	Stop shaving

After the service

This section looks at the disposal of waste after the service and advice you may give to the client about intervals between shaves, and products to use at home. It is essential to complete the service as professionally as you have carried it out to provide the client with an all-round first-class service.

You will cover:
- disposal of waste
- recommended intervals
- after-care advice.

Disposal of waste

Following a shave service, you will have some waste materials that need to be disposed of in line with both legislation and the salon's procedures. It is imperative to dispose of used razor blades in a sharps bin; if your salon does not have one, you are in breach of government legislation. A sharps bin should be clearly labelled to identify its purpose and should be stored safely with the lid closed at all times. Also, any hazardous waste such as chemicals must be diluted before being disposed of down the sink. If you have lather that you have not used, it should be washed down the sink and not re-used on another client; this will prevent the risk of cross-infection. Used towels should be placed in a covered towel bin and any used tissue also placed in a covered litter bin. Failing to adhere to strict rules on safe disposal of waste not only leaves you open to the risk of prosecution and legal action, but also shows unprofessionalism in your work.

Check it out

In order to ensure that everyone is following salon procedures and are in line with legislation, create a table detailing how different waste should be disposed of safely and display it in your staff room as a reminder for all staff to follow daily.

 Key Skills Links: Level 2 Communication

Recommended intervals

The time between shaving services will vary for each client. If the client has a dense growth, then it is likely that he will require shaving more often. If the facial hair is fine and sparse, then less frequent services will be required. In the same way, a client with dark facial hair will require more regular shaving than a client with lighter hair, as the dark growth will be more noticeable. In either case, you should recommend to the client what you feel is adequate, as they will be able to judge themselves from the apparent visible growth.

After-care advice

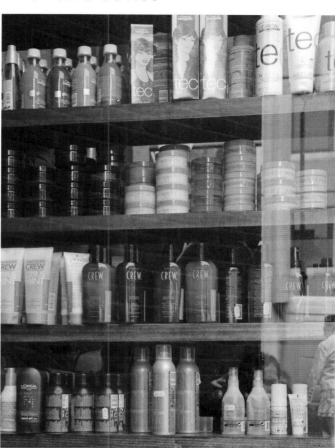

After-care advice must always be given to complete a professional service. You must check with your client that they know how and when to shave at home. Give them a small demonstration if necessary and always inform them of how often it should be carried out. This will differ with each client, depending on the type of facial hair the client has. The advice you give to the client should also take into account any problems that may arise at home, for example, shaving rash or in-growing hairs. An in-growing hair is when the hair grows back on itself and continues to grow under the skin; this is more likely to occur on curly hair. Exfoliating should be advised to help alleviate this problem. However, if this does not suffice, then the skin will have to be broken with a sterile needle to release the trapped hair. Shaving rash can occur when the skin is irritated and should be treated with sensitivity. Moisturising the skin will help to prevent discomfort and the use of strong astringents such as aftershave should be avoided. You should also advise your client on the use of a good cleanser and give advice on the type most suitable for their skin. For example if the skin is oily, use water-based products, and if the skin is dry, use oil-based products.

	When	**How**
Cleanse	Cleansing the skin should be carried out daily and particularly before the shave	There are many types of cleansers available such as creams that are wiped over the face, or washes that are rubbed over the face and washed off
Exfoliate	In between shaves, a couple of times a week	Rubbed into the skin and then removed by washing off
Moisturise	Daily, either once or twice a day	Moisturisers can be either creams or milks that are massaged onto the skin and absorbed

Retailing products and equipment for home use will not only improve your profile but also extend the service you provide into the client's home. You can increase your revenue while ensuring your clients are using reputable, good-quality products or equipment.

Advise the client on their correct use and explain all the benefits of buying your products and equipment; discuss the disadvantages of using cheap razors and products and the damage they can cause to the skin. Good-looking skin helps to boost confidence and this is what you are selling to your clients!

Be professional ★★★

Never send a client away with products or equipment unless they fully understand how to use them correctly, as incorrect use could result in injury to the skin – this is your responsibility.

You may also be required to give your client advice on how to maintain the look at home and how the look can be changed if necessary. If you have shaved a new shape into the facial hair, then it is important that the client understands how to shave the outline to maintain the look or how to change the shape if needed. Demonstrate how this is done and question the client to check their understanding. Remember that the client is a walking advertisement for your salon – he may leave the salon with a professional finish, but will it still look so good in a few weeks? This should have also been discussed at the initial consultation to ensure the look is achievable for the client at home. Further information on effective communication can be found on pages 29–32 of Unit G21.

Check your knowledge

The following questions will help you to check your understanding of this unit. The answers can be found on page 420. Take care, as there may be more than one correct answer for some questions.

1 Why is it important to wear gloves during the shaving service?
   a To prevent the spread of infection
   b To prevent your skin from coming into contact with shaving products
   c So you don't break a nail
   d So that the client cannot see if your hands are dirty

2 What safety considerations should be taken into account during the shaving service?
   a Your client should be wearing a clean gown
   b You should be wearing a clean gown
   c The floor should be freshly mopped
   d The client should be positioned correctly

3 Why is it important to keep your work area clean and tidy?
   a In case a health and safety inspector passes by
   b To prevent any accidents due to untidiness
   c To give the junior staff something to do
   d To prevent the spread of bacteria

4 Why must you use a new blade on every client?
   a To waste money
   b To save money
   c To prevent cross-infection
   d To impress your boss

5 Why is it necessary to apply a warm towel to the face before lathering?
   a To soften the hair and cleanse the face
   b So the service takes longer
   c So the client thinks you are professional
   d To open the follicle and lift the hair

6 Why must tension be applied to the skin during the shaving process?
   a To see how much elasticity the skin has
   b So that the client can feel you pulling his skin
   c To make sure you have put enough lather on
   d To prevent the blade from cutting the skin

7 When might it be necessary to carry out a sponge shave?
   a If the hair is coarse or stubborn
   b If the hair is fine
   c If the hair is very short
   d If the client insists upon it

8 What effect will a cool towel have on the face after the shaving process?

   a Prevent the skin from burning

   b Cool the skin

   c Close the follicle

   d Cleanse the skin

9 What action should you take if you accidentally cut the skin during shaving?

   a Stop immediately and administer first aid and only continue if bleeding stops

   b Ignore it unless it bleeds heavily

   c Ask your boss to come over and deal with it

   d Put a plaster on

10 How should used blades be disposed of safely?

   a In the general waste bin

   b Thrown to the floor to be swept up by the assistant

   c In a clearly labelled sharps box

   d Wrapped in tissue and put in a covered bin

Assessment guidance

You will have to prove that you can professionally shave clients in your everyday work. You will be assessed shaving a client on at least three separate occasions and simulation is not allowed for any activity within this unit.

You will have to demonstrate competence in:
- shaving full facial hair and beard outlines
- using all the types of tools and equipment
- taking into account all the factors
- using all the lathering products
- using all the shaving techniques
- using all the finishing products
- giving all the advice listed in the range.

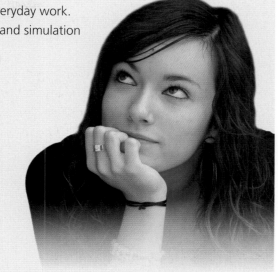

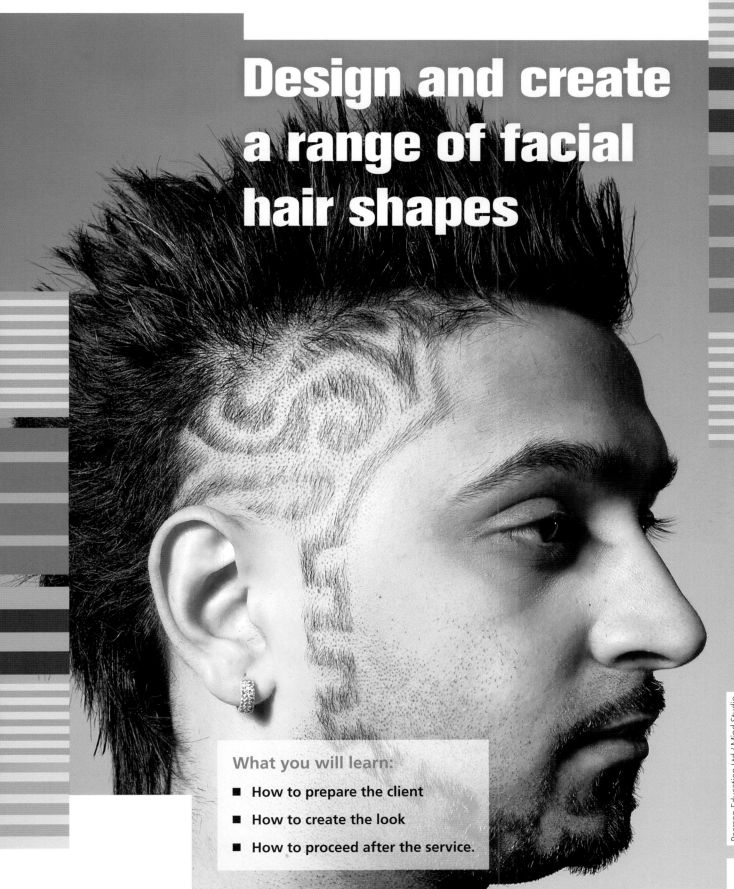

Unit GB7

Design and create a range of facial hair shapes

What you will learn:

- How to prepare the client
- How to create the look
- How to proceed after the service.

Pearson Education Ltd / Mind Studio

Introduction

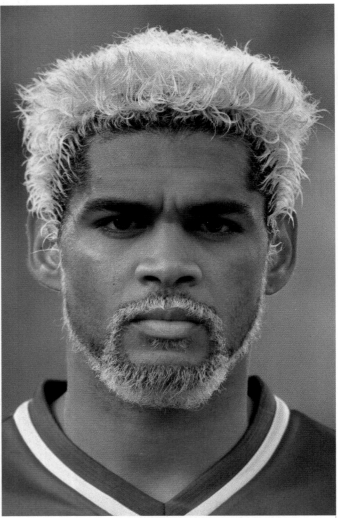

Beard and moustache shapes create a personalised look for each client

This unit is concerned with the trimming and redesigning of beards and moustaches. There are three different types of looks that you need to be competent in achieving:

1 Moustache only
2 Partial beard and moustache
3 Full beard and moustache.

While undertaking the cutting of beards and moustaches, you will use several of the cutting techniques that you have already learnt, for example, scissor-over-comb, clipper-over-comb and free hand. You will need a high level of skill in all three of these cutting techniques in order to create the looks required by men. You must consider that you are using your cutting tools near to the face and the risk of cutting the skin is greater.

You the stylist

The ability to concentrate and your **manual dexterity** will be vital in assisting you to produce a variety of looks. This unit will help you to appreciate the tremendous versatility in the designs of beards and moustaches.

Manual dexterity

using your hands with swift and precise movements.

Preparing the client

This section covers everything that is important when preparing the client for any facial hair cutting services. Being thoroughly prepared reflects your own professionalism and the salon's image, and is an essential part of the process.

Thorough consultation

The initial consultation plays a crucial part in determining the final outcome (see also Unit G21). As the stylist, it is your responsibility to determine the client's requirements and advise the client accordingly. He may require a traditional look or something more **avant-garde**. The use of visual aids to assist you in this task may be necessary, for example, a stylebook or picture from a magazine. If you feel confident enough, drawing the style you are thinking of creating could be beneficial. During your consultation there are several factors that you must consider and these are known as influencing factors.

Avant-garde

a look which is out of the ordinary, not really seen on the high street.

Influencing factors

Although influencing factors have been greatly covered in Unit G21, there are several points that are purely relevant to cutting facial hair.

Head and face shape

When designing a look for a beard or moustache, the client's personal preferences must be considered as well as his head and face shape. The size of the beard or moustache should correspond with the facial features. The rule of thumb is a larger, thicker beard or moustache for heavy or large facial features, and a smaller design for fine, smooth facial features. You must also consider the following points:

- The size of the mouth, for example, a small mouth should have a narrow, short moustache.

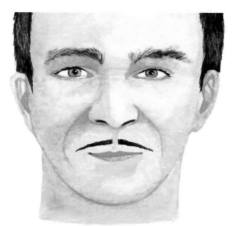

- The size of the nose, for example, a prominent nose should have a large or thick moustache.

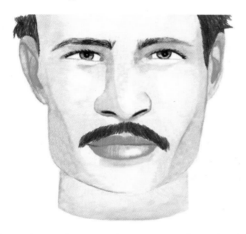

- The face shape, for example, a square face should have a curved beard or moustache. A round face should have a square-edged design.

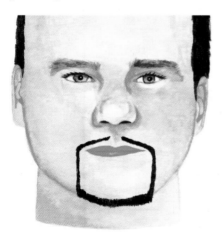

Any unusual features can be cleverly disguised with the use of a beard or moustache, particularly any facial scarring.

Hair growth patterns

You should be looking all over the facial hair for any deviance in the way the hair grows. This can play a vital part in the finished outcome. For example, if a client has a **whorl** in the growth pattern, it will affect the finished shape.

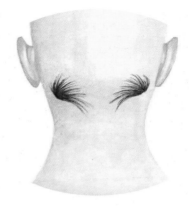

Whorls can look untidy as they begin to grow out, which makes the design harder for the client to maintain. There may be some areas of baldness in the facial hair, which can affect your choice of design. For example, if the client required a full beard and moustache but no hair grew at the sides of the mouth, you would suggest a moustache without the beard connected.

> **Whorl**
>
> an usual growth pattern where the hair grows in a circular direction.

Hairstyle

The way the client wears his hair will have an effect on the look and design of the facial hair. Although there are no set rules on what can or cannot be worn well together, it would be beneficial for the client to have a design that complemented his hairstyle. If the client has little or no hair, then a large, thick beard and moustache can look out of place. Alternatively, if a client has thick, long hair, then a fine, small moustache can also look misplaced. As the stylist, you should work with your client to find a design that suits both his personal preference and the overall look.

> **Check it out**
>
> Take a look at men with facial hair, both in the media and in public, and note the hairstyle that is worn with it. Do you notice any patterns or trends? If you are looking at magazines, you could cut out the pictures to make a stylebook. Alternatively, you could invest in a digital camera and take some photographs of your own work to produce a stylebook.
>
> **(KS) Key Skills Links**: Level 2 Communication

Unit GB7 Design and create a range of facial hair shapes

Adverse skin conditions

It is imperative that on the initial consultation you look carefully for any suspected infections or infestations as these may prevent you from continuing with the service (see Unit G21 for more on this topic).

Be professional ★★★

If a client has heavy facial hair growth at the start, you must be extra vigilant. Take time to comb through the hair, parting it and looking at the skin. It can be difficult to spot a cold sore on a lip if the client has a thick moustache.

If you begin a service and then discover something that you suspect to be infectious, you should inform the client and give any advice you feel is necessary. You may have to finish the service you are carrying out, but be sure to thoroughly clean and sterilise any tools and equipment you have used to prevent the risk of cross-infection. (Refer to Unit G22, pages 13–14 for the correct methods of sterilisation.)

Hair density

The thickness of the facial hair will affect the choice of style and cutting technique used. For example, if a client has very dense facial hair, then a fine, narrow moustache may not be possible. You also need to consider that if the hair is thicker, then you may have to use the clippers to cut the beard or moustache, as a scissor-over-comb technique may take too long.

Be professional ★★★

As clippers remove more hair and move through the hair more easily, they are not only quicker to use, but also a more comfortable option for the client. Trying to comb through thick hair when using a scissor-over-comb technique can cause discomfort to the client.

Facial piercing

It is essential that you discover all facial piercings and ask the client to remove them before you carry out any facial hair cutting. It will not only hinder the close scissor or clipper work that needs to be done, but, more importantly, if you were to catch the piercing, it could tear the skin. If your client does have any facial piercing, take note of when it was carried out and if it looks inflamed or infected. It may be that if it is relatively new, the skin may still be inflamed, in which case you would advise the client to leave the treatment and re-book at a later date.

Facial contours

You should take note of facial contours and balance the design of the beard and / or moustache to complement these. Also facial contours may affect the way you cut the hair, for example, if the client has a dimple in his chin and you need to cut the hair that grows within it, you must ask him to place his tongue over his bottom teeth to try and push out the skin, making the hairs protrude.

Client's wishes

You should consider your client's wishes in all the decisions you make about the service. You may need to advise the client on another option if you feel what he requires is not suitable, but remember to do this with tact and professionalism.

Lifestyle

Taking your client's lifestyle into consideration is vital. You must consider:

- the amount of time he has to spend on his facial hair each day
- whether he can commit to the maintenance of the chosen look
- whether the proposed service complements his occupation
- whether the proposed service is achieveable with the type of facial hair he grows.

All of the above should be addressed during the consultation to ensure the client will be able to manage his hair between visits. You must ensure he can commit to the upkeep of the chosen style and fully explain what this will entail, for example, time spent grooming each day and how often he needs to revisit the salon for maintenance.

Sterilisation

Cleaning, **disinfecting** and **sterilisation** of tools and equipment is essential to prevent the spread of infection or infestation. There are several methods that you can use in the salon, all of which have been covered in great detail in Unit G22.

Disinfecting

the method of inhibiting growth of bacteria or germs.

Sterilisation

the method of killing bacteria or germs.

Check it out

List the tools and equipment that you use in the cutting and designing of facial hair and write next to each one the method of disinfecting and sterilisation that you currently use in the salon. You should check that what you are using is sufficient by looking at Unit G22. Could your methods be adapted to improve the disinfecting and sterilisation routines that you use in the salon?

KS **Key Skills Links**: Level 2 Communication

Personal hygiene

As with all hairdressing services, you will be working in close proximity to your client. You must ensure that your body and breath are fresh. Regular washing and bathing is essential as is the use of a good deodorant to prevent body odour. After a cigarette or lunch break, make sure that your breath smells fresh by either brushing your teeth or using a breath freshener. Clients may take offence at strong odours and it is very unpleasant for them. Your own health is important when you are working in the salon. If you do not feel one hundred per cent, the quality of your work may reflect this. Also, if you are infectious or contagious, you may spread germs to your clients and colleagues.

Personal protective equipment

The personal protective equipment that you use when cutting facial hair is essential to provide protection to the client from small, sharp hair cuttings. The facial hair is often coarser and can cause infection by entering the skin. Removing loose hair as you progress through the cut will help to prevent this and taking special care at the end to ensure all hair is correctly removed is also beneficial. Care needs to be taken to ensure that hair cuttings do not fall onto the client's clothing by correctly gowning him. The gown should also be checked regularly to ensure it has not slipped and is still providing a high level of protection. You can place small, round cotton wool pads over the client's eyes to protect them. This will also help to keep their eyes closed, but remember to let the client look, when needed, for an opinion on the length or shape of the beard, or moustache.

Preparing the facial hair for the cutting service

You should thoroughly detangle the facial hair before you begin the cut and it may be necessary to cleanse the facial hair as well. While you are carrying out the initial consultation, you should be combing the beard or moustache looking for any adverse skin conditions. If your client is returning home from work, the hair may contain dirt or debris. Removing grease, dirt or dandruff from the facial hair will prevent any damage to your cutting tools. It will also show your professionalism by preparing the hair correctly for the cutting service.

Cleansing the facial hair can be done using a variety of methods. If you are shampooing the client's hair, then it can be carried out during this process. Alternatively, you may ask the client to wash his face, or if it is only a small moustache, then a facial cleansing wipe could be used.

Be professional ★★★

If you are carrying out a complete re-design of the facial hair, drawing an outline on the facial hair growth will assist you, as you will be able to follow a guideline. On lighter hair, you could use an eyebrow pencil; alternatively, on very dark hair you could use a white pencil. Remember to remove any leftover pencil on completion of the cut.

Creating the look

In this section you will find all the information that will assist you in carrying out facial hair cutting. You will need to be aware of the cutting tools available for use and the various techniques you can adopt to achieve a variety of looks. There are several safety considerations that you must bear in mind; remember that you are working in close proximity to the skin on the face and extra care will need to be taken. You will need to research (media is a good option) and find a variety of designs of beards and moustaches for you to use on clients in the salon. Being aware of the trends and designs of facial hair is paramount to your success.

Cutting tools and their uses

Of all the cutting tools available for use on the hair, there are only two that we use on facial hair. These are scissors and clippers.

Scissors

The scissors that you use on a client need to be extremely sharp and great care must be taken when cutting hair on the face. Scissors can be used to trim or re-design either a beard or a moustache. They can be used for both scissor-over-comb work to reduce the bulk of the beard or moustache or for freehand work when outlining.

Be professional ★★★

When you are using a pair of scissors, they are just an extension to your hand and should feel very comfortable to hold. If not, they can become clumsy to use, causing carelessness and possible cutting of the client's skin. If you are not happy with the scissors you are using, then change them for a different pair that feel more comfortable.

Clippers

When using clippers on facial hair, the smaller, trimmer clippers are more commonly used. They are particularly good for removing the hair on the outline of the beard or moustache as they cut very close to the skin. This will assist anyone who is not confident enough to use a razor to shave off the excess hair.

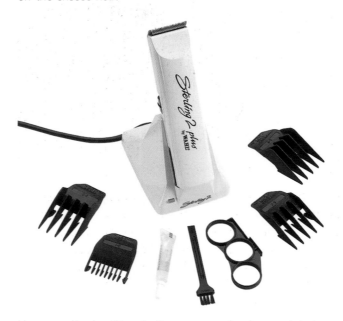

However, the traditional clippers may also be used, but as they are larger and more bulky, it is much harder to work in finer detail.

Clippers are used to remove bulk from a beard or moustache, especially if the facial hair is thick or very long. It will save time to use clipper-over-comb, as this technique will remove the hair at a quicker rate. Both types of clippers work in the same way with a set of two serrated-edge blades, one of which moves rapidly over the other. It is an essential requirement that after each use you thoroughly clean the clippers, using a small brush to remove any loose hair cuttings. The blades should also be oiled regularly to prevent them from seizing up. Manufacturers of clippers provide the brush and oil for maintenance and a hygiene spray can be purchased in order to disinfect.

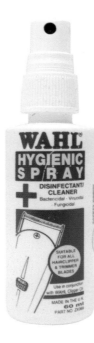

Hygiene spray for clippers

Remember

Clippers are electrical and should be used in line with the Electricity at Work Regulations. Refer to Unit G22 to remind yourself of these responsibilities.

Cutting techniques used in facial hair cutting

There are three cutting techniques that you will be using when cutting beards and moustaches and they are scissor-over-comb, clipper-over-comb and free hand.

Scissor-over-comb

The scissor-over-comb technique will allow you to carry out fine graduation on short beards and moustaches. When using this technique, you place the comb into the hair against the skin and by moving the comb away from the face, cutting the hair that protrudes through the teeth of the comb, you will cut the hair to the required length.

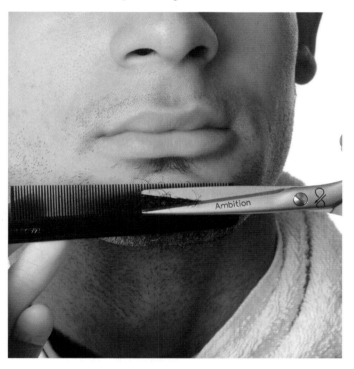

Remember

Any scissor-over-comb work that you carry out requires a great deal of skill and accuracy. Caution needs to be taken, as you will be working around the soft tissue of the face, for example, the lip area.

Clipper-over-comb

This technique produces the same effect as scissor-over-comb but cuts the hair at a much quicker rate, making it ideal to use if you are busy in the salon. Generally, you would use the smaller, trimmer clippers, not only to allow you to work more freely in the confines of the facial curves, but also to produce finer gradation. As previously stated, if as a barber stylist you are not yet confident enough to use a razor to shave off excess facial hair, then trimmers will cut very close to the skin. Clipper-over-comb work is carried out in the same way as scissor-over-comb. The comb is placed against the skin and moved away from the face, with the hair protruding through the teeth of the comb being cut by the clippers.

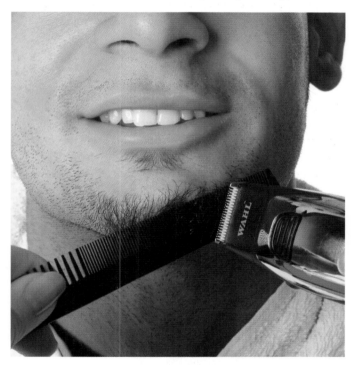

Clippers have a lever on the side that allows you to open or close the blades at varying degrees. If you are working on coarse, dense hair, then it is beneficial to open the blade out to allow the clippers to cut through the hair without dragging, causing discomfort to the client. Alternatively, if you are cutting fine hair, or wish to cut close to the skin, then closing the blades will ease cutting the hair.

Types of beards and moustaches

Beards and moustaches have been worn in various forms for centuries. They can signify religious beliefs or just serve as a fashion statement. In recent times, facial hair has once again grown in popularity, with many celebrities wearing goatees or sideburns in a range of shapes and designs.

Moustaches

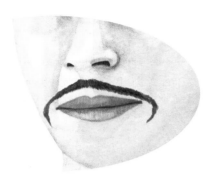
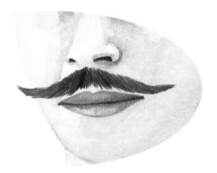

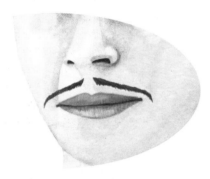
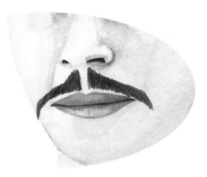

Beards

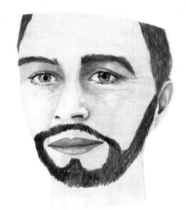
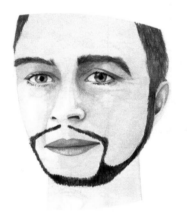

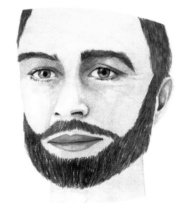
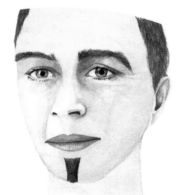

Be professional ★★★

The type of beard or moustache that you recommend to a client will be strongly influenced by their facial features, as discussed earlier in the section on 'Preparing the client'. You will need to adopt a keen eye for recognising facial features and styling the facial hair accordingly.

Procedure for facial hair cutting

Check it out

Before you begin the service, you should be aware of your salon's expected service times for the cutting of facial hair. The service time may differ from salon to salon and can vary by as much as fifteen minutes. Find out the expected service times in your salon for several facial hair cutting services, including a full beard and moustache trim, a moustache trim, and a complete re-design.

Whether you are carrying out a complete re-design or just a trim on the facial hair, it is crucial for you as the barber stylist to know where to begin the cut and how. The type of beard or moustache you are working on will determine the cutting techniques you use. For example, if it is a fine, narrow moustache, then scissor work will suffice; however, if you are cutting a coarse, dense beard, then using the clippers is preferable.

Before you begin, you must be aware of what you are trying to achieve and how to reach that point. Always ask the client, 'When did you last have your beard or moustache cut?' This will give you a good indication of how much hair needs to be removed. If you consider that the hair grows on average 1 to 2 cm per month, this will allow you to determine how much the hair has grown since the last cut.

It is usual to remove the bulk first and then to outline the shape of the beard or moustache afterwards. By removing the bulk of hair it will allow you to see clearly the outline shape. While carrying out the cutting service, remove any loose hair cuttings as you go along, not only for your client's comfort, but also to allow you to see a clear picture of your design. Even if your client's eyes are closed and covered, ask them to look as you go along to ensure you are achieving a design they are happy with. When you are satisfied with the finished look, you must remove the hair that is left outside the outline. You may use the trimmer clippers for this, or alternatively, shave off the hair with a razor.

Remember

You should be checking with the client throughout the cut that they are happy with the shape that you are creating and that they are comfortable in the position you have placed them in for cutting.

The table below shows the types of problems that you may encounter and how to overcome them. It can be used as a quick reference guide.

Types of problem	Possible remedy
Cutting the skin	Administer first aid immediately
Bald patch in the facial hair	Style in a way to avoid exposure of the bald area
Adverse skin conditions	If infectious, do not carry out the service and advise to seek medical attention
Unusual growth patterns in the facial hair	Avoid styling in a way that will look uneven when growing out
Uneven result on completion	Use a pencil to draw the outline and re-style to even out the design

Be professional ★★★

If you have used an outline pencil, always check to ensure it has all been removed during the cut. It looks unprofessional if you let the client leave the salon with markings on the facial hair.

Trimming facial hair: a step-by-step guide

1 Before the beard trim.

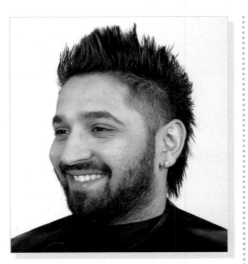

2 Once the overall beard length has been reduced using a clipper over comb technique, cut in the outline shape all around the beard design.

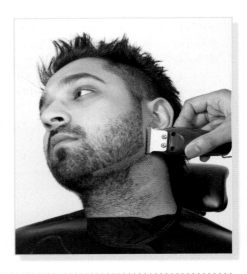

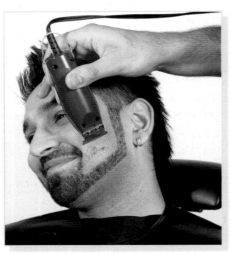

3 Again, take out the excess hair above the beard design over the cheek area (this can also be done by shaving).

4 Begin to add a pattern, taking out the hair in the required areas using the no-guard and the small taper clippers.

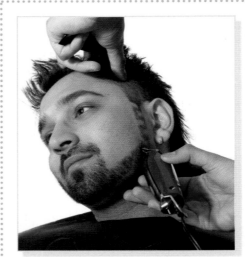

5 Continue patterning into the hairline using the corner of the small clippers for finer detail.

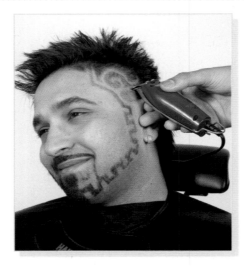

6 The finished look.

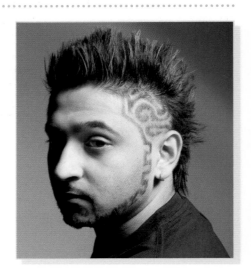

Safety considerations

Extreme caution must be taken at all times when using sharp implements next to the client's skin. Your concentration must never falter and you should not be distracted from your work. If your hand is hovering over a client's face holding a pair of scissors or a razor and you are looking away to talk to someone else, this will prove to be a very uncomfortable experience for the client. If you do cut a client's skin, you must follow strict health and safety procedures when dealing with the incident.

Procedure for dealing with a cut

- Use a steri-wipe to clean over the area; if doing this yourself, you must be wearing gloves to prevent the risk of cross-infection. This will remove any loose hair cuttings and prevent them from entering the skin.
- Applying pressure to the cut will stem the flow of blood.
- You should continue with the service only when the cut has stopped bleeding.
- When you continue with the service, give the client a clean tissue to keep wiping around the area to prevent any hair from entering the skin.

The tools you are using against the skin need to be clean and sterile for each use. Never re-use a razor on another client's skin, as there is a high risk of cross-infection. Using clean, sterile tools will also prove your ability to the client and demonstrate your high level of professionalism.

After the service

This section looks at completing the service with your client by offering after-care advice and recommending when he should return. It is essential to complete the service as professionally as you have carried it out, to provide the client with an all-round first-class service.

After-care advice and recommended intervals between cuts

Clients will have a preferred time interval between the cuttings of their facial hair. However, you should be advising three to five weeks, which usually falls in line with their haircut but not always. You must stress the importance of coming back into the salon to maintain the look otherwise they may become a poor advert for your salon with a grown-out look! In between visits to the salon, the client will have to maintain the look by removing hair outside of the outline, usually carried out by shaving. You may need to give advice on this, for example, how often and in which areas.

Ensuring that your client is fully informed about how to look after the design of his facial hair is important; make sure he also understands the potential for style change. If the client cannot take care of the design at home, then you may find that when he returns to the salon he has changed the shape completely, or even shaved off his beard or moustache. Even though the client may have been happy when leaving the salon, unless the maintenance of the look has been fully explained, dealing with the design at home may prove difficult and leave the client feeling frustrated. If this happens, the chances of the client returning to you will be greatly reduced.

Home-care products and equipment

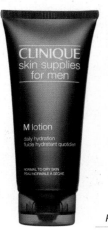

Clinique

Products for home use

Salon life

Left with a scar!

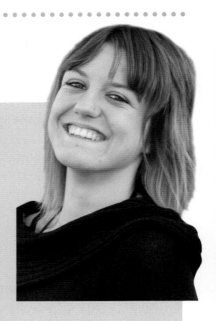

Janine's story

As my regular client Jay approached me I noticed a fresh scar on his nose and during the initial consultation I jokingly asked him, 'What have you been up to, then?' I half expected some tale about a football injury but the reply he gave me wasn't what I expected at all. He explained that a couple of days after his last appointment, which had been three weeks ago, his nose became red, swollen and sore. By the third day, there was a painful boil forming on his nose. He told me that he went to see the nurse at his doctor's surgery and during treatment the nurse pulled out a small, sharp hair from the skin. It was obvious that it had entered the skin during the moustache trim he had a few days previously. Once the hair had been removed, the boil took another week to clear up, which is why the scar still looked so fresh. I was horrified to think it was my fault – if I had taken more care to remove all the hair cuttings from his face, then this would not have happened. I was extremely apologetic and told him that his appointment this time would be free! Luckily he was happy to accept my apology, even though he had been through this bad experience. He even said he would still come to the salon as my client.

Be professional ★★★

- As facial hair is often strong and coarse in texture, short hairs can feel like sharp needles. Always brush hair away gently so as not to push the hair down into the skin.
- If any problems do arise out of a service that you have given to a client, then always offer a suitable remedy or an incentive, such as a free treatment. This should appease the client and hopefully help to maintain your professional reputation.

ASK THE PROFESSIONALS

Q *Why do you think the hair entering the skin caused this type of reaction?*

A The human body would view this hair as a foreign body and try to remove it as quickly as possible, therefore causing an infection of this kind.

Q *What measures could you take to prevent this from happening to clients?*

A You could use a face cloth to protect the client's exposed skin during the facial hair trimming or alternatively keep brushing away any loose hairs throughout the cut and be extremely careful when the cut is complete to remove all traces of loose hair.

Unit GB7 Design and create a range of facial hair shapes

It is important to advise your client about the benefits of looking after their facial hair and skin. Nowadays there is much less stigma attached to men using facial products. This is evident by the number of products available on the market. You have a responsibility as the barber stylist to educate your clients and inform them of how to look after their skin.

Exfoliation of the skin is essential to remove the dead skin cells from the top layer of the epidermis. It will not only improve the texture of the skin, but will also help to prevent in-growing hairs from forming. The action of exfoliating also stimulates the circulation, which provides the much-needed blood supply and nourishment for the skin. Exfoliating not only brightens the skin, but also makes it more receptive to moisturising products, helping the skin to hold its elasticity and youthful glow. If you are selling the benefits of regular exfoliating and moisturising in this way, how can the client resist buying the products?

> **Exfoliating**
>
> the method of removing dead skins cells with an abrasive product.

You should also stress the importance of using the correct equipment for maintaining the style at home. If you sell trimmers for home use, then not only can the client purchase them from you but you can demonstrate their use ensuring that he will be using them correctly.

Disposal of waste materials

Disposal of waste should always be carried out in line with any health and safety legislation. The most likely waste to be disposed of after facial hair cutting would be:

- hair cuttings
- used razor blade
- eye pads
- empty product containers.

Each of these must be disposed of safely and **hygienically** following salon procedure.

> **Hygienically**
>
> maintaining healthy practices.

Check it out

Looking at the list of disposable items, write down the key points about how each should be disposed of correctly (see page 7 of Unit G22 for more information). Compare your salon's procedures for disposal of waste to current health and safety legislation.

 Key Skills Links: Level 2 Communication

In the salon

Waheed's story

At Waheed's salon, the staff were complaining that, as they were all so busy carrying out services on clients, there was not enough time to clean up properly. He decided to give them a helping hand and employed a cleaner for a few hours per week. Shirley had been cleaning at the salon for a couple of weeks and all was going well. The staff were much happier as they did not feel under as much pressure, knowing that Shirley would do the jobs they did not have time for.

One Friday evening, after a busy day at the salon, Shirley was getting on with the cleaning and Waheed was cashing up. Suddenly Shirley screamed and Waheed looked up to see her holding her hand with blood running out of a wound. He rushed over and immediately administered first aid. Shirley told him she had been pulling some rubbish out of the small pedal bin to put into the large bin bag for disposal. She could see only some tissues and did not notice that there was a used razor blade in the bin. On closer inspection, Waheed could see that the wound was quite deep and would need further medical attention. He locked up the salon and took Shirley straight to hospital.

The next day in the salon, Waheed called an emergency staff meeting to discuss the incident and find out how it could have happened. It appeared that the salon assistant had thrown the used blade into the bin and was oblivious to the hazard she had created. In fact, it was the salon's fault for not educating her in the use of a sharps box and its importance.

- By cutting herself on a used razor blade, what risks has Shirley been exposed to?
- Who do you think was negligent: Waheed, Shirley, or all the staff?
- How could this incident have been avoided?

Check your knowledge

The following questions will help you to check your understanding of this unit. The answers can be found on page 420. Take care, as there may be more than one correct answer for some questions.

1 The minimum requirements for PPE. for your client would be:
   a gown and gloves
   b gown, gloves and apron
   c gown and towel
   d towel and cotton wool pads

2 Where must you dispose of used sharps?
   a In the waste bin
   b In the sharps bin
   c In the outside bin
   d At home

3 Why should you protect your clients from hair clippings?
   a To maintain client comfort both throughout and following the service
   b To keep the salon clean
   c To make good use of the gowns
   d To protect the client's hair

4 By what method would you sterilise your gowns?
   a Chemical
   b UV rays
   c Vapour
   d Moist heat

5 What is the average growth rate for facial hair?
   a ½ cm per month
   b ¾ cm per month
   c 1–2 cms per month
   d 2–3 cms per month

6 Why should you establish and follow guidelines?
   a So that you look professional
   b To ensure methodical progression of the facial haircut
   c To make the hair uneven
   d So that the cut takes more time

7 Why should clients be encouraged to exfoliate the outline after the facial haircut?
   a To soften the skin to prevent in-growing hairs
   b To allow you to sell more products
   c To prevent 'shadowing'
   d To prevent cross-contamination

8 Why is it important to consult with the client throughout the facial haircut?
  a To check the progress of the facial haircut meets the client's expectations
  b To ensure he is comfortable
  c To find out where the client is going on holiday
  d To find out what the client's occupation is

9 How long should you advise a client to leave between cuts?
  a Every couple of months
  b Once a week
  c From 2–4 weeks depending on the chosen style
  d He shouldn't need to come back

10 Why are eye pads sometimes used during the facial haircut?
  a To help the client relax
  b To protect the eyes from hair clippings
  c So the room appears darkened
  d So that the work area looks clean

Assessment guidance

You will have to prove your competence in cutting a variety of facial hair shapes. You will be assessed cutting one moustache only shape and three beards with moustaches. Simulation is not allowed for any activity within this unit.

You will have to demonstrate competence in:

- cutting moustaches only, partial beards and moustaches and full beard and moustaches
- using clippers and scissors
- taking into account all the factors that may affect the cut
- using scissor and clipper-over-comb techniques and cutting freehand
- giving thorough and comprehensive advice

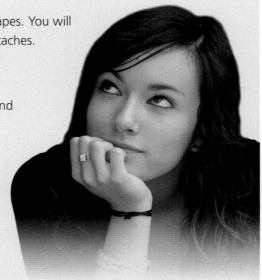

Unit GB7 Design and create a range of facial hair shapes

Creatively cut hair using a combination of barbering techniques

What you will learn:

- How to prepare the client
- How to create the look
- How to proceed after the service.

Pearson Education Ltd / Mind Studio

Introduction

Cutting hair, whether it is men's or women's, requires a high level of skill to be successful. This unit focuses on using and combining an extensive range of cutting techniques to creatively re-style men's hair. You will use the cutting techniques you have previously learnt but will adapt them to create a diverse range of men's styles. The principles of cutting are the same for men and women; the differences lie in the outline and neckline shapes.

You the stylist

You need to be skilled in creating a variety of men's hairstyles involving the use of many cutting techniques. The step-by-step photographs in this unit demonstrate how to re-style a current look.

Preparing the client

In this section you will learn about the fundamental principles of preparing a client for the cutting service.

You must always observe and follow the salon's code of practice including any relevant health and safety laws, for example, the correct gowning procedure and the safe disposal of used sharps. With thorough preparation, not only will you present a professional image but also ensure the best use of the time available.

> **Be professional ★★★**
>
> In order to present a professional image, you should always shampoo a man's hair prior to cutting. This will prevent any damage to your cutting tools by removing dirt or debris from the hair. Your client may have come straight from work and his hair may be dirty, or it may have product build-up which needs to be removed. It will also show your professionalism by preparing the hair correctly for the cutting service, ensuring that your cutting tools are used effectively on the hair.

Thorough consultation

The consultation you carry out with your client will determine your client's requirements. It also creates an opportunity for you to use your imagination and recommend what you think will be suitable. There are certain factors that you must consider when creating a style for a client (Unit G21, pages 58–60, covers this in much greater detail). However, when consulting with a male client, there are other factors that must be considered such as:

- the presence of male pattern baldness
- the presence of added hair.

Both these factors, if present, need to be addressed in your consultation.

Male pattern baldness

If a client has **male pattern baldness**, then your styling of the hair will need to be adapted to take account of this. Male pattern baldness is caused when activity in the dermal papailla (often referred to as the growing factory) stops and therefore results in no more hair growing. This condition is usually passed on in a hereditary gene, therefore if a client's father or grandfather had thinning hair, the likelihood of their hair starting to recede is much higher.

> **Male pattern baldness**
>
> the term used to describe a receding hairline or thinning of the hair.

> **Check it out**
>
> Revisit Unit G21, pages 39–40, to remind yourself how hair grows.

Unit GB8 creatively cut hair using a combination of barbering techniques

Typical patterns of male pattern baldness

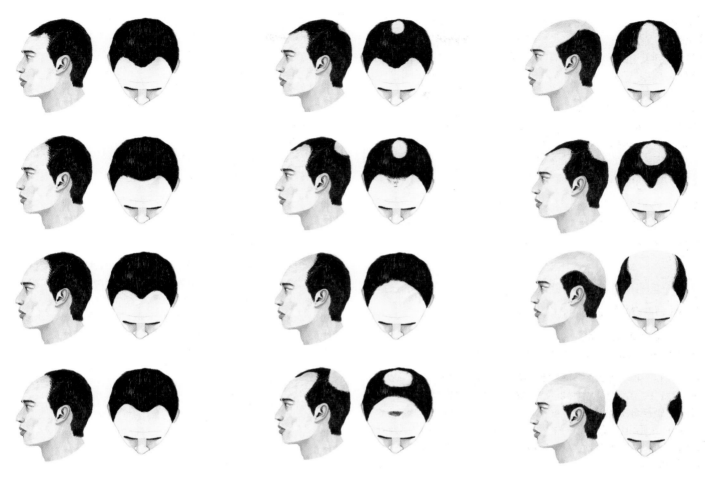

Some men prefer the hair to be cut very short or even shaved off completely to help disguise any thinning areas. However, some men prefer to leave the hair longer and comb across the thinning area. As the stylist, it is your responsibility to determine the client's requirements and advise on whichever is the most suitable option.

If the client has added hair, for example, a toupee, then when you cut the hair you must take account of this and blend the two together, keeping it as natural looking as possible. However, the specialist who supplies the hairpiece usually carries out this type of cutting. Your client may wear a full wig and may require you to cut the hair very short to prevent any hair from showing beneath; this must also be taken into consideration.

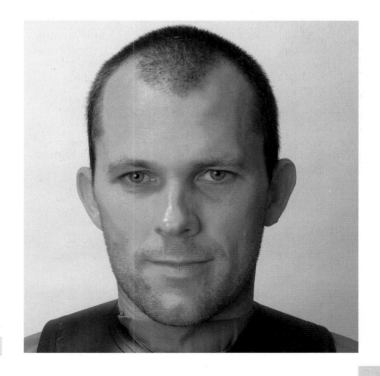

A crew cut can help to disguise a thinning hairline

Unit GB8 Creatively cut hair using a combination of barbering techniques

Other considerations

The age of your client is something that you should consider. For example, children often need short, easy-to-manage styles that require little or no styling. You must also check to see if your client is wearing spectacles or a hearing aid. Both can present problems as they interfere with the lie of the hair after the cut and you will need to take this into account.

Be professional ★★★

- Take the time to have a thorough discussion with your client and find out their exact requirements.
- Use a stylebook to help to clarify the look you and your client have in mind. This will ensure there are no misunderstandings between you regarding the final outcome.

Checking for contra-indications and influencing factors

Contra-indications

something which you must take account of that could prevent you from continuing with the service

There are several contra-indications and influencing factors that you must consider. Each one has different effects on the haircut that you are creating.

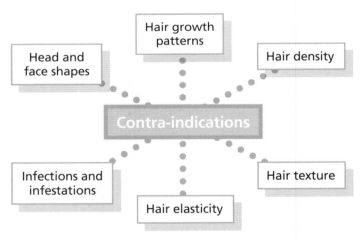

Each of these contra-indications and influencing factors has been addressed in greater detail in Unit G21, pages 34–57.

As the majority of men have their hair cut short, the growth pattern in the nape area will determine the type of neckline you can achieve. The client will have great difficulty maintaining the style if the growth pattern conflicts. For example, if a strong nape whorl is present, then it would create a problem for the client when the hair begins to grow, especially if cut into a round neckline.

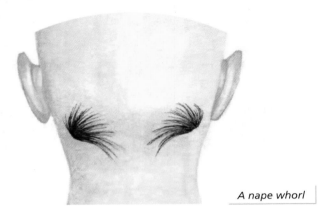

A nape whorl

Looking for infections and infestations is very important (see Unit G21, pages 45–7). If you suspect the presence of these, you must inform the client of your suspicions immediately. You should then thoroughly clean and sterilise any tools and equipment that you have used to prevent the risk of cross-infection.

Personal hygiene

It is imperative to present a professional image at all times. This can be achieved only by maintaining high standards within the salon. You need to consider your own standards of hygiene as well as those of the salon. Washing regularly and using a good deodorant will ensure you always smell fresh. As you are working in close proximity to your client, your body odour and breath will be unmistakable. It is therefore essential to have fresh breath at all times, especially after lunch or a cigarette break. Strong odours such as onions or nicotine can be offensive to a client. Check that your hands and nails are also clean, as dirty fingernails will not convey a high standard of hygiene.

Check it out

List the methods of sterilisation used in your salon. Next, look at Unit G22, pages 13–14, to remind yourself of the all the methods available and decide if you are using the correct methods for your salon's requirements.

(KS)

Key Skills Links: Level 2 Communication

Remember

If you follow strict rules of health and hygiene in the salon, the chances of passing on an infection or infestations will be greatly reduced.

Personal protective equipment

Protecting yourself and the client should always be a high priority. When cutting a male client's hair, it is essential to ensure that you adequately protect his clothes from loose hair cuttings. The only protective equipment needed will be for the client's benefit, for example, the gown, cutting collar, or neck strip. You must be sure before you begin the cut that the gown covers all the clothing and no areas are left exposed that may become covered in hair. Secure the gown properly to prevent it slipping off. Always use some other type of protection over the gown, following your salon's requirements. For example, using a towel, cutting collar, or neck strip around the shoulders will provide added protection and help to prevent any loose hair from falling down the neck of the gown.

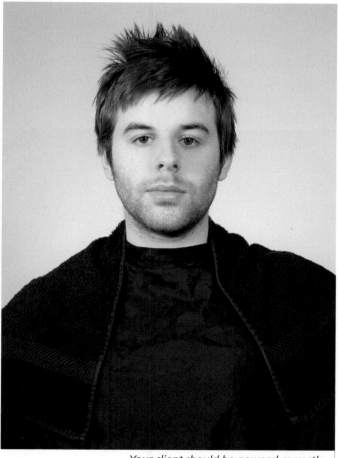

Your client should be gowned correctly

Be professional ★★★

You must continue checking throughout the haircut that the personal protective equipment used still effectively covers your client. This will continue to protect the client's clothing from hair cuttings.

Preparing your work area

It is essential that you be fully prepared for the service that you are carrying out. The salon junior will play a vital role in ensuring that your work area is ready for you. Their training is of great importance and should be initially taught by watching you prepare the work area.

Check it out

What are the salon's rules regarding correct storage and handling of cutting tools and equipment?

There are several aspects of preparation that must be checked prior to commencement.

- Make sure you have everything you will need with you.
- Check all tools and equipment are clean and fit for purpose.
- Visually check any electrical equipment prior to use.
- Sterilise any necessary tools and equipment.
- Check the surrounding work areas are clean, tidy and free of excess hair.

Being fully prepared for your client will save you time in the long run. It also presents a professional image to the client if you are ready for the service. Having to excuse yourself to find something you forgot not only slows you down but can also irritate the client.

Creatively cut hair using a combination of barbering techniques **Unit GB8**

Salon life

A quick trim

Simon's story

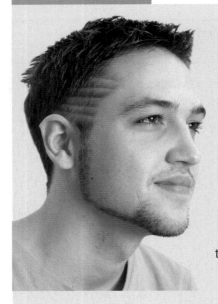

Today at lunch I was in the staff room eating my sandwich when a guy that I have never seen in the salon before came in asking for a quick trim. It had been a quiet week and so I thought rather than refuse him I would offer to do the cut. I offered him a seat at my workstation and nipped into the back to finish my sandwich, which only took a minute or so. When I came back he stressed that, as it was his break from work, he would have to be quick and time was of the essence. I went to get a gown for him from reception and whilst there quickly answered the phone and took a booking for later in the week; this really didn't take long though. When I went back to him he again stressed his limited time and asked me to be as quick as possible. When I had put the gown on the client, I realised that I had left my tool wrap and equipment on the workstation at the other side of the salon where I had been working last. I again excused myself and went to retrieve them. However, I couldn't believe what happened next, the client jumped up from the chair, threw the gown to the floor and left the salon looking rather angry!

Be professional ★★★

- When you finish a client, always tidy up and return tools and equipment to their correct place as this will save on preparation time for your next client.
- Allow for a proper lunch break in your working day when you sit down. Have a rest and do not work. Even if this is only 20 minutes it is not only a requirement of law under the 'working time directive' but is essential for you to maintain stamina and good health.

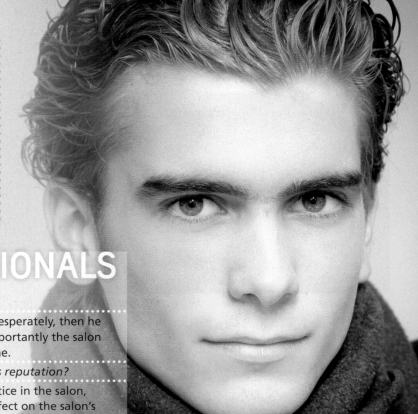

ASK THE PROFESSIONALS

Q *What should Simon have done differently?*

A Firstly, if he really wanted to eat his lunch that desperately, then he should have turned the client away, but most importantly the salon should always be prepared for a client at any time.

Q *What could a situation like this do for the salon's reputation?*

A If this type of unprofessionalism is common practice in the salon, then without doubt it will have a detrimental effect on the salon's reputation and ultimately revenue.

Creating the look

In this section you will be looking at how to carry out re-styling on men's hair, which includes traditional and current looks.

The act of cutting hair, whether it is men's or women's, demands a high level of skill. When cutting men's hair, you must be able to meet the demands of your client, whatever style he requires. To be successful, you need to have a sound knowledge of all the cutting tools available. You must also be able to achieve a variety of looks by adapting cutting techniques.

Cutting tools and their uses

There are many cutting tools available for use. You need to be familiar with each one and the effects you can achieve using them. Below is a table showing cutting tools and their uses.

Cutting tools	Uses	Illustration
Scissors	Used for a variety of techniques, e.g. club cutting, slicing, texturising or thinning	
Thinning scissors	Used to remove bulk but not length, only on dry hair	
Razors	Used to remove bulk or length, especially good for texturising. Only used on wet hair	
Clippers	Used for club cutting, especially good for creating very short styles	

Scissors

The scissors you use must be extremely sharp to function correctly. A good-quality pair need not be the most expensive, but always choose a pair that feels comfortable to use. When cutting men's hair, the majority of haircuts that you carry out are on short styles that require a lot of scissor-over-comb work. The length of the blade on your scissors is therefore very important. You will find it much easier to carry out good scissor-over-comb work using a pair of scissors with longer-length blades. As a guide, a minimum of 15 cm should be used. If you use scissors with a short-length blade, then it may cause 'steps' within the haircut. Although these 'steps' are often removable, it will prolong the time that you spend on carrying out the haircut.

Remember

Any scissors that you use must be handled with care and well maintained in order to prolong their working life and to ensure they give you the best possible results with each cut. Blunt scissors can cause damage to the hair ends by splitting them. Each time you use your scissors, wipe them when you have finished the cut. Using light oil on the hinge regularly will prevent them from rusting or seizing up. You must sterilise them to prevent the passing on of infection or infestation. Due to the fact you are using them so close to the hair and skin, it is inevitable that they pick up bacteria from one client that could easily be passed on to another.

Thinning scissors

As well as straight-edged scissors, there are thinning scissors with serrated edges; these can also be called **aesculaps** or texturising scissors. This type of scissor is used to remove bulk but not length from the hair and should be used only on hair that is dry. They can be bought in a variety of styles, with either one or both of the blades having a serrated edge. The degree of serration may also vary and this will allow you to produce a variety of different effects. For example, thinning scissors with only one blade serrated will remove less bulk from the hair. However, if both blades are serrated then more bulk can be removed and, if the degree of serration is increased, a very textured look can be achieved.

Aesculap

initially a brand name of a company that developed thinning scissors. Because of their popularity it became the most common name used for this type of scissor.

Be professional ★★★

- Thinning scissors can be used to remove 'steps' within the haircut if used on the ends of the hair.
- Never use thinning scissors around the hairline, crown or near a parting. It may leave exposed, short spiky hairs that protrude off the head.
- Thinning scissors are especially good for use on thick hair but do not produce particularly good results on fine hair.

Razors

Razors are used in hairdressing to remove bulk and length and should be used only on wet hair. They are especially good at thinning the hair ends, producing particularly stylish textured looks and when used to cut wavy or curly hair will encourage the curl or wave. There are a variety of razors available for use and you will have to decide which one is right for you. The table below shows the types of razors available, with a description of each.

Type of razor	Information	Illustration
Safety razor	This type of razor has removable blades, which is therefore more hygienic	
Shaper	This type of razor is only used in hair cutting and favoured in cutting women's hair	

It is essential that you hold and use a razor correctly, not only for your own and your client's safety, but also to prevent damage to the hair.

Check it out

Look at this photo of the correct method of holding a razor. You must practise holding the razor this way to ensure safety of use.

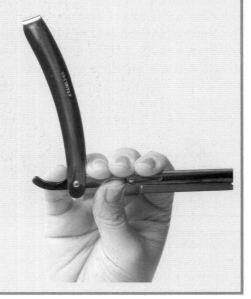

The blade of the razor must be extremely sharp; this will prevent any damage to the hair ends or discomfort to the client. The hair must be kept thoroughly wet whilst cutting to allow the razor to slice into the hair more easily and again to prevent discomfort to the client.

In the salon

Asia's story

Asia was carrying out a short razor cut on a man's hair one day in the salon. He was a regular client and they were also friends socially. They were chatting and laughing about a recent night out they had both been on. Asia was telling her client a story about one of their mutual friends and she was being quite animated in her description. Unfortunately, whilst demonstrating the actions, she flung out her arms and dropped the razor from her hand. As it fell to the floor, it cut her leg quite deeply. She had to receive medical treatment for the wound and was unable to carry on at work that day.

- Was Asia taking the care necessary with her use of the razor?
- How could she have avoided this accident?

Check it out

Try using your razor to shave off a few hairs on your arm or leg whilst the hair is dry. Take care not to cut yourself! It feels like the hair is being ripped out and is most uncomfortable. This is what your client is feeling on their head if you razor cut dry hair.

You should always inform the client of the risk of **in-growing hairs** after close razor or even clipper work. This can happen if the hair curls as it is growing and starts to grow back into the skin. It would be evident from a small lump in the skin that can become infected. They are, however, usually easy to remove by piercing the skin with a sterile surgical needle, allowing the hair to be freed. In-growing hairs are more likely to happen to a client with curly or African type hair.

In-growing hair

hair that doesn't grow out of the opening of the follicle but begins to grow under the skin.

Remember

- Great care must be taken when using a razor; the risk of cutting the skin when using sharp implements must never be forgotten. This must also be remembered when cutting short hair around the eye or ear area. You will need to concentrate and not allow yourself to be distracted from your work.
- You must follow the salon's rules regarding the disposal of used sharps. This will prevent the risk of harm or injury and also cross-infection.

Unit GB8 creatively cut hair using a combination of barbering techniques

Clippers

Clippers are used a great deal in the cutting of men's hair, as they can produce very short styles. Clippers have two blades with serrated edges and during use one of the blades moves over the other to cut the hair.

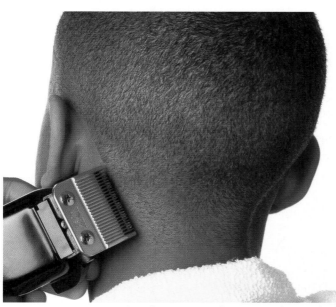

Using clippers to produce a very short style

Due to the style of the blades, it is essential that specialist services carry out the sharpening of the clipper blades (usually the manufacturer). The clipper blades must be cleaned after each use and are usually supplied on purchase with a cleaning kit, containing a small hard bristle brush and lubricating oil. The brush should be used to remove any loose hair cuttings and occasional use of the oil will ensure smooth running of the equipment.

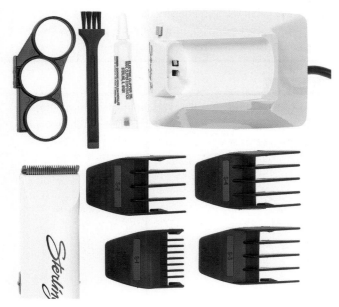

Be professional ★★★

If you are using clippers on thick or curly hair, you must open the blades using the lever on the side. This will allow the clippers to glide through the hair and will prevent pulling or dragging, which causes discomfort.

Cutting combs

There are two different types of cutting comb used in men's hairdressing. The traditional cutting comb is probably the most commonly used.

However, the barber styling comb is also used for cutting and is particularly useful for fine graduation, for example, tapering in the neckline or sides of the head. This is due to the fine teeth, which allow close-up work in confined areas, such as around the ears.

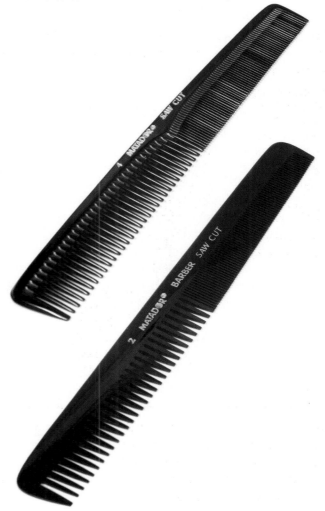

Cutting techniques and effects

There are several cutting techniques used in the cutting of men's hair that you will need to become familiar with. The cutting techniques used in men's and women's hairdressing are exactly the same. It is the overall style produced that differs.

Club cutting

This technique removes the hair length only and gives the hair ends a very blunt look. Clubbing or blunt cutting allows you to cut very straight and precise lines. When club cutting, it is the angle at which you hold the hair that determines the finished effect. For example, if you wish to produce graduation, you will need to over direct the hair and hold at an angle above 45 degrees to achieve this. You have to hold the hair firmly between the fingers with even tension and ensure each section is thoroughly combed; this will produce an even cut. You can club cut on wet or dry hair, but it is more precise on wet. Also, when cutting on wet hair you should maintain the dampness of the hair at all times otherwise the end result will be uneven! When you clipper cut the hair, you are also club cutting.

Scissor- and clipper-over-comb

Scissor-over-comb is most commonly used in men's hairdressing. It allows you to cut the hair very short and is especially good for blending short areas of graduation. To carry out this technique, you place the comb into the hair at the root area and pull out the comb away from the scalp up to the desired length. It is important to keep a flowing movement as you cut the hair that protrudes through the teeth of the comb. The scissors must open and close to cut at the same pace up the haircut or else lines will develop, known as 'steps'. Again, this type of cutting requires accuracy and a great deal of practice. Clipper-over-comb is done in exactly the same way, except the clipper blades are run over the hair protruding through the teeth of the comb. Clipper-over-comb is better used on thick hair or when there is a lot of bulk to be removed. This technique is quicker and saves time.

Check it out

You can practise the movement of scissor-over-comb in the workstation mirror. Make sure that the comb follows the movement of the opening and closing scissor action and that you hold your comb in a way so that you can flip it over to comb down each section that you have just cut.

Tapering

This technique is used when you want to remove bulk or join together short and long layers. It can be done on wet hair if using a razor and dry if using scissors. The scissors slide into the hair and as you slightly open and close the blades care must be taken not to close the blade together or the hair will be cut straight across. With the razor method, you scoop into the hair sections and apply pressure according to the amount of hair you want to remove. This method requires a great deal of accuracy and skill so as not to cut off too much hair. Tapering will produce a textured look on short hair or blend short to long layers as in feathering.

Thinning

This method of cutting is used to remove bulk from the hair but not length. It is more commonly carried out with thinning scissors; however, there are scissor-thinning techniques that you can use. For instance, chipping into the hair at the root area will remove bulk and the shorter hairs will help to provide style support to the longer lengths.

When barber stylists are seen using thinning scissors on longer length hair, instead of sectioning the hair off, they use the end of the blades to lift the hair up before placing the comb into the section. You must be sure that the blades are fully closed to prevent them cutting the hair if using this method.

Be professional ★★★

- Thinning scissors should be used only on dry hair to prevent too much hair from being removed. They should not be used on partings or around hairlines, as short hairs can be seen protruding once the hair has been styled.
- Thinning scissors are not suitable for use on fine or thinning hair, but are good for very thick or coarse hair. You can use the thinning scissors at any point along the hair length depending on the amount of hair you wish to remove and the effect you want to create.

Remember

If you have cut hair very short and there are 'steps' in the haircut that you cannot remove, a good tip is to use thinning scissors to go over the hair ends to remove them.

Unit GB8 creatively cut hair using a combination of barbering techniques

Razoring

Razor cutting can be done anywhere in a haircut and removes bulk or length, depending on where you use the technique. With razor cutting, the hair is held between the fingers and can be cut either on top or below the section, with the razor held at a slight angle to the hair shaft. The amount of pressure you apply will determine the amount of hair removed, so take care — it is much safer to remove a little at a time than to take off too much. Razor cutting is especially good for creating very textured looks or for blending short layers into very long layers.

> **Check it out**
>
> Visit your council offices and look up the local by-laws for the use of razors. This should give you information on safe practice.
>
> **Key Skills Links**: Level 2 Communication

Freehand

Cutting the hair without holding it between the fingers or comb is known as freehand cutting. Freehand can be carried out on wet or dry hair. The hair is combed into place and cut without any tension being applied. It is particularly useful when cutting around an unusual growth pattern, for example, around a nape whorl. You must allow the hair to lie as it will without applying any pressure, and then cut. This will allow the hair to fall into its natural lie and will not look uneven when finished.

Texturising

Texturising is used to remove both length and bulk and can be carried out on wet or dry hair. The ends of the scissors are used to cut into the hair anywhere along the hair shaft, from mid-lengths to ends, depending on the effect you are trying to create. You can use it to produce a much more choppy, uneven finish or just to give softer broken edges. It can be incorporated into many different styles; for instance, when cutting a straight-edged one-length look, you can texture the ends to soften the edges.

Fading

This technique is used when you want the design to really fade out on the head to a very short, almost bald look. The clippers are used to cut the hair shorter to a no guard length. Look at the photo on page 385 of clippers being used to see an example of fading.

Disconnecting

This technique is used when you want to achieve a look that contains shorter and longer sections within the haircut. Instead of blending the shorter lengths to the longer lengths, they are left disconnected which gives a more dramatic effect and has become increasingly popular. It is also useful for taking bulk out of a cut and cutting shorter layers underneath for style support.

Layering and graduating

Now that you have looked at all the cutting techniques, you need to familiarise yourself with the effects you will be creating by cutting angles. They fall into two main types: layering and graduation. You will no doubt be familiar with the terminology, but do you fully understand the difference between the two?

Firstly, you will layer most haircuts, except for one-length cuts. The most common layering technique is the uniform layer — this is where the hair is cut at a 90-degree angle to the scalp and is cut to the same length all over the head.

Graduation is when the hair is cut to varying lengths throughout the haircut; this is used in the majority of men's haircuts. For example, the layers on top will be longer than the layers underneath, with the style tapering into the neckline to much shorter layers, as with a short back and sides design.

Men's re-style: a step-by-step guide

1 Before the cut.

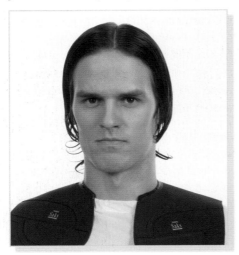

2 Create a square horseshoe section from the high recession area and divide in two above the ear area and over the head.

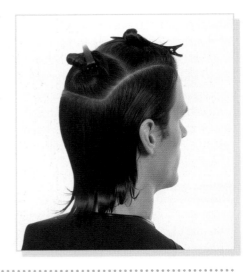

3 Take a profile line section of approximately ½ inch in the back section of the horseshoe section. Proceed to elevate the hair parallel to the head shape and use a blunt cutting technique.

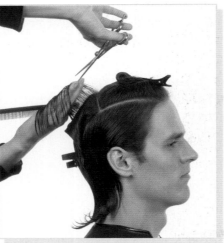

4 Continue by elevating parallel and pivoting from the top of the profile line section to the ear area. The last section is over directed back to the previous section, by holding the section horizontally and blunt cutting.

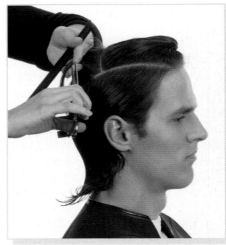

5 Continue cutting through this section using the previous section as your cutting guideline.

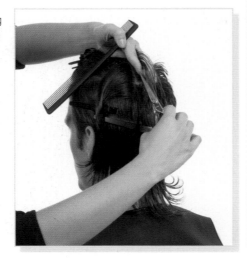

6 On the last section, over direct back to the previous section, holding the section on a diagonal angle. Cross check to ensure balance.

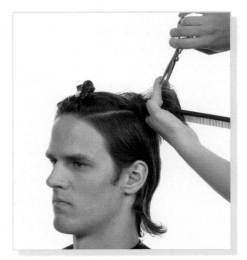

7 The right side is cut first. Using the back section as a guideline, elevate horizontal sections to a horizontal angle and blunt cut. Continue to use the previous section as a guideline until section is complete.

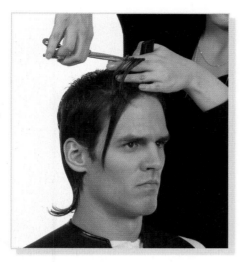

8 The left side of the top section is blunt cut, using the previous back section as a guideline. Elevate horizontal sections to a diagonal angle.

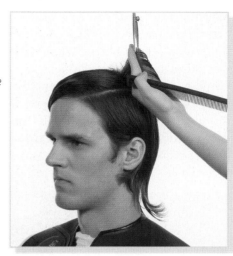

9 Draw a vertical section on both corners of the head shape to divide the hair underneath the horseshoe section. Starting at the high recession area, below the horseshoe section, hold the hair in the comb at a horizontal angle. Use the previous section above as a guideline and proceed to point cut.

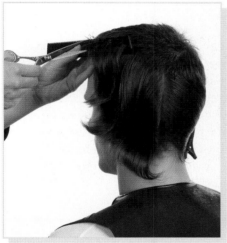

10 Work sections towards the back of the head in the same manner.

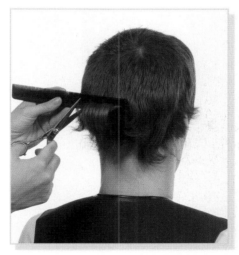

11 At the front hairline, using a blunt cutting technique, elevate the section parallel to the head shape. Continue by pivoting from the recession area across to the opposite recession area.

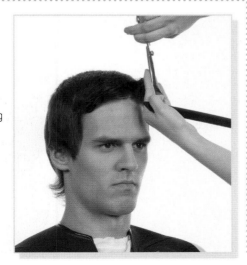

12 The finished look.

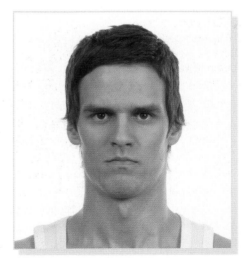

Creatively cut hair using a combination of barbering techniques **Unit GB8**

Creating traditional looks

When creating traditional looks you will use traditional cutting techniques: scissor- and clipper-over-comb and club cutting. A commonly requested traditional look is a short back and sides. This style requires the barber stylist to cut the back and the sides to a much shorter length than the top sections. On the shorter lengths (the back and side sections) you will use scissor- or clipper-over-comb and for the longer lengths (the top sections) use the club cut technique. If the hair is thick, then consider using the thinning scissors through the top to reduce bulk.

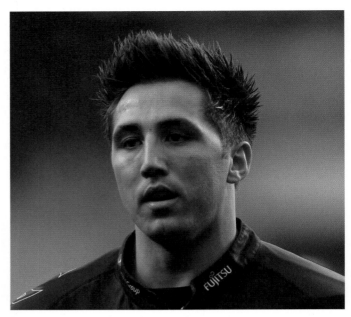

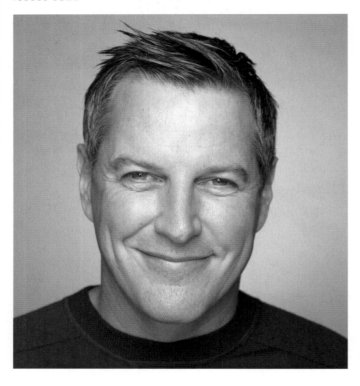

Creating current looks

When creating current looks you will need to use a variety of cutting techniques depending on the look you want to create. You can take your inspiration for current looks from the media; a lot of celebrities change their hair frequently to stay current, for example, Johnny Depp, David Beckham and Gavin Henson. To create really up to the minute looks it will be necessary to adapt your cutting techniques to allow for imagination in your work, for example, using a razor to produce extremes of short to longer lengths within a cut. All of the cutting techniques within the range can be used in a variety of ways to produce creativity and flair in your work, such as using clippers freehand to cut patterns into the hair, but this takes a lot of skill and practice to ensure accuracy.

Neckline shapes

When cutting men's hair, there are a variety of **neckline shapes** that can be created. They can be used together and separately to create many different effects. For example, a client may require a square neckline that has also been tapered. It is usually the client's choice that determines the neckline shape, as most men have a personal preference. However, other influencing factors must be considered, for example, hair growth patterns. The most common have been listed in the table below.

Neckline shape
the shape the hair is cut into at the neckline.

Neckline shape	Illustration
Square	
Round	
Tapered	

Be professional ★★★

When cutting the neckline shape, always cut the sides of the neckline first and then across the neckline to join the two sides. This will allow you to judge the correct height at which to cut the neckline length.

Cutting angles, guidelines and outlines

It is extremely important that throughout the cut you are aware of the **cutting angles** you are using, as they will affect the finished shape and balance of the hair. It is also important that you are accurate in the way that you section the haircut. It is not always necessary to start at the back, but be sure to section off the hair and follow neat and even sections throughout the cut. Good sectioning will allow you to follow your **guideline** and ensure that no areas are missed; this looks professional to the client and results in the haircut being even at the end.

Cutting angle

the angle at which the hair is cut.

Guideline

the line of the hair cut that you follow as you progress through the cut.

Below are some examples of the cutting angles used.

Most men's haircuts can be divided into three sections, as shown in the illustration below.

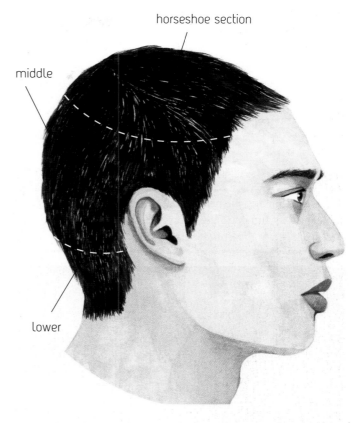

Men's haircuts can be divided into three sections

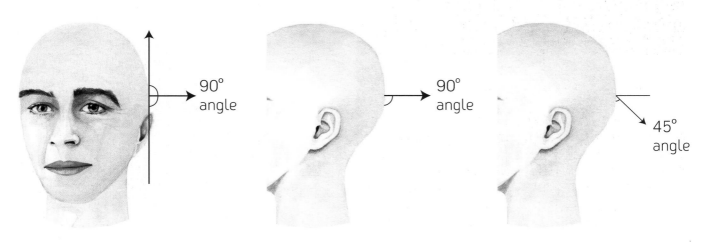

Different cutting angles

Unit GB8 creatively cut hair using a combination of barbering techniques

The lower section, into the nape of the head, is usually cut first, followed by the middle section, and then finally the horseshoe section from the temple, round the crown, and back to the temple on the other side. Each of these sections is blended into the other during cutting. **Outlining** a short- or medium-length man's cut is essential to create a professional finish. Cutting around and over the ears is known as the arching technique and this arched look is visible in the photo below. Any hair below the outline must be removed by using either the clippers or a razor to shave the hair away. If using the clippers, then the small taper clippers are ideal as they cut closer to the skin.

Outline

the outer shape of the haircut that follows from the nape, over the ears and up to the temples, including the shape of the sideburns, if present.

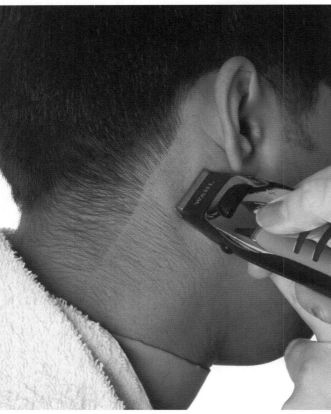

Using taper clippers to remove hair below the outline

Remember

When using a razor blade on a client, the blade must be disposed of after each use in line with your salon's policies. This will reduce the risk of cross-infection.

Check it out

What is your salon's policy for the safe disposal of used sharps? Does it adequately cover the lawful requirements of safe disposal?

Correct positioning of self and client

The correct position of your client is extremely important whilst carrying out the haircut. You must ensure that you position your client and their head in the correct way. This will prevent you from being restricted whilst cutting in difficult-to-reach areas such as the nape. You must make certain that your client is seated upright and not slouching. As you work your way around the haircut, be sure to position the client's head in a way that will assist you, without causing him any discomfort. If your client is not positioned correctly, it will not only restrict your cutting but could produce an uneven finished result.

Your own stance while working must also be considered at all times. The way that you stand to work will affect your posture and can lead to muscle fatigue if incorrect. Think about balancing the weight over your body when you stand and not leaning to one side for long periods. It is far too easy to put unnecessary strain on muscles and ligaments by over-reaching or stretching. However, this can be avoided by taking the time to adopt a good posture whilst working. Eventually it will become habit to stand in the correct position and you will soon do it without realising.

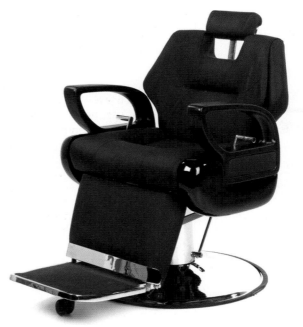

A good quality chair will aid your posture and keep the client comfortable

Look back at the 'In the salon' feature on Luca on page 130 of Unit GH16. This is a good example of how poor posture can affect you over a period of time; you must take your posture seriously.

Timings

The time that you spend on a haircut will differ from client to client. However, the salon you work in will usually have expected service times and it is important that you are aware of these and work within them.

Check it out

> Find out the expected service times in your salon for cutting services. Do both senior and junior staff work to the same expected service times?

Solving cutting problems

If any problems arise during the cutting service, it is essential that you are aware of the methods used to solve them. Usually problems arise because your consultation was not accurate. For instance, you begin the cut and then find that there is a conflicting hair growth pattern that is preventing you from getting the look you require. You will have to deal with problems such as these whenever they occur, but keep the client informed, use your professional judgement, and be tactful in explaining the situation. You must remain confident in your approach, stay calm, and never panic. Panic will serve only to alarm your client and he in turn will lose confidence in your ability. Below is a table of cutting problems and possible remedies that you may come across during the cutting process.

Cutting problem	Possible remedy
Sides are not even on finished cut	Cross-check, use the mirror and remove the longer length to even up
Can't get close enough into the nape to cut to required length	Adjust the way you hold the hair for cutting, or use a different cutting technique
Hair won't lie correctly around hairline	Adjust the finished style to incorporate the hairline's natural lie
Cut the client's or own skin	Stop immediately and clean the wound so it's free from hair and apply pressure to stop bleeding. Use a band-aid if continuing

Another common problem is loose hair cuttings being allowed to fall onto the client's clothing. This can easily be avoided by securely fastening the gown and checking it throughout the cut to ensure it is still in place. Removing the cut hair during the cutting process also helps to prevent a build-up around the neckline.

Remember

> A good tip if the cut hair is wet and sticking to the skin is to use a little talcum powder on your neck brush to help to remove it.

Thorough preparation and staying focused on the service you are carrying out will help to prevent any problems arising.

Be professional ★★★

- Be aware of critical influencing factors, such as growth patterns, at all times.
- If cutting wet hair, keep it wet throughout, especially if using a razor.
- Always take neat, even sections.
- Ensure that your tension is good and even throughout the cut.
- Make sure you can see your guideline before you cut a section.
- Never cut shorter than your guideline.
- Check regularly throughout the cut that it is level.
- Always cross-check your cut.
- Do not cut off too much hair when cross-checking, only the hair you have missed.
- Maintain the consultation throughout with the client to check what you are doing is to his requirements.
- If things go wrong, do not let the client see you are panicking.
- Remember, if you cut the hair too short, there is nothing you can do about it!

Use this table of cutting techniques as a quick reference.

Technique	Effect	Cut on wet, dry or either	Best suited on straight or curly hair
Clubbing	Gives a blunt, straight edge to the hair ends	Either, but more precise on wet hair	Either, but will help to reduce curl
Clippering	Gives a blunt straight edge to the hair ends	Dry	Can be used on either, but open the blades slightly to aid cutting on curly hair
Thinning	Removes bulk but not length	Dry	Either, but will encourage curl
Razoring	Removes bulk and length, good for texturising	Wet	Either, but will encourage curl
Freehand	Removes length and bulk	Either	Either
Texturising	Produces softer, broken edges	Either	Either
Tapering	Removes bulk, gives texture	Wet with razor and dry with scissors	Either
Scissor-over-comb	Club cutting on short hair	Either	Either
Fading	Cutting the hair very short to a blend out to no hair	Dry	Either
Disconnecting	Creates long and short lengths that do not blend together	Either	Either

After the service

This section is about completing the service in a manner that ensures the client leaves the salon fully satisfied. This may involve making recommendations for styling products for home use or making further appointments.

Using styling products to finish

It is likely that the salon has a particular product range that you use and are familiar with. However, you must keep abreast of new developments within the styling range in order to ensure that your knowledge is up to date. There are several ways of doing this, for example, reading trade magazines, checking at the wholesale suppliers when you visit, or talking to technical representatives when they call into the salon with information on offers and developments.

There are several product companies that are dedicated to selling only men's styling products, but if your salon is unisex, you may wish to stock a range that caters for both men and women. Men are less likely to ask about how to maintain the style at home and it is your responsibility as the stylist to recommend the correct product for them to use. There are many styling products available and they each serve a different purpose; however, they can usually be categorised into whether they provide hold and / or shine for

the hair. A client may have a preference as to the look they require or they may be looking for advice from you. Discuss your client's requirements and determine what the finished look requires the product to do — you will then be able to recommend something suitable.

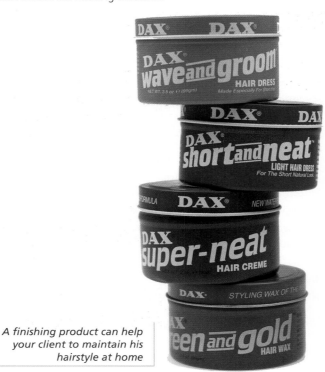

A finishing product can help your client to maintain his hairstyle at home

The table below lists several men's styling products available for use and the effects they will help you to achieve.

Styling product	Effect achieved
Wax	Gives texture and will define curl
Dressing / styling cream	Will add shine to the hair, reduces static and will define curl
Hairspray	Will hold the hair in place. Natural to ultra firm hold
Gel / gel spray	Will provide extreme hold. Ranges from firm to ultra

Confirmation of the finished look

Confirming your client's satisfaction with his finished look is no less important than the rest of the service. Take the time to show the client the back and sides of the cut, using the back mirror. Check to be sure the client can see through the back mirror and adjust the angle of the mirror if necessary. Usually, if you can see through the mirrors, then your client will also.

If the cut needs adjusting to the client's specific requirements, do not take this as a dislike of your finished work. You must look at it from the client's point of view — he wants the finished look to meet his expectations. Minor adjustments should be made but never a re-cut of the whole head. This should be left to another appointment. Do not be afraid to correct any mistakes, for example, a few longer hairs left above the ear. The client will thank you in the long run if he leaves the salon with a perfect cut.

Correct removal of the protective clothing

When removing the gown, always take care to take it off properly. Unfasten it correctly and ensure that any cut hair is thrown from the gown onto the floor and not over the client's clothing. If you do find there is some on his clothes, offer him a clothes brush to remove it but never let him leave the salon with hair on his clothes. This looks unprofessional and does not give a good impression of the salon. Remember that a client is looking for an all-round excellent service; he may think that although you have given him a fabulous haircut, your customer service skills leave a lot to be desired.

Recommendations and intervals between cuts

Never be afraid to give the client advice on styling, as it is a reflection on your salon's good name if his hair always looks good. He is, after all, a walking advertisement for you out on the streets. As you are finishing off, you can discuss with your client the styling techniques you are using and why and how the products are helping you to achieve the final look. Ensure you have a selection of brushes and tools available for retail sale. A client may find it easier to style his hair at home using the tools that you use and it is another good selling opportunity. Straighteners are very popular to use as a styling aid and a small pair with thin plates are especially effective to use on short men's styles. Always ensure you demonstrate their use for your client before they purchase.

Advise the client on when he will need to return to the salon for his next appointment. This may be for a service other than cutting, but generally clients have their haircut maintained between every three to six weeks, unless they are growing their hair at which point they may want to leave a longer gap. Usually, no more than ten weeks is advised. If it is left any longer, the ends of the hair become more susceptible to splitting.

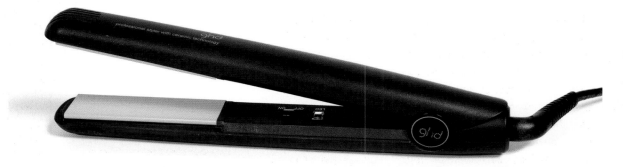

Disposal of waste, including sharps

There are different types of waste that must be disposed of safely in the salon. However, after a cutting service it is only likely to be hair cuttings, used sharps, and empty product containers. Hair cuttings left on the floor can cause a slippery surface and this then becomes a **hazard** in the salon, to both you and the client when he stands up. Salons dispose of hair cuttings in different ways, but it is more hygienic to ensure that they are placed in a covered bin and put in the outside bin in a tied-up bag to prevent them spilling out.

Hazard

something likely to cause injury.

Remember

Aerosol containers, even when they feel empty, can still contain flammable materials. There is also a risk of them exploding if punctured or overheated so care must be taken with regards to their safe disposal.

Check it out

Using a selection of pictures or photographs of your own work, describe how you achieved the overall look and incorporated different cutting techniques. In your descriptions, indicate the cutting angles and list the tools and equipment you used. State which products you used to create the looks.

 Key Skills Links: Level 2 Communication

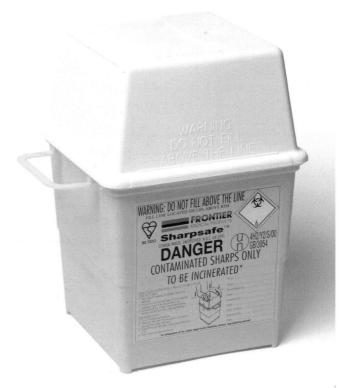

A sharps bin

Used sharps must be disposed of with extreme care due to the risk of injury or cross-infection. A sharps bin must be used and this should be a sealed container with a clear label stating its purpose. You must follow the salon policy for the safe disposal of empty product containers; usually they are placed in a covered bin and put outside for refuse collection. However, in today's environmentally friendly society, recycling is becoming increasingly popular and your salon should be adopting a policy for this.

Check your knowledge

The following questions will help you to check your understanding of this unit. The answers can be found on page 421. Take care, as there may be more than one correct answer for some questions.

1 Where would you find information on the use limitations of open blade razors?
  a Your local council offices
  b Your salon policies and procedures booklet
  c A trade magazine
  d The product supplier's website

2 What safety considerations must be taken into account when cutting men's hair?
  a Use the correct personal protective equipment
  b Ensure the client relaxes at all times
  c Check if the client needs a drink
  d Visually check electrical equipment before use

3 What visual aids may be used during consultation to help ascertain the client's requirements?
  a Watching television
  b Looking through the local newspapers
  c Stylebooks
  d Photos that the client brought in

4 What are thinning scissors used for?
  a To remove length
  b To remove bulk and length
  c To remove bulk but not length
  d To remove split ends

5 Why is it important to cut to the client's natural hairline?
  a To avoid discomfort
  b So the hair grows back evenly
  c So the haircut looks neat and tidy
  d To prevent the client from cutting it themselves

6 Why do you need to establish, and follow, a guideline during cutting?
  a To ensure you achieve a balanced cut
  b To ensure the finished result is even
  c So that the haircut takes longer
  d To prevent you from using the wrong cutting techniques

7 What are the commercially expected service times for cutting men's hair?
  a An hour
  b 2 hours
  c ½ an hour
  d 1 and ½ hours

8 What are the recommended time intervals between men's haircuts?

  a About 4 weeks depending on the client's hair length

  b At least 2 months

  c 7 or 8 weeks

  d Every fortnight

9 How should clippers be maintained correctly?

  a Wash them thoroughly every month

  b Brush off any hair after each use and oil regularly

  c Use hygiene spray regularly to prevent the spread of bacteria

  d Visually check the wires before each use for faults

10 How should cutting tools be stored safely?

  a Kept on the reception desk

  b Put away in the correct holder or case after each use

  c Kept in the stock room

  d In your pocket so you always have them to hand

Unit GB8 creatively cut hair using a combination of barbering techniques

Assessment guidance

Unit GB8 is about the use of advanced cutting skills to re-style men's hair in a way that enhances their personal image. A high level of professionalism and strict following of health and safety procedures is essential.

Whilst completing this unit you will have to demonstrate competence in a variety of cutting techniques:

- club cutting
- scissor-over-comb
- clipper-over-comb
- thinning
- texturising
- freehand
- razor cutting
- tapering
- fading
- disconnecting.

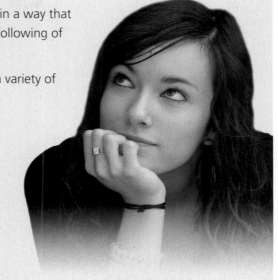

You must also be able to use safely a variety of cutting tools to achieve these looks:

- scissors
- clippers
- razors.

However, use of clipper attachments is not allowed at Level 3.

You must prove your ability in graduating and layering on both current and traditional looks, as these are the looks you will mainly deal with in your everyday work as a barber stylist.

Unit AH35

Design and create patterns in hair

Pearson Education Ltd / Mind Studio

What you will learn:

- **How to prepare the client**
- **How to create the look**
- **How to proceed after the service.**

Introduction

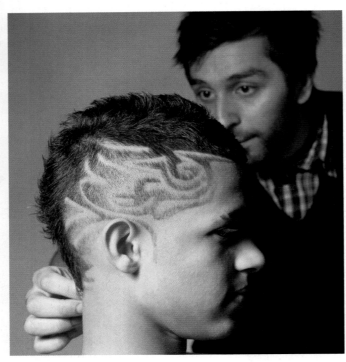

In order to design and create patterns in hair you will need a certain amount of artistic flair. You will be using all the cutting techniques you have previously learnt but using them creatively to cut patterns into the hair. You will have to be inventive in your work and be able to create a variety of different designs in order to fulfil the needs of your clientele.

You the stylist

You will need to be skilled in creating patterns that are: **3D-pictorial**, **repeated** and **symmetrical** over both a full head and a partial head to meet the needs of you clients. You should stay up to date with the latest design ideas and be able to adapt these to put your own individual stamp on them. If you are creative in this way, then you can become very successful in your work.

3D pictorial

a pattern that looks 3D in effect and is illustrative, using symbols or graphics to produce a picture.

Repeated

a pattern that is repeated over and over.

Symmetrical

a pattern that is identical throughout.

Preparing the client

This section looks at everything that is important when preparing the client for the service. Being prepared and ready with everything to hand reflects not only your own level of professionalism, but also that of the salon. If you are fully prepared it will also save you time and increase the client's confidence in your ability.

Thorough consultation

The consultation you carry out with your client will determine your client's requirements. It also creates an opportunity for you to use your imagination and recommend what you think will be suitable. You must be able to communicate well with your client, not only to extract the right information from him, but also to ensure he fully understands your perceptions of this. Using visual aids is essential to make sure that both you and the client fully understand how the pattern will look.

Check it out

Produce a portfolio of designs that you can use with your clients in the salon whilst carrying out the consultation. You can add photos of your own work, or take them from magazines, or even drawings of the patterns you have designed.

 Key Skills Links: Level 2 Communication

All the information taken during consultation and regarding the service should be written down on the client's record card. This keeps an accurate and up-to-date account of exactly what the client wants and what you offered / carried out. This would be especially useful if you need to refer back to clear up any discrepancies. For more detailed information on record keeping refer to page 31 in Unit G21.

Contra-indications and influencing factors

'Influencing factors' are all the points that must be considered during the consultation; you must ask appropriate questions to determine these, in order to discover any contra-indications. These may affect the service you provide or even prevent you from continuing!

Influencing factors are things such as scars, head and face shape and hair length; all of these should be discussed with your client and it should be made clear how they may affect the finished look. Contra-indications such as skin disorders should be identified visually and then questions asked to determine if you can proceed with the service, for example: 'I suspect you have a skin condition. Are you aware of this?' 'Are you receiving any medical treatment for the condition?'

Be professional ★★★

- You should always inform your client of how any influencing factors may affect the finished look and ensure your client fully understands this.
- You need to inform the client of the expected length of the service and this should fall within the expected service times for your salon. Remember that these will differ according to the type of service required, for example, full or partial head pattern.

Head and face shape

It is vital that, to ensure a neat and balanced design, you take a good look at the client's head and face shape. It's important to make sure that the finished pattern you are creating will complement the client's head and face shape and so suit the client. The head shape may clash with the design the client has chosen, it is up to you during consultation to advise on what is appropriate and what is achievable with the head shape the client has. For example, you would not want to give a client with a sharp angular face shape an extreme angular pattern; you should try to soften the look for them with a swirling, softer design.

Hair growth patterns

The way in which the hair grows over the head must be looked at in great detail prior to commencing the design. You should look for problem areas, for example, **whorls** or bald patches, as these will affect the pattern.

Whorls

an usual growth pattern where the hair grows in a circular direction.

Hair density

The thickness of the hair will affect the choice of design and cutting technique used. How thick or sparse the hair is over the head will need to be considered in order to ensure that the finished design is shown off to good effect. If the hair is finer or lighter, then stick with bigger, bolder patterns using straight lines and square designs to increase sharpness; if the pattern is too intricate, it will lose its definition.

Hair length

You will always need to ensure that the hair is of a suitable length before you begin to cut the pattern into the hair. If the hair is too long, you will not be able to cut the pattern in with

accuracy, and if the hair is too short, then the pattern won't have good definition. Aim to begin with the hair at a length of 1 ½ guard, although you can use a 1 guard length if the hair is dark and thick.

Hair texture

The hair texture affects your choice of design and cutting techniques in much the same way as density of hair. If your client has fine-textured hair, then you may struggle to define the pattern well; alternatively, if the hair is very coarse, then you may find it difficult to cut enough hair away for the pattern to be clearly seen. However, generally on darker, thicker hair it is much easier to create a vivid design.

Presence of male pattern baldness / scarring

If your client has areas of baldness, then you would never cut patterns over this area as the bald areas would interfere with the overall design. This same principle applies for areas with scarring – if you were trying to cut in a design over a scar where no hair grows, it will obviously affect the finished look. You must always discuss this with your client and make sure they fully understand how the final look will be affected by the areas with no hair.

Skin disorders

Skin and scalp disorders may prevent you from carrying out the service and should be given careful consideration. If the client is suffering from an infection or infestation, you must not continue with the service as there is a high risk of **cross-infection**. It is crucial that these are found on initial consultation and not during the service.

Cross-infection

when bacteria or germs are passed from one person to another.

Personal hygiene

It is imperative to present a professional image at all times. This can be achieved only by maintaining high standards within the salon. You need to consider your own standards of hygiene as well as those of the salon. Washing regularly and using a good deodorant will ensure you always smell fresh. As you are working in close proximity to your client, your body odour and breath will be unmistakable. It is therefore essential to have fresh breath at all times, especially after lunch or a cigarette break. Strong odours such as onions or nicotine can be offensive to a client. Check that your hands and nails are also clean, as dirty fingernails will not convey a high standard of hygiene.

Personal protective equipment

Protecting yourself and the client should always be a high priority. When cutting a male client's hair, it is essential to ensure that you adequately protect their clothes from loose hair cuttings. The only protective equipment needed will be for the client's benefit, for example, the gown, cutting collar or neck strip. You must be sure before you begin the cut that the gown covers all the clothing and no areas are left exposed that may become covered in hair. Secure the gown properly to prevent it slipping off. Always use some other type of protection over the gown, following your salon's requirements. For example, using a towel, cutting collar or neck strip around the shoulders will provide added protection and help to prevent any loose hair from falling down the neck of the gown and causing client discomfort.

Be professional ★ ★ ★

You must continue checking throughout the haircut that the personal protective equipment used still effectively covers your client. This will continue to protect the client's clothing from hair cuttings.

Safe working practices

While working in the salon, it is a requirement of law that you comply with health and safety legislation. The tools you use must always be thoroughly cleaned, disinfected, sterilised and fit for purpose. The methods of cleaning, disinfection and **sterilisation** you use will depend upon what is available in the salon; however, it may be that you have other options to consider. (Refer back to pages 13–14 of Unit G22.)

Sterilisation

the method of killing bacteria or germs.

Check it out

List the tools and equipment that you use in the salon while cutting and write next to each one the method of sterilisation that you currently use. You should check that what you are using is sufficient by looking at Unit G22, pages 13–14. Could your methods be adapted to improve your sterilisation routine?

KS **Key Skills Links**: Level 2 Communication

Be professional ★ ★ ★

- Before sterilising any tools or equipment you should thoroughly clean them with soap and water and, if it is electrical, a suitable cleaning lotion or spray. Blades may be wiped over with spirit before sterilising.
- You also need to consider your responsibilities under the Electricity at Work Regulations. Do you visually check all electrical equipment before use? Is all the electrical equipment tested regularly for faults? You must be sure that both you and the staff for whom you have responsibility, are complying with the safe use of electrical equipment.

Check it out

Go to your local council offices and look up any local by-laws that affect the work you do in the salon, particularly regarding the use of open blade razors. You have a duty to follow these, and remember, if you move to another salon in a different area, the relevant by-laws may be different.

Preparing your work area

It is essential that you are fully prepared for the service that you are carrying out. The salon junior will play a vital role in ensuring that your work area is ready for you. Their training is of great importance and should be initially taught by watching you prepare the work area.

Check it out

List the salon's rules regarding correct storage and handling of cutting tools and equipment.

There are several aspects of preparation that must be checked prior to commencement.

- Make sure you have everything you will need with you.
- Check all tools and equipment are clean and fit for purpose.
- Visually check any electrical equipment prior to use.
- Sterilise any necessary tools and equipment.
- Check the surrounding work areas are clean, tidy and free of excess hair.

Being fully prepared for your client will save you time in the long run. It also presents a professional image to the client if you are ready for the service. Having to excuse yourself to find something you forgot not only slows you down but can also irritate the client.

Creating the look

In this section you will find all the information that will assist you in carrying out the design and cutting of patterns in hair. You will need to be aware of the cutting tools available for use and the various techniques you can adopt to achieve a variety of designs.

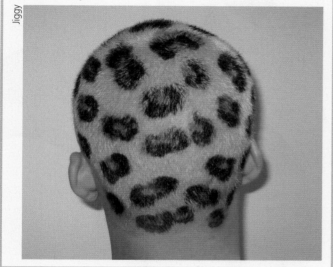

Jiggy

Cutting tools and their uses

There are three cutting tools available for use and you need to be familiar with each one and the effects you can achieve using them. Below is a table showing cutting tools and their uses.

Cutting tools	Uses	Illustration
Scissors	Used for scissor-over-comb work, fading and outlining	
Razors	Used to shave out hair to define the pattern	
Clippers	Used for clipper-over-comb work, fading and outlining. Also for cutting the pattern into the hair	

Scissors

The scissors you use must be extremely sharp to function correctly. A good-quality pair need not be the most expensive, but always choose a pair that feels comfortable to use. You will find it much easier to carry out good scissor-over-comb work using a pair of scissors with longer-length blades. As a guide, a minimum of 15 cm should be used. If you use scissors with a short-length blade, then it may cause 'steps' within the cut. Although these 'steps' are often removable, it will prolong the time that you spend carrying out the haircut.

Clippers

Clippers are used a great deal in the cutting of men's hair, as they can produce very short styles; taper clippers or trimmers are especially useful for 'drawing' patterns in hair. Clippers have two blades with serrated edges and during use one of the blades moves over the other to cut the hair.

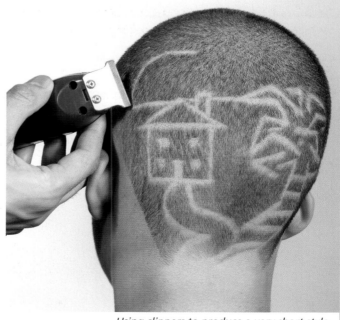

Using clippers to produce a very short style

Due to the style of the blades, it is essential that specialist services carry out the sharpening of the clipper blades (usually the manufacturer). The clipper blades must be cleaned after each use and are usually supplied on purchase with a cleaning kit, containing a small hard bristle brush and lubricating oil. The brush should be used to remove any loose hair cuttings and occasional use of the oil will ensure smooth running of the equipment.

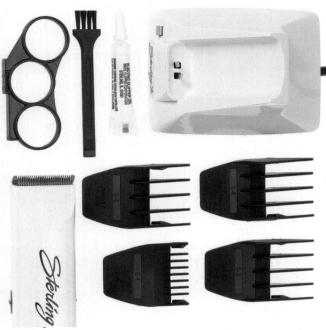

Clippers with attachments

Remember

As clippers are electrical, they must be used in line with the Electricity at Work Regulations.

Be professional ★★★

If you are using clippers on thick or curly hair, you must open the blades using the lever on the side. This will allow the clippers to glide through the hair and will prevent pulling or dragging, which causes discomfort.

Razors

Razors are used to define the lines of the pattern and to shave out the hair in certain areas. You should always use a clean and sterile razor for each client. Using razors with disposable blades and a new one for each client is essential these days to prevent the spread of infection. It is not only the risk of HIV but, more commonly, hepatitis that you should be aware of, and your working practices should take this into consideration.

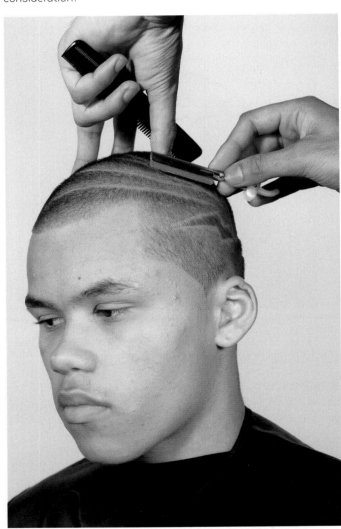

Cutting techniques

Clipper-over-comb

This technique produces the same effect as scissor-over-comb but cuts the hair at a much quicker rate, making it ideal to use if you are busy in the salon. To carry out this technique, you place the comb into the hair at the root area and pull out the comb, away from the scalp, to the desired length and then cut the hair that protrudes through the teeth using the clippers.

Clippers have a lever on the side that allows you to open or close the blades to varying degrees. If you are working on coarse, dense hair, then it is beneficial to open the blade out to allow the clippers to cut through the hair without dragging, causing discomfort to the client. Alternatively, if you are cutting fine hair, or wish to cut close to the skin, then closing the blades will ease cutting the hair.

Scissor-over-comb

Scissor-over-comb allows you to cut the hair very short and is especially good for blending short areas of graduation. To carry out this technique, you place the comb into the hair at the root area and pull out the comb away from the scalp to the desired length. It is important to keep a flowing movement as you cut the hair that protrudes through the teeth of the comb. The scissors must open and close to cut at the same pace up the haircut to avoid lines, known as 'steps'. This type of cutting requires accuracy and a great deal of practice.

> **Check it out**
>
> You can practise the movement of scissor-over-comb in the workstation mirror. Make sure that the comb follows the movement of the opening and closing scissor action and that you hold your comb in a way so that you can flip it over to comb down each section that you have just cut.

Razor work

Razors are used extensively when creating patterns in hair and a great deal of accuracy and attention to detail is required. Accurate use of the razor will develop the more you use it and as your dexterity improves. You may use the razor to take out hair and create the pattern and to clean outlines, but also in the cutting of the style if the client has a partial design and the rest of the hair cut into shape.

You should always inform the client of the risk of in-growing hairs after close razor or clipper work; this happens when the hair curls as it is growing and starts to grow back into the skin. It would be evident from a small lump in the skin that can become infected. They are, however, usually easy to remove by piercing the skin with a sterile surgical needle allowing the hair to be freed. Also, a client with dark skin will need to be advised about the changes that can happen to the skin with repeated use of razor work or even close clipper work. The area of skin that has been clippered or razored may start to thicken or darken, causing discolouration of the skin that will be very noticeable below the hairline; this is known as '**shadowing**'.

> **Shadowing**
>
> when the skin becomes darkened through continued use of close clipper or razor work.

Freehand

Cutting the hair without holding it between the fingers or comb is known as freehand cutting. The hair is combed into place and cut without any tension being applied. It is particularly useful when cutting around an unusual growth pattern, for example, around a nape whorl. You must allow the hair to lie as it will without applying any pressure, and then cut it. This will allow the hair to fall into its natural lie and it will not look uneven when finished.

Fading

This technique is used for two reasons; first, when you want the design to really fade out on the head to a very short, almost bald look. The clippers are used to cut the hair shorter to a no-guard length. Second, fading is the technique used to create the difference between 2D or 3D effect, adding fading to the pattern gives the illusion of depth and a more dramatic effect.

Designing patterns in hair — full head: a step-by-step guide

1 Before the service.

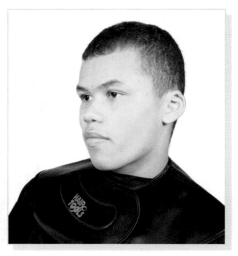

2 Reduce the length of the hair to a 1 1/2 guard length using the clipper over comb technique.

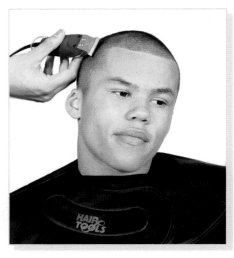

3 Begin the pattern with the beach hut design using the corner of the trimmers.

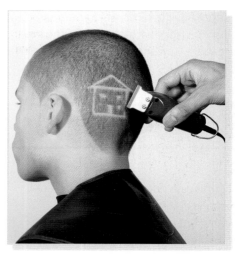

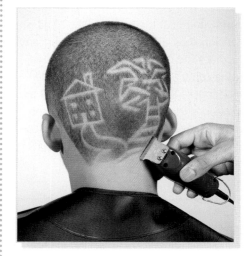

4 Use the trimmers freehand to design the palm tree.

5 Add the sun, again using the corner of the clippers for fine detail.

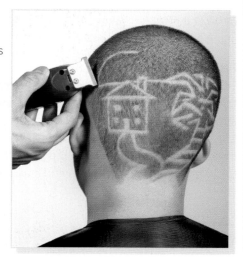

6 Then add the sun's rays.

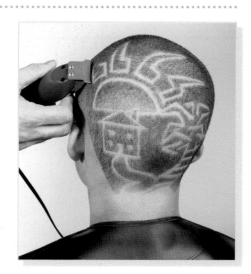

7 Remove any loose haircuttings with a soft but stiff bristle brush.

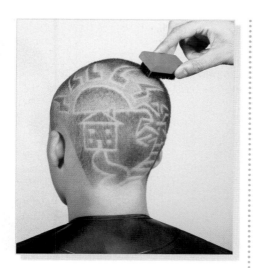

8 Use the clippers freehand on no-guard length to add fading over the design (this gives a 3D effect).

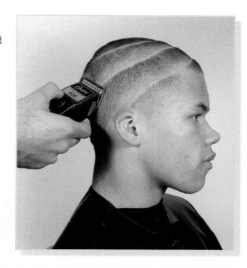

9 Define the lines using a razor with an open blade, using tension.

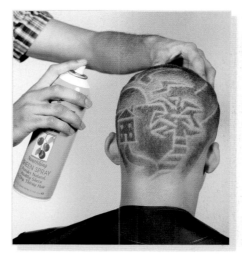

10 Apply olive oil spray to add sheen to the finished look and define the pattern.

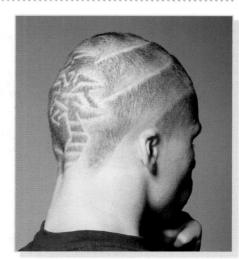

11 The finished look.

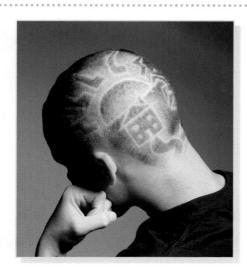

12 The finished look.

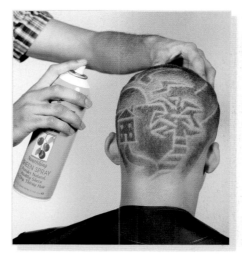

Design and create patterns in hair Unit AH35

Designing patterns in hair — partial head: a step-by-step guide

1 Before the service.

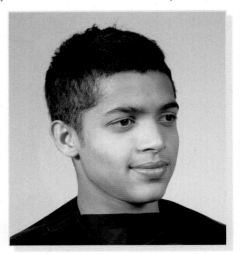

2 Cut the hair to the desired shape and length, using the trimmers to neaten off the front hairline.

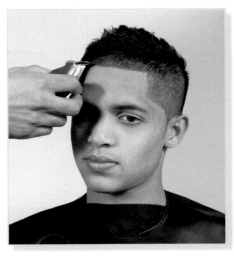

3 Use the corners of the trimmers to cut the design in the side of the head.

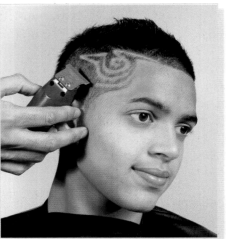

4 Continue with the pattern over all the area you are designing into.

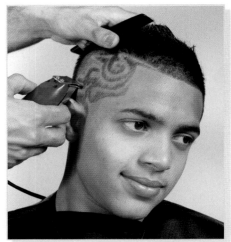

5 Use the razor, open blade, to define the lines and outside edges, using tension.

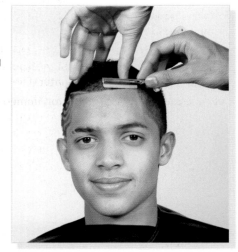

6 The finished look.

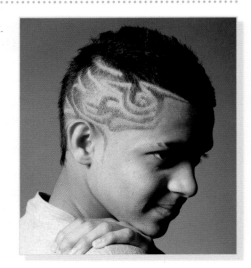

There are many design possibilities available and with experience you will become expert at choosing the right ones every time; but you must also be aware of limitations not only of the work you are initially capable of producing but also of the client's head and hair. Always consider lumps and bumps over the head shape, as these will affect the finished look, and never forget the importance of texture and density as this will also affect the finished look!

Over time you will become adept at looking at designs and being able to visualise what will work and how to scale a pattern up or down. Take time to really look at both the pattern and the client's head to imagine the finished look; this is where your artistic flair will come into force.

> **Be professional** ★★★
>
> Always look carefully at the space on the head where you will create the pattern and visually plan the size and proportion of how it will all fit onto the head before you begin. Make mental notes to yourself and use various points over the head, for example, top of the ear or below the ear as markers.

Correct positioning of self and client

The correct position of your client is extremely important whilst carrying out the design. You must ensure that you position your client and their head in the correct way. This will prevent you from being restricted whilst cutting in difficult-to-reach areas such as the nape. You must make certain that your client is seated upright and not slouching as you work your way around the haircut, and be sure to position the client's head in a way that will assist you, without causing him any discomfort. If your client is not positioned correctly, it will not only restrict your cutting but could also produce an uneven finished result.

Your own stance while working must also be considered at all times. The way that you stand to work will affect your posture and can lead to muscle fatigue if incorrect. Think about balancing the weight over your body when you stand and don't lean to one side for long periods. It is far too easy to put unnecessary strain on muscles and ligaments by over-reaching or stretching. However, this can be avoided by taking the time to adopt a good posture whilst working. Eventually it will become habit to stand in the correct position and you will soon do it without realising.

Look back at the 'In the salon' feature on Luca on page 130 of Unit GH16. This is a good example of how poor posture can affect you over a period of time; you must take your posture seriously.

> **Check it out**
>
> Is your posture good or could it be improved? Ask a colleague to check how you stand while working over the day and report back anything that they think could be improved upon. Ensure they know what to look out for!

Solving cutting problems

If any problems arise during the service, it is essential that you are aware of the methods used to solve them. Usually problems arise because your consultation was not accurate. For instance, you begin the cut and then find that there is a conflicting hair growth pattern that is preventing you from getting the pattern you require. You will have to deal with problems such as these whenever they occur, but keep the client informed, use your professional judgement, and be tactful in explaining the situation. You must remain confident in your approach, stay calm and never panic. If you panic you will only alarm your client and they in turn will lose confidence in your ability. Below is a table of cutting problems and possible remedies that you may come across during the cutting process.

Cutting problem	Possible remedy
Symmetrical pattern is not even on finished look	Cross-check, use the mirror and change the pattern to even out
Can't get close enough into the nape to cut to required length	Adjust the client's position or your own, or use a different cutting technique
Hair won't lie correctly around hairline	Adjust the finished design to incorporate the hairline's natural lie
Cut the client's or own skin	Stop immediately and clean the wound so it's free from hair and apply pressure to stop bleeding. Use a band-aid on yourself if continuing

Salon life

To colour or not to colour!

Rick's story

I was busy designing a pattern in the hair of a regular client; he was going to a music festival for the weekend and wanted a really funky design to show off. We had had a good chat about how he wanted the design to look and together we had a chosen dramatic 3D picture of a beach scene. As I finished the pattern I showed him the look and then began to explain where I was going to lift the colour so the beach looked like sand. I couldn't believe his reaction, he said, 'No way! I have only had colour on my hair once and had a really bad allergic reaction – never again!' I was shocked as I'm sure I explained in the consultation that I would need to colour this design to finish the look off. I was really disappointed now as the pattern just didn't look right, there was too much beach in the design and adding colour would have given it some emphasis. I decided to add a few waves just to break it up and the client seemed really happy with the finished look, but I wasn't and felt that I had let myself down by not getting it right this time.

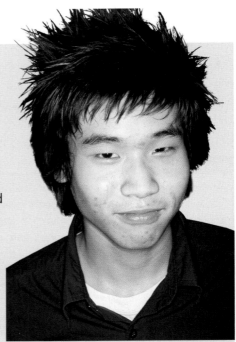

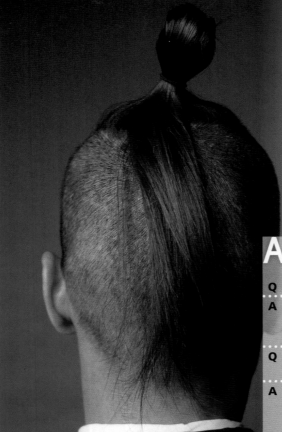

Be professional ★★★

- Always use images of the type of look you are going to create to make sure your client can visualise the finished look.
- Always make absolutely sure your client has understood your recommended service during the initial consultation.
- If you are using permanent colour, don't forget to skin test!

ASK THE PROFESSIONALS

Q *Why is the initial consultation so important?*

A To ensure that both you and the client fully understand the look you are about to achieve and that you know before you begin that it is achievable. This will avoid any disappointment for the client.

Q *Why can't you apply colour to the client's hair without discussing it with them first?*

A You must always ask the client about previous allergic reactions to colour and, if it is permanent colour, do a skin test first to avoid allergic reaction. A client may take legal proceedings against you if you were to harm them in any way.

After the service

This section looks at completing the service with your client by offering after-care advice and recommending when he should return. It is essential to complete the service as professionally as you have carried it out to provide the client with an all-round first-class service.

After-care advice

Clients will have a preferred time interval between the cuttings of the pattern in their hair. However, you should be advising every 7–10 days. You must stress the importance of coming back into the salon to maintain it otherwise he may become a poor advert for your salon with a grown-out look!

Ensuring that your client is fully informed about how to look after the design is important. Make sure he also understands the potential for style change, which can realistically be every 10–14 days. If the client cannot take care of the design at home, then you may find that when he returns to the salon he has changed the shape completely, or even shaved off his hair. Even though the client may have been happy when leaving the salon, unless the maintenance of the look has been fully explained, dealing with the design at home may prove difficult and leave the client feeling frustrated. If this happens, the chances of the client returning to you will be greatly reduced.

Home-care products

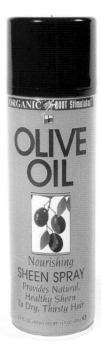

Olive oil spray

It is likely that the salon has a particular product range that you use and are familiar with. However, you must keep abreast of new developments within the styling range in order to ensure that your knowledge is up to date. There are several ways of doing this, for example, reading trade magazines, checking at the wholesale suppliers when you visit, or talking to technical representatives when they call into the salon with information on offers and developments.

There are several product companies that are dedicated to selling only men's styling products, but if your salon is unisex, you may wish to stock a range that caters for both men and women. Men are less likely to ask about how to maintain the style at home and it is your responsibility as the stylist to recommend the correct product for them to use. There are many styling products available and they each serve a different purpose; however, they can usually be categorised into whether they provide hold and / or shine for the hair. A client may have a preference as to the look they require or they may be looking for advice from you. Generally though, when advising on products to use over patterns, you should advise a product that provides shine and gloss to help define the pattern, especially on lighter hair.

Disposal of waste materials

There are different types of waste that must be disposed of safely in the salon. However, after a cutting service, it is only likely to be hair cuttings, used sharps and empty product containers. Hair cuttings left on the floor can cause a slippery surface and this then becomes a **hazard** in the salon, to both you and the client when they stand up. Salons dispose of hair cuttings in different ways, but it is more hygienic to ensure that they are placed in a covered bin and put in the outside bin in a tied-up bag to prevent them spilling out.

> **Hazard**
>
> something likely to cause injury.

> **Remember**
>
> Aerosol containers, even when they feel empty, can still contain flammable materials. There is also a risk of them exploding if punctured or overheated, so care must be taken with regards to their safe disposal.

Check your knowledge

The following questions will help you to check your understanding of this unit. The answers can be found on page 421. Take care, as there may be more than one correct answer for some questions.

1 Why is it important to keep your work area clean and tidy?
   a In case a health and safety inspector passes by
   b To prevent any accidents due to untidiness
   c To give the junior staff something to do
   d To prevent the spread of bacteria

2 What safety considerations must be taken into account when cutting hair?
   a Use the correct personal protective equipment
   b Ensure the client relaxes at all times
   c Check if the client needs a drink
   d Visually check electrical equipment before use

3 What visual aids may be used during consultation to help ascertain the client's requirements?
   a Watching television
   b Looking through the local newspapers
   c Stylebooks
   d Photos that the client brought in

4 How should clippers be maintained correctly?
   a Wash them thoroughly every month
   b Brush off any hair after each use and oil regularly
   c Use hygiene spray regularly to prevent the spread of bacteria
   d Visually check the wires before each use for faults

5 How should cutting tools be stored safely?
   a Kept on the reception desk
   b Put away in the correct holder or case after each use
   c Kept in the stock room
   d In your pocket so you always have them to hand

6 The minimum requirements for personal protective equipment for your client would be:
   a gown and gloves
   b gown, gloves and apron
   c gown and towel
   d towel and cotton wool pads

7 Where must you dispose of used sharps?
   a In the waste bin
   b In the sharps bin
   c In the outside bin
   d At home

8 How long should you advise a client to leave between cuts?
  a Every couple of months
  b Once a week
  c From 2–4 weeks depending on the chosen style
  d He shouldn't need to come back

9 Can you still design a pattern in the hair if a client has scars?
  a No, never over scars
  b Yes, but avoid the area
  c Yes, you may be able to design a pattern that hides the scar
  d Not unless they really demand it

10 What action should you take if you accidentally cut the skin with the razor?
  a Stop immediately and administer first aid and only continue if bleeding stops
  b Ignore it unless it bleeds heavily
  c Ask your boss to come over and deal with it
  d Put a plaster on

Assessment guidance

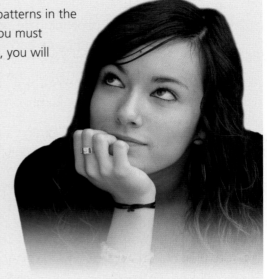

You will have to demonstrate in your work that you can design and create patterns in the hair and your assessor will observe you carrying out work on your clients. You must follow all necessary health and safety legislation and rules of the salon. Plus, you will have to prove competence in the following:

- using all the tools and equipment
- taking into account all the factors
- using all the cutting techniques listed
- producing designs over a full and a partial head
- creating patterns that are 3D pictorial, repeated and symmetrical
- advising your client on maintenance and home care.

No simulation is allowed for any of your practical skills in this unit.

Answers to check your knowledge questions

Unit G22 Answers

1   c.   something that has the potential to cause harm
2   b.   COSHH;   d. Personal Protective Equipment at Work Regulations
3   b.   Ultra-violet cabinet;   d.   Autoclave
4   a.   move the boxes somewhere else;   b.   tell the manager
5   a.   reduce the risk of accidents;   b.   ensure you are fulfilling your health and safety obligations
6   a.   prevent contact dermatitis;   b.   prevent scratching the client
7   b.   ask for help from a colleague;   c.   make sure you keep your back straight and lift using your leg muscles;   d.   empty some of the items out of the box until you can lift it easily
8   b.   make sure it's logged in the accident book;   c.   apologise to the client
9   b.   get her a pair of gloves to use;   c.   speak to her afterwards, explaining the reasons why gloves should be worn
10 b.   if the salon acquires a new piece of equipment;   d.   if a new member of staff starts work

Unit G21 Answers

1   a.   Cortex;   d.   Cuticle
2   a.   Anagen
3   d.   the tensile strength of the cortex
4   b.   its shiny appearance
5   c.   Impetigo;   d.   Folliculitis
6. c.   a sebaceous cyst
7   a.   ensure you can offer the requested service;   b.   maintain satisfied clients
8   a.   services that are time consuming;   c.   Christmas and/or New Year's Eve;   d.   clients that regularly default (don't turn up)
9   b.   accurate and up to date;   c.   legible
10 a.   reading trade magazines;   b.   attending hair shows and exhibitions;   c.   watching fashion-related programmes on TV;   d.   attending courses run by product manufacturers

Unit G18 Answers

1   a.   It will make more money for the salon;   b.   The clients will have great hair;   c.   The staff can become competitive at selling
2   b.   So that staff and clients feel that they have a voice;   c.   To ensure there are no misunderstandings between anyone;   d.   So the client gets the best service possible
3   b.   open questions
4   b.   Advertising on local radio;   c.   Advertising in local papers;   d.   Word of mouth
5   d.   planning, implementation, evaluation
6   a.   Client's name and address;   d.   Client's service details
7   b.   In case they would have to be used in legal proceedings;   c.   So that you can read clearly and understand exactly what a client wants for next time
8   b.   Smiling at clients;   c.   Making positive eye contact
9   a.   Clearly spoken at a normal pace
10 b.   Yes, always

Unit G19 Answers

1   b.   Staff have good knowledge of the products that they use;   d.   The staff are highly trained with excellent communication skills
2   c.   Sending and receiving of information between people using various methods
3   d.   To ensure that you provide for your market which will increase revenue
4   a.   To ensure you are providing a service that suits the needs of your clients;   d.   To show your clients that you value their opinion of the service you provide
5   b.   Informal means you don't record it, e.g. just a chat with a client, and formal means something recorded, e.g. on a customer survey
6   a.   Client suggestion box;   c.   Feedback via the salon website
7   a.   Client age group;   c.   Where clients live or work;   d.   Whether clients use/like the salon products
8   b.   To ensure you present a positive, united campaign to clients;   c.   So that all staff feel valued and important
9   b.   To show clients that you feel these are of benefit to the salon and them

10 a. By believing in and staying focused on the positives of the changes made; b. By encouraging staff and clients to see the benefits of the changes

Unit G11 Answers

1 b. So all stock can be monitored and recorded; c. To make sure there is always sufficient stock
2 b. Client dissatisfaction
3 b. The Trade Descriptions Act; c. COSHH
4 a. To prevent litigation; b. To maintain a professional image
5 a. To maximise profits; b. To reduce waste; c. To set a good example to the other staff members
6 c. To maximise your own earning potential; d. To maximise the salon's profits
7 a. Seasonal promotions; b. Promoting new products and services
8 a. To ensure the stylist remains focused; c. To allow regular contact with the manager; d. To help with the development of reflective skills
9 a. The clients may not understand the information they have been given; b. The wrong products may be used; d. Clients may be offended
10 a. clients being kept waiting until resources become available; c. client dissatisfaction

Unit GH16 Answers

1 b. Electricity at Work Regulations 1989
2 a. To prevent discomfort; b. It looks professional
3 a. To save time; d. To prevent accidents
4 d. To ensure you fully understand the client's requirements
5 d. Hair may start to in-grow
6 a. To prevent damage to your cutting tools; d. So the hair is clean which aids the cutting process
7 b. Wet only
8 c. To highlight any mistakes that need to be corrected; d. It helps to provide a professional service
9 b. quietly inform the client; c. clean and sterilise all tools and equipment immediately when finished
10 b. To ensure the client can look after her hair at home; c. To open up a retail sale opportunity; d. To show professionalism in your work

Unit GH17 Answers

1 a. A warm room will speed up the development of lightening products; d. The use of added heat will speed up the development of lightening products.
2 d. open the cuticle
3 b. the colour not being left on long enough
4 a. To avoid damage to the hair and scalp; c. To stop any further development taking place
5 d. To raise the cuticles of resistant hair
6 a. To restore lost pigment to pale hair that needs to be made darker or warmer; c. To keep warm tones on porous hair
7 a. Tightly packed cuticles; c. Product build-up
8 a. Identify the depth and tone of colouring products; c. identify the hair's natural depth and tone; d. help choose the colour
9 a. to help prevent colour fade; b. to close the cuticles; c. to add moisture to the hair; d. to restore the natural pH balance of the hair
10 a. to ensure good coverage; c. to enable you to work methodically

Unit GH18 Answers

1 a. the hair to be lightened because it's too dark; c. the hair to be darkened because it's too light; d. a change of tone
2 a. oxygen
3 c. permanent colour; d. bleach / lightening products
4 c. apply hydrogen peroxide to the resistant areas, then apply heat to open the cuticles
5 b. To find out whether the client is allergic to the products to be used
6 b. prevent accidents or electrocution; c. make sure it's working properly
7 d. Diluted with plenty of cold water, and then flushed down the drain
8 a. ensures you are complying with the Data Protection Act; b. will help the next stylist when the client returns; c. may be used in a case of litigation
9 d. mix 1 part hydrogen peroxide to 1 part water
10 d. help to prevent colour fade

Unit GH19 Answers

1 b. protect the hair from the effects of humidity;
   d. keep the style in longer
2 c. allow the curl to set in its new shape;   d.   give a longer-lasting curl
3 b. root to point
4 c. produce waves with specific direction
5 b. increased volume;   c.   A firmer curl
6 b. off base
7 b. the temperature of the tools used;   c.   the amount of tension to be applied
8 a. trailing flexes;   b.   scalp burns
9 d. has the ability to absorb atmospheric moisture
10 d. hair that has been stretched and dried into a new shape

Unit GH20 Answers

1 a. whether it conducts heat;   d.   whether it has sharp edges
2 c. straightening;   d.   blow-drying
3 a. it's easier;   c.   it's quicker
4 c. brushed and thoroughly de-tangled
5 b. prevent sagging;   d.   Ensure the style is well balanced
6 b. the cuticle scales being roughened;   c.   added volume
7 b. brush the hair starting at the points and work gradually up towards the roots
8 b. fragilitis crinium;   c.   trichorrhexis nodosa
9 a. scorched;   c.   discoloured
10 a. a receding hairline;   d.   raised follicles

Unit GH21 Answers

1 a. To make sure you don't go over budget;   d.   To make sure you have all the necessary resources
2 a. the Internet;   b.   the local library;   c.   TV
3 a. photographs;   b.   sketches
4 b. ensure that excessive spending doesn't occur;
   c. ensure that the activity doesn't end up costing too much
5 a. confirm the historical period;   d.   portray a futuristic image
6 a. increase your professional profile;   c.   create potential job opportunities
7 a. questionnaire;   d.   asking relevant people

8 a. whether your objectives were met;   c.   areas for improvement
9 c. To make sure there are no misunderstandings
10 a. Spillages caused by using basins not designed for shampooing;   c.   Trailing wires and flexes

Unit GH22 Answers

1 c. To be sure that there is no misunderstanding;
   d. In case the information has to be reviewed at a later date
2 a. The hair's condition;   d.   If the client has any open wounds on the scalp
3 a. An elasticity test;   c.   A porosity test
4 c. Gown;   d.   Cotton wool
5 d. Disulphide linkages
6 a. If the hair is already very porous;   b.   If the perm lotion is left on too long
7 c. To even out porosity along the hair length;
   d. To help prevent damage to the hair
8 d. It restores moisture and pH balance to the hair
9 a. To ensure that the added curl or wave is maintained;
   d. To keep the hair in the best condition possible
10 b. Only if the hair's condition allows

Unit GH23 Answers

1 c. traction alopecia;   d.   a sensitive scalp
2 b. To ensure the hair's internal structure is in good enough condition to carry out the process
3 a. To ensure they blend correctly with the natural hair;
   b. To make sure the extensions are as natural as possible
4 d. Finishing spray
5 a. Braid spray;   b.   Serum;   c.   Wax
6 d. loss of hair at the root area
7 b. always return to the salon for professional removal of the extensions
8 c. About 1 centimetre a month
9 a. use the manufacturer's recommended removal solution
10 a. hair that has been cut from the head and the cuticles are all lying in the same direction

Unit H32 Answers

1 a. increase salon business and enhance salon image
2 b. Salon website;   d.   Via media
3 c. The salon owner
4 a. No fire exits;   d.   Overloading electrical sockets
5 c. Smart, measurable, achievable, realistic, time-bound
6 c. To assess any hazards and minimise risk
7 c. Put measures in place to deal with it
8 a. To ensure you look knowledgeable and professional;   d.   To comply with consumer law
9 b. Client asks for prices;   c.   Client wants to smell and feel the products
10 d. To determine whether or not you have achieved your stated objective

Unit AH28 Answers

1 b. To make sure you can control the hair effectively;   c.   So you can achieve the required style
2 a. Keep the floor clear of loose hair;   b.   Ensure the client is positioned correctly to ensure you are both comfortable throughout the service;   c.   If using bands to secure the ends of the braids, make sure you use professional bands;   d.   Use products following manufacturers' instructions
3 c. To avoid product build-up
4 c. By visually checking the hair as you work
5 c. You must make sure the style complements the head and face shape
6 a. The hair becomes less dense;   c.   A receding hairline
7 b. Keep away from the braiding service until normal hair growth resumes;   d.   To see a trichologist
8 a. Kanekalon;   b.   Human hair;   c.   Yak
9 b. The hair becomes dry;   c.   The scalp becomes itchy;   d.   The natural hair may become damaged
10 a. Braid spray;   b.   Wax;   c.   Oil;   d.   Sheen spray

Unit AH30 Answers

1 a. Store, handle, use and dispose
2 a. To prevent it from scorching;   c.   To prevent it from discolouring
3 c. Stop and administer first aid immediately
4 b. To prevent the build-up of product and carbon on the equipment;   d.   To ensure they run at optimum efficiency
5 b. Able to absorb moisture from the atmosphere

6 b. To prevent hair breakage
7 a. To present a professional image of your salon;   b.   To ensure your client's hair stays in optimum condition;   c.   To improve your retail sales income;   d.   To ensure the new style lasts as long as possible for the client
8 b. Avoid getting the hair wet or damp;   c.   Use correct products to maintain the style;   d.   Cover the hair with a silk scarf or durag when sleeping
9 b. If the hair is very thick;   d.   When the client wants a hard press
10 b. wound on base

Unit GB6 Answers

1 a. To prevent the spread of infection;   b.   To prevent your skin from coming into contact with shaving products
2 a. Your client should be wearing a clean gown;   d.   The client should be positioned correctly
3 b. To prevent any accidents due to untidiness;   d.   To prevent the spread of bacteria
4 c. To prevent cross-infection
5 a. To soften the hair and cleanse the face;   d.   To open the follicle and lift the hair
6 d. To prevent the blade from cutting the skin
7 a. If the hair is coarse or stubborn
8 b. Cool the skin;   c.   Close the follicle
9 a. Stop immediately and administer first aid and only continue if bleeding stops
10 c. In a clearly labelled sharps box

Unit GB7 Answers

1 c. gown and towel
2 b. In the sharps bin
3 a. To maintain client comfort both throughout and following the service
4 d. Moist heat
5 c. 1–2 cms per month
6 b. To ensure methodical progression of the facial haircut
7 a. To soften the skin to prevent in-growing hairs
8 a. To check the progress of the facial hair cut meets the client's expectations;   b.   To ensure he is comfortable
9 c. From 2–4 weeks depending on the chosen style
10 b. To protect the eyes from hair clippings

Unit GB8 Answers

1   a. Your local council offices;   b.   Your salon policies and procedures booklet
2   a. Use the correct personal protective equipment;
     d. Visually check electrical equipment before use
3   c. Stylebooks;   d.   Photos that the client brought in
4   c. To remove bulk but not length
5   b. So the hair grows back evenly;   c.   So the haircut looks neat and tidy
6   a. To ensure you achieve a balanced cut;   b.   To ensure the finished result is even
7   c. ½ an hour
8   a. About 4 weeks depending on the client's hair length
9   b   Brush off any hair after each use and oil regularly;
     c   Use hygiene spray regularly to prevent the spread of bacteria;   d   Visually check the wires before each use for faults
10 b. Put away in the correct holder or case after each use

Unit AH35 Answers

1   b. To prevent any accidents due to untidiness;
     d. To prevent the spread of bacteria
2   a. Use the correct personal protective equipment;
     d. Visually check electrical equipment before use
3   c. Stylebooks;   d.   Photos that the client brought in
4   b. Brush off any hair after each use and oil regularly;
     c. Use hygiene spray regularly to prevent the spread of bacteria;   d.   Visually check the wires before each use for faults
5   b. Put away in the correct holder or case after each use
6   c. gown and towel
7   b. In the sharps bin
8   c. From 2—4 weeks depending on the chosen style
9   c. Yes, you may be able to design a pattern that hides the scar
10 a. Stop immediately and administer first aid and only continue if bleeding stops

Index